Application of Nursing Process and Nursing Diagnosis

An Interactive Text for Diagnostic Reasoning

Application of Nursing Process and Nursing Diagnosis

An Interactive Text for Diagnostic Reasoning

FIFTH EDITION

Marilynn E. Doenges, *APRN, BC-retired*

Adult Psychiatric/Mental Health Nurse, retired
Adjunct Faculty
Beth-El College of Nursing & Health Science
CU-Springs
Colorado Springs, Colorado

Mary Frances Moorhouse, *RN, MSN, CRRN, LNC*

Nurse Consultant
TNT-RN Enterprises
Adjunct Faculty
Pikes Peak Community College
Colorado Springs, Colorado

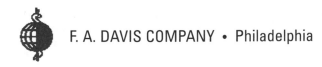

F. A. DAVIS COMPANY • Philadelphia

F. A. Davis Company
1915 Arch Street
Philadelphia, PA 19131
www.fadavis.com

Printed in the United States of America

Last digit indicates print number: 10 9 8 7 6 5 4 3 2

Publisher, Nursing: Joanne Patzek DaCunha, RN, MSN
Director of Content Development: Darlene D. Pedersen
Project Editor: Meghan K. Ziegler
Manager of Art & Design: Carolyn O'Brien

As new scientific information becomes available through basic and clinical research, recommended treatments and drug therapies undergo changes. The author(s) and publisher have done everything possible to make this book accurate, up to date, and in accord with accepted standards at the time of publication. The author(s), editors, and publisher are not responsible for errors or omissions or for consequences from application of the book, and make no warranty, expressed or implied, in regard to the contents of the book. Any practice described in this book should be applied by the reader in accordance with professional standards of care used in regard to the unique circumstances that may apply in each situation. The reader is advised always to check product information (package inserts) for changes and new information regarding dose and contraindications before administering any drug. Caution is especially urged when using new or infrequently ordered drugs.

Library of Congress Cataloging-in-Publication Data

Doenges, Marilynn E., 1922-
    Application of nursing process and nursing diagnosis : an interactive text for diagnostic reasoning/Marilynn E. Doenges, Mary Frances Moorhouse. — 5th ed.
        p. ; cm.
    Includes bibliographical references and index.
    ISBN 978-0-8036-1909-8 (pbk. : alk. paper)
    1. Nursing. 2. Nursing assessment. 3. Nursing diagnosis.   I. Moorhouse, Mary Frances, 1947-
II. Title.
    [DNLM: 1. Nursing Process. 2. Nursing Diagnosis—methods. 3. Patient Care Planning.
WY 100 D615a 2008]
    RT41.D54 2008
    610.73—dc22   2008005127

DavisPlus Resources

Diagnosis Resource Center—online **resources open to students and faculty!**

Student and Instructor Resources:

- Concept Map Generator
    - **Design a concept map in minutes with easy drag-and-drop boxes.**
    - **Dynamic full-color concept maps, individualized for each patient.**
    - **Students create, print, and e-mail as many as they like.**
- Assessment Tool
    - **An interactive form that allows users to enter assessment data selectively.**
    - **Print and e-mail functionality.**
- Eight Case Studies
    - **Featuring interactive learning exercises.**
- Care Plan Template
    - **A quick and user-friendly format for creating care plans.**
    - **Includes print and e-mail functionality.**
- New and Revised Nursing Diagnoses
    - **Updated to reflect the 2007–2008 changes.**
    - **A quick list that can be printed or e-mailed.**

Instructor Resources:

- Instructor Resources—**password-protected online resources available upon adoption.**
    - **Answers to case study questions from student CD.**
    - **Suggestions on how to use concept maps.**
    - **PowerPoint presentation.**

http://davisplus.fadavis.com

Notes to the Educator

The nursing process has been used for over 35 years as a systematic approach to nursing practice. The process is an efficient and effective method for organizing nursing knowledge and clinical decision making in providing planned client care. Although it has been undergoing re-evaluation and revision, the concepts within the process still remain central to nursing practice.

Healthcare accrediting agencies and nursing organizations have developed standards of nursing practice that focus on the tenets of the nursing process; that is, assessing, diagnosing, planning, implementing, evaluating, and documenting client care. Although the formats used to document the plan of care may change with the interpretation and evaluation of standards and advances in technology, the nursing responsibilities and interventions required for planned client care still need to be learned, shared, performed, evaluated, and documented.

The nursing process is by its nature interactive. This text mirrors that interactive focus by presenting a step-by-step problem-solving design to help students develop an understanding of the meaning and language of nursing. We have included definitions and professional standards that will serve as a solid foundation for your students to understand and apply the nursing process. The vignettes, practice activities, work pages, and case studies provide an opportunity to examine and scrutinize client situations and dilemmas in practice, consider alternatives, and evaluate outcomes. The worksheets serve as graphic summaries that provide students with criteria to evaluate their decisions and demonstrate their understanding of the concepts and integration of the material presented. Tear-out pages for independent learning provide an opportunity for practical application and beginning mastery of the nursing process. These pages can be taken to the clinical area to reinforce selected aspects of the nursing process. Finally, review of client situations and the Code for Nurses can serve as a catalyst for philosophical and ethical discussions. All these activities encourage the student to actively seek solutions rather than passively assimilate knowledge, thus stimulating the student's critical thinking ability.

Chapter 1, The Nursing Process: Delivering Quality Care

This introductory chapter presents an overview of the nursing process. Students are introduced to the definitions of nursing and nursing diagnosis and the American Nurses Association's Standards of Practice.

Chapter 2, The Assessment Step: Developing the Client Database

This chapter introduces students to the first step of the nursing process. Organizational formats for constructing nursing assessment tools are discussed, and both the physical and psychosocial aspects of assessment are blended into the interview process. Examples of client data assist students to identify categories of nursing diagnostic labels.

Chapter 3, The Diagnosis Step: Analyzing the Data

The definition and concepts of nursing diagnosis are presented in this chapter. We use the term *Client Diagnostic Statement* to describe the combination of the NANDA-I (formerly the North American Nursing Diagnosis Association)-approved label, the client's related factors (etiology), and associated defining characteristics (signs/symptoms). A six-step diagnostic reasoning process is presented to assist students in their beginning efforts to analyze the client's assessment data accurately. The remainder of this chapter focuses on ruling out, synthesizing, evaluating, and constructing the client diagnostic statement.

Chapter 4, The Planning Step: Creating the Plan of Care

Information on developing the individualized outcomes for the client is provided in this chapter. A focus on writing measurable outcomes correctly is presented. In addition, examples from the standardized nursing language for outcomes, Nursing Outcomes Classification (NOC), are also presented. Nursing interventions are defined, and acknowledgment of the work by the Iowa Intervention Project's Nursing Interventions Classification (NIC) is included. The topics, priorities of interventions, discharge planning, and selecting appropriate nursing interventions are discussed along with examples of a fourth standardized language, the Omaha System. A practice activity for recording the steps of the nursing process learned thus far is included to provide the student with a realistic application. An interactive plan of care worksheet is used to present examples and guidelines for developing the client's outcome statement, selecting nursing interventions, and providing rationales for nursing interventions. Finally, information about the use of mind or concept mapping to stimulate right-brain activity to facilitate the planning process is presented along with a sample plan of care.

Chapter 5, The Implementation Step: Putting the Plan of Care Into Action

Information is presented about the validation and implementation of the plan of care. Concerns regarding the day-to-day organization of the nurse's work is used creatively in a practice activity in which students use time management to plan the day's client care interventions. Change-of-shift reporting principles are also discussed and practiced.

Chapter 6, The Evaluation Step: Determining Whether Desired Outcomes Have Been Met

The crucial step of evaluation and its accompanying reassessment and revision processes are presented in this chapter on the last step of the nursing process. A practice activity is provided to help students evaluate the plan of care partially constructed in Chapter 4. Revisions to the plan of care are necessary, and the activity provides a realistic exercise for this final step. The plan of care worksheet, available for download on the DavisPlus Web site, is designed to ask your students questions about their clients' progress and the effectiveness of their implemented nursing interventions.

Chapter 7, Documenting the Nursing Process

This chapter introduces students to ways of documenting successfully their use of the nursing process. Communication, legal responsibilities, and reimbursement are a few of the topics introduced in this chapter. The documentation systems of SOAP and FOCUS CHARTING™ are presented to show two possible methods of documenting the nursing process. The last section of the interactive worksheet focuses the students' attention on three important aspects of documentation: the reassessment data, interventions implemented, and the client's response.

Chapter 8, Interactive Care Planning: From Assessment to Client Response

This final chapter provides an evaluation checklist that can be used to evaluate your students' progress in all aspects of the nursing process. The checklist is designed to include the criteria listed on the Interactive Care Plan Worksheets, ANA Standards of Practice, and the JCAHO nursing standards. The chapter ends with a case study that gives your students an opportunity to apply all the steps of the nursing process. The evaluation checklist, along with the TIME OUTS included in the plan of care worksheets, provides the students with the required guidance when constructing their first complete plan of care.

Appendixes

Appendix A, Code for Nurses, has been included for your use both in the classroom and during clinical rounds to share with your students the values that guide nursing practice today. A reference to the Code and a discussion of beliefs that affect nursing practice are contained in Chapter 1, and an ethical activity is presented in Chapter 5.

Appendix B provides an adult medical-surgical nursing assessment tool as referenced in Chapter 2, along with excerpts from assessment tools developed for the psychiatric and obstetric settings. The tools are helpful to students in their assessment of the client's response to health problems and life processes as well as their gathering of physical assessment data.

Appendices C and D provide tools for the student to measure the accuracy of their choice of nursing diagnosis labels. The Ordinal Scale of Accuracy of a Nursing Diagnosis assigns a point value to a diagnosis that is consistent with the number of cues and disconfirming cues identified. This tool aids students in validating their analysis of the collected data and choice of nursing diagnosis. The Integrated Model for Self-Monitoring of the Diagnostic Process provides direct feedback to students but can also be shared with you to demonstrate the students' progress in data analysis and diagnosis.

Appendix E is a sample of a Clinical (Critical) Pathway, providing you with the opportunity to address alternate forms for planning and evaluating care.

Appendix F provides a glossary of common terms.

Appendix G defines the seven axes of the NANDA-I Taxonomy II.

Appendix H organizes the NANDA-I diagnostic labels within Maslow's hierarchy of needs to aid in visualizing and determining priorities for providing client care.

A listing of the NANDA-I nursing diagnoses are included in Appendix I. Each nursing diagnosis's definition, related/risk factors, and defining characteristics are provided to assist the student in selecting the appropriate nursing diagnosis.

Some commonly accepted charting abbreviations, which may be useful in your discussion of the documentation process, can be found on the end pages.

Finally, the Keys to the Practice Activities and Work Pages (practice activities within chapters and end-of-chapter work pages) are also included on the Student CD bound into this book.

The National League for Nursing emphasizes the need for graduates of nursing programs to think critically, make decisions, and formulate independent judgments. To achieve this outcome, you as an instructor are encouraged to use teaching strategies that will "stimulate higher-order critical thinking in both theory and practice situations" (Klaassens, 1988). These strategies include: questioning, analysis, synthesis, application, writing, problem-solving games, and philosophical discussions.

It is our hope that the interactive features of this text, CD, and Web suite will provide the strategies to assist you in sharing with your students the meaning and language of the nursing process and in making a smooth and effective transition from the classroom to any clinical setting.

Marilynn E. Doenges

Mary Frances Moorhouse

Notes to the Student

The nursing process will be described by your instructors as a systematic approach to the practice of nursing. Shortly, you will find that this process is an efficient and effective method for organizing both nursing knowledge and practice. The process will also assist you in accurately performing clinical decision-making activities in planning your client's care. The process has been continually refined since its inception in the 1960s. However, to date, the concepts within the process still remain central to nursing practice. Through the use of this text, your instructors will share with you the meaning of the concepts and this evolving nursing practice language.

The nursing process is an interactive method of practicing nursing, with the components fitting together in a continuous cycle of thought and action. This interactive focus was used in developing and writing this text for you. The text focuses on the steps of the nursing process and provides information and exercises to aid your understanding and application of the process. Included are practice activities, ongoing reference to simulated clinical experiences through the use of vignettes, and end-of-chapter work pages to promote your understanding. Definitions of nursing and the nursing process, along with the American Nurses Association's (ANA) Standards of Practice, are presented to provide a solid foundation for you to build an understanding of the language and knowledge of nursing and application of the nursing process.

In addition, a six-step diagnostic reasoning/critical thinking process is presented for analyzing your clients' assessment data. It will assist you in ruling out, synthesizing, evaluating, and constructing the client diagnostic statement, which is pivotal for developing individualized plans of care for your client. A practice activity for writing a nursing plan of care was developed to provide a realistic application of your newly learned knowledge. An example of a typical day's work requirement is used in a practice activity in which you are given the opportunity to use time management principles and skills to plan your client's care within an 8-hour shift. A third practice activity is provided to give you a chance to choose client information you would include in a change-of-shift report to communicate the outcomes of your use of the nursing process.

Next, you are given an opportunity to test your initial skills in developing a complete plan of care. A set of step-by-step forms is provided for you to document your clinical judgment by selecting client diagnostic statements, developing the goals/outcomes, and identifying the nursing interventions. Finally, an evaluation checklist is provided to serve as a valuable self-assessment of the appropriateness and accuracy of your comprehension of the planning exercise and future plans of care that you will design for your clients.

At the end of the chapters, a bibliography and list of suggested readings are included to guide you in further and future reading and understanding of both nursing knowledge and the nursing process. In Chapter 1, a suggested reading list provides a listing of publications from an historical perspective. The listing should be helpful to you in searching out the meaning of nursing and the nursing process. The list may also prove valuable in writing varied required papers on similar topics. The second section gives you the most current listing of publications at the time of the printing of this edition. Once again, the selected publications are provided to assist you in this learning process.

The work pages, downloadable care plan worksheets, and the evaluation checklist were especially designed for your independent learning. The care plan worksheets are on the student CD accompanying this book. These worksheets can be printed and taken to the clinical area to reinforce selected aspects of the nursing process. It is our hope that the interactive features of this text, student CD, and Web suite will assist you in making the successful and effective transition from the classroom to your assigned clinical setting. We wish you well in this beginning phase of your new profession.

Marilynn E. Doenges

Mary Frances Moorhouse

Acknowledgments

To our families, who support us in all we do and who continue to support our dreams, fantasies, and obsessions.

With special thanks to:

The Doenges family: the late Dean, whose support and encouragement are sorely missed; Jim; Barbara and Bob Lanza; David, Monita, Matthew, and Tyler; John, Holly, Nicole, and Kelsey; and the Daigle family: Nancy and Jim; Jennifer, Brandon, Annabelle, Will and Henry Smith-Daigle, and Jonathan, Kim, and Mandy JoAnn.

The Moorhouse family: Jan; Paul; Jason, Thenderlyn, Alexa, and Mary Isabella.

Alice Murr, for being available when we need help.

The staff at Memorial Hospital library, for cheerfully filling in all the blanks and by helping us find those elusive references.

To the nursing students of Beth-El College of Nursing at UCCS and of Pikes Peak Community College, who continue to challenge us to make the nursing process and nursing diagnosis understandable.

To our colleagues, who continue to provide a sounding board and feedback for our professional beliefs and expectations. We hope this interactive text will help you and your students at all stages clarify and apply these concepts.

To our F. A. Davis family, especially our publisher and friend, Robert (Bob) Martone; Joanne DaCunha; and all who facilitated the revision process to get this project completed in a timely fashion.

To NANDA and the international nurses who are developing and using nursing diagnoses. And to the nurses who have patiently awaited this revision, we hope it will help in applying theory to practice and will enhance the delivery and effectiveness of their care.

Contents

Chapter 5

The Implementation Step: Putting the Plan of Care Into Action 103

Chapter 6

The Evaluation Step: Determining Whether Desired Outcomes Have Been Met 117

Chapter 7

Documenting the Nursing Process 131

Chapter 8

Interactive Care Planning: From Assessment to Client Response 155

Appendix A

Code for Nurses 177

Appendix B

General Assessment Tool 179

Appendix C

Lunney's Ordinal Scale for Degrees of Accuracy of a Nursing Diagnosis 187

Appendix D

Self-Monitoring of Accuracy Using the Integrated Model: A Guide 189

Appendix E

Clinical (Critical) Pathways: A Sample 191

Appendix F

Glossary 197

Appendix G

NANDA-I Taxonomy II: Definitions of Axes 201

Practice Activities and Work Pages

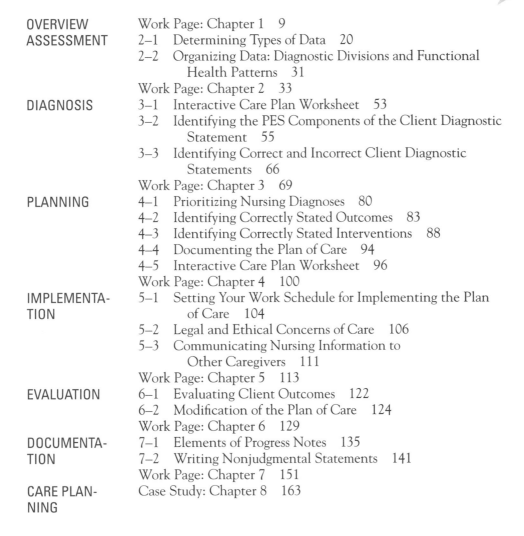

Practice Activities
and Work Pages

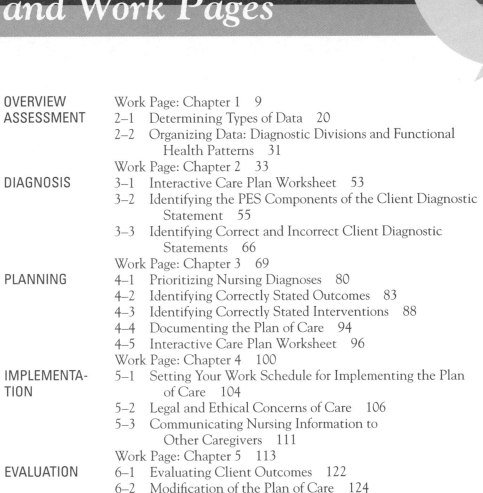

Chapter 1

The Nursing Process: Delivering Quality Care

The Nursing Profession

DEFINITION OF NURSING

The essence of nursing is characterized by the protection, promotion, and optimization of health and abilities, prevention of illness and injury, alleviation of suffering through the diagnosis and treatment of human response, and advocacy in the care of individuals, families, communities, and populations (American Nurses Association, 2003).

Nursing is both a science and an art involving the physical, psychological, sociological, cultural, and spiritual concerns of the individual. The *science* of nursing is based on a broad theoretical framework, whereas its *art* depends largely on the individual nurse's skills and ability to care. The importance of the nurse within the healthcare system is being recognized in many positive ways, and the profession of nursing is itself acknowledging the need for its practitioners to be professional and accountable.

In its early developmental years, nursing did not seek nor have the means to control its own practice. Florence Nightingale, in discussing the nature of nursing, observed that "nursing has been limited to signify little more than the administration of medicines and the application of poultices" (Nightingale, 1859). Although this attitude still persists in some cases, the nursing profession has identified what makes nursing unique and defined a body of professional knowledge.

Thus, barely a century after Nightingale noted that "the very elements of nursing are all but unknown" (Nightingale, 1859), the American Nurses Association (ANA)

1

developed the first Social Policy Statement (1980) defining nursing as "the diagnosis and treatment of human responses to actual or potential health problems." In 1995 the statement was revisited, updated, and entitled *Nursing's Social Policy Statement* (ANA, 1995). That policy statement acknowledged that, since the release of the original statement, nursing had been influenced by many social and professional changes as well as by the science of caring. Nursing integrated these changes with the 1980 definition to include treatment of human responses to health and illness.

The statement identified four essential features of contemporary nursing practice:

1. Attention to the full range of human experiences and responses to health and illness without restriction to a problem-focused orientation
2. Integration of objective data with knowledge gained from an understanding of the client's or group's subjective experience
3. Application of scientific knowledge to the processes of diagnosis and treatment
4. Provision of a caring relationship that facilitates health and healing (ANA, 1995)

The 2003 revision of *Nursing's Social Policy Statement* recognizes nursing's commitment to meeting the broader needs of society and the necessity of adapting to changes in healthcare environments and within the profession. This includes addressing organizational, social, economic, legal, and political factors within the healthcare system and society (ANA, 2003).

In the modern world of nursing, human responses, defined as people's experiences with and responses to health, illness, and life processes across the lifespan, are the phenomena of concern for nurses. Thus, nursing's role includes health promotion as well as activities that contribute to recovery from or adjustment to illness. Also, nurses support the right of clients to define their own health-related goals and engage in care that reflects their values.

There are other well-known nursing resources (some included in the "Suggested Readings" section) that offer additional definitions of nursing. As your knowledge and experience develop, your definition of nursing may change to reflect your focus on a particular care setting or population—or on your specific role. For example, although the definition of nursing developed by Erickson, Tomlin, and Swain (1983) is 25 years old, it remains viable and timely because it combines the concepts noted previously and today's holistic approach to care. Their definition includes what nursing is, how it is accomplished, and its goals: "Nursing is the holistic helping of persons with their self-care activities in relation to their health. This is an interactive, interpersonal process that nurtures strengths to enable development, release, and channeling of resources for coping with one's circumstances and environment. The goal is to achieve a state of perceived optimum health and contentment."

In your journey to discover, understand, and apply this body of knowledge, each chapter presents and guides you through the knowledge of nursing diagnoses, nursing interventions, and client outcomes. These three components of nursing knowledge are applied in practice activities and end-of-chapter work pages to further your understanding and correct application of this knowledge.

You will be introduced to the language described in the nursing process. This introduction includes the classification of nursing diagnoses published by **NANDA INTERNATIONAL** (formerly the North American Nursing Diagnosis Association), the Iowa Intervention and Outcome Projects: Nursing Interventions Classification

(NIC) (McCloskey & Bulecheck, 2004) and the Nursing Outcomes Classification (NOC) (Johnson, 2004), and the Omaha Classification Sys-tem (Martin, 2004). NANDA, NIC, and NOC have combined their classification systems (NNN Alliance); the Omaha Classification System also combines all three aspects of the language to provide comprehensive nursing languages. The four client scenarios presented in the text use examples from NANDA, NIC, NOC, and the Omaha Classification to provide you with differing ways of seeing the nursing process in action.

The *nursing process* provides an orderly, logical, problem-solving approach for administering nursing care so that the client's needs for such care are met comprehensively and effectively.

The Nursing Process

Nursing leaders have identified a process that "combines the most desirable elements of the art of nursing with the most relevant elements of systems theory, using the scientific method" (Shore, 1988). This process incorporates an interactive/interpersonal approach with a problem-solving and decision-making process (Peplau, 1952; King, 1971; Travelbee, 1971; Yura & Walsh, 1988).

The **NURSING PROCESS** was introduced in the 1950s as the three steps of assessment, planning, and evaluation, all based on the scientific method of observing, measuring, gathering data, and analyzing the findings. Years of study, practice, and refinement have led nurses to expand the nursing process to five steps, which provide an efficient method of organizing thought processes for clinical decision making, problem solving, and delivery of higher quality, individualized client care:

> *Assessment*—systematic collection of data relating to client
> *Diagnosis*—analysis of collected data to identify the client's needs or problems
> *Planning*—two-part process of identifying goals and the client's desired outcomes to address the assessed health and wellness needs and selecting appropriate nursing interventions to assist the client in attaining the outcomes
> *Implementation*—putting the plan of care into action
> *Evaluation*—determining the client's progress toward attaining the identified outcomes and monitoring the client's response to and the effectiveness of the selected nursing interventions, for the purpose of altering the plan as indicated.

Because these five steps are central to nursing actions, the nursing process is now included in the conceptual framework of nursing curricula and is accepted as part of the legal definition of nursing in the nurse practice acts of most states.

When a client enters the healthcare system, whether as an acute-care, clinic, or home-care client, the steps of the nursing process are set in motion. The nurse collects data, identifies client needs (nursing diagnoses), establishes goals, identifies outcomes, and selects nursing interventions to assist the client in achieving these goals and outcomes. Following the implementation of the intervention, the nurse evaluates the client's responses and the effectiveness of the plan of care in reaching the desired goals and outcomes to determine whether the needs or problems have been resolved and the client is ready to be discharged from the care setting. If the identified needs or problems remain unresolved, further assessment, additional diagnoses, alteration of goals and outcomes, and/or changes in interventions are required.

Definition of Nursing Process
The nursing process consists of five steps:
1. Assessment
2. Diagnosis/Analysis
3. Planning
4. Implementation
5. Evaluation

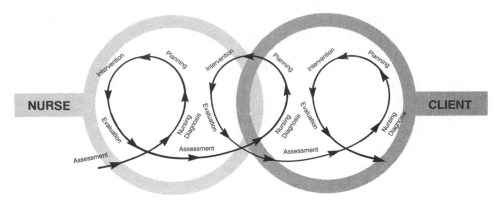

FIGURE 1–1. Diagram of the nursing process. The steps of the nursing process are interrelated, forming a continuous circle of thought and action that is both dynamic and cyclic.

Although the terms *assessment, diagnosis, planning, implementation,* and *evaluation* are used as separate, progressive steps, in reality they are interrelated. These steps form a continuous circle of thought and action that recycles throughout the client's contact with the healthcare system. Figure 1–1 shows a model of how this cycling process can be visualized. The nursing process uses the nursing diagnosis—the clinical judgment product of critical thinking—as the initial platform for subsequent planning. Based on this judgment, nursing interventions are selected and implemented. These two products of critical thinking—clinical judgment and implementation of selected nursing interventions—are reviewed in later chapters.

Figure 1–1 also shows how the progressive steps of the nursing process create an understandable model of both the products and processes of critical thinking contained within the nursing process. The model graphically emphasizes both the dynamic and cyclic characteristics of the nursing process.

How the Nursing Process Works

The scientific method of problem solving, mentioned in the previous section, is used by most people without conscious awareness.

> **FOR EXAMPLE:** You have celebrated completion of your semester finals with a very spicy, late-evening pizza. You awaken during the night with a burning sensation in the center of your chest. You are young and in good health and note no other symptoms **(assessment).** You decide that your pain is the result of the spicy food you have eaten **(diagnosis).** You then determine that you need to relieve the discomfort with an over-the-counter preparation before you will be able to return to sleep **(planning).** You take a liquid antacid for your discomfort **(implementation).** Within a few minutes, you note the burning sensation is relieved, and you return to bed without further concern **(evaluation).**

This is a process, which you routinely use to solve problems in your own life, that can be readily applied to client-care situations. You only need to learn the new terms describing the nursing process rather than having to think about each step **(assessment, diagnosis, planning, implementation,** and **evaluation).**

To use the nursing process effectively, the nurse must possess and be able to apply some basic abilities. Particularly important is a thorough knowledge of science and theory, as applied not only in nursing but also in other related disciplines such as medicine and psychology. Creativity is also needed in the application of nursing knowledge as well as adaptability in handling the many unexpected changes that may occur. As a nurse, you must make a commitment to practice your profession in the best possible way, trusting in yourself and your ability to do your job well and displaying the necessary leadership to organize and supervise as your position requires. In addition, intelligence, well-developed interpersonal skills, and competent technical skills are essential.

FOR EXAMPLE: A client's irritable behavior could be a sign of anger or a sense of helplessness regarding life events; it could also be the result of low serum glucose or the effect of excessive caffeine intake. A single behavior may have varied causes. It is important that your nursing assessment skills identify the underlying etiology so that you can provide appropriate care.

In addition to these abilities, several fundamental beliefs (Box 1–1) provide guidance for applying the nursing process and enhancing the quality of nursing care. To further increase your knowledge and clinical decision-making skills, Appendix A contains the nine statements of the ANA *Code of Ethics for Nurses* (ANA, 2001). Take time to read, think about, and incorporate these nine statements into your professional practice, and refer to the complete work for interpretation of the code statements.

The practice responsibilities presented in the definitions of nursing and the nursing process are explained in *Nursing: Scope & Standards of Practice* (ANA, 2004). The standards provide workable guidelines to ensure that the practice of nursing can be carried out by each nurse. Box 1–2 presents an abbreviated description of the standards of clinical practice. With the ultimate goal of quality health care, the effective use of the nursing process will result in a viable nursing-care system that is recognized and accepted as nursing's body of knowledge that can be shared with other healthcare professionals.

BOX 1–1

Fundamental Philosophical Beliefs in Nursing

Several fundamental philosophical beliefs are essential to the practice of nursing and need to be kept in mind when using the nursing process.

- The client is a human being who has worth and dignity.
- Humans manifest an essential unity of mind/body/spirit (ANA, 1995).
- Health and illness are human experiences, and the presence of one does not preclude the other (ANA, 1995).
- There are basic human needs that must be met (see Chapter 4, Maslow's hierarchy).
- When these needs are not met, problems arise that may require intervention by another person until the individual can resume responsibility for self.
- Human experience is defined contextually and culturally (ANA, 1995).

Continued

Fundamental Philosophical Beliefs in Nursing (Continued)

- The interaction between nurse and client occurs within the context of the values and beliefs of the nurse and client (ANA, 2003).
- Clients have a right to quality health and nursing care delivered with interest, compassion, and competence, with a focus on wellness and prevention.
- The therapeutic nurse-client relationship is important in the nursing process in order to promote a safe environment in which the client can freely talk about his/her concerns.
- The relationship between nurse and client involves participation of both in the process of care (ANA, 2003).

BOX 1-2

ANA *Standards of Nursing Practice*

Standards of Care

Describe a competent level of nursing care as demonstrated by the nursing process, which encompasses all significant actions taken by the registered nurse (RN) in providing care, and form the foundation of clinical decision making.

1. **Assessment:** the RN collects comprehensive data pertinent to the patient's health or situation.
2. **Diagnosis:** the RN analyzes the assessment data to determine the diagnoses or issues.
3. **Outcome identification:** the RN identifies expected outcomes for a plan individualized to the patient or the situation.
4. **Planning:** the RN develops a plan that prescribes strategies and alternatives to attain expected outcomes.
5. **Implementation:** the RN implements the identified plan.
6. **Evaluation:** the RN evaluates progress toward attainment of outcomes.

Standards of Professional Performance

Describes roles expected of all professional nurses appropriate to their education, position, and practice setting.

7. **Quality of Care:** the RN systematically enhances the quality and effectiveness of nursing practice.
8. **Education:** the RN attains knowledge and competency that reflects nursing practice.
9. **Professional Practice Evaluation:** the RN evaluates one's own nursing practice in relation to professional practice standards and guidelines, relevant statutes, rules, and regulations.
10. **Collegiality:** the RN interacts with and contributes to the professional development of peers and colleagues.

11. **Collaboration:** the RN collaborates with patient, family, and others in the conduct of nursing practice.
12. **Ethics:** the RN integrates ethical provisions in all areas of practice.
13. **Research:** the RN integrates research findings into practice.
14. **Resource Utilization:** the RN considers factors related to safety, effectiveness, cost, and impact on practice in planning and delivering nursing services.
15. **Leadership:** the RN provides leadership in the professional practice setting and the profession.

Practice Advantages of the Nursing Process

Practice Advantages of the Nursing Process:
Organizing framework
Human response focus
Structured decision making
Client involvement
Common language
Economic contributions

Using the nursing process has many advantages:

- The nursing process provides a framework for meeting the needs of the individual client, the client's family/significant other(s), and the community.
- The steps of the nursing process focus the nurse's attention on the individual human responses of a client/group to a given health situation, resulting in a holistic plan of care addressing specific needs.
- The nursing process provides an organized, systematic method of problem solving, which may minimize dangerous errors or omissions in caregiving and avoid time-consuming repetition in care and documentation.
- The nursing process promotes the active involvement of the client in his or her own health care, enhancing consumer satisfaction. Such participation increases the client's sense of control over what is happening, stimulates problem solving, and promotes personal responsibility, all of which strengthen the client's commitment to achieving identified goals.
- The nursing process enables you as a nurse to have more control over your own practice. This enhances the opportunity for you to use your knowledge, expertise, and intuition constructively and dynamically to increase the likelihood of a successful client outcome. This, in turn, promotes greater job satisfaction and professional growth.
- The nursing process provides a common language for practice, thus unifying the nursing profession. Using a system that clearly communicates the plan of care to coworkers and clients enhances continuity of care, promotes achievement of client goals, provides a vehicle for evaluation, and aids in the development of nursing standards. In addition, the structure of the process provides a format for documenting the client's response to all aspects of the planned care.
- The nursing process provides a means of assessing nursing's economic contribution to client care. The nursing process supplies a vehicle for the quantitative and qualitative measurement of nursing care that meets the goal of cost-effectiveness while still promoting holistic care.

Summary

The nursing profession has identified a body of knowledge that contributes to the prevention of illness and to the maintenance or restoration of the client's health (or relief of pain and provision of support when a return to health is not possible). The nursing process is the basis of all nursing actions and is the essence of nursing. It can be applied in any healthcare or educational setting, in any theoretical or conceptual framework, and within the context of any nursing philosophy. The process is flexible and yet sufficiently structured to provide a base for nursing actions.

The following chapters identify, discuss, and clarify each step of the nursing process. Inclusion of the standards of clinical nursing practice in the appropriate chapters provides additional information to reinforce your understanding. There are opportunities to apply your knowledge by means of practice activities and a work page at the end of each chapter.

Four clients help you in your learning process by sharing their personal experiences. The term *client* is used throughout rather than *patient* to reflect the philosophy that the individuals or groups with whom you work are legitimate members of the decision-making process and have some amount of control over the planned regimen. They are able, active participants in the planning and implementation of their own care (Erickson, Tomlin, & Swain, 1983).

- Robert is a 72-year-old African-American male admitted to a medical acute-care unit for a recurrence of bilateral lower lobe pneumonia. He is a retired truck driver who has been living alone since his wife's death 5 years ago. He is concerned about his future and about losing control of his life, which presents you with ethical concerns and challenges in dealing with family dynamics.
- Sally is a 30-year-old female who is pregnant and experiencing the onset of labor—this is her third pregnancy. Sally completed her evening shift as a respiratory therapist, although she noted early signs of labor at 8:00 p.m. You will follow Sally through labor, delivery, and home visits by a public health nurse in order to enhance your understanding of the continuity of care.
- Michelle is a 14-year-old female who has suffered multiple injuries in a mountain bike accident. She is a ninth-grader at the local high school and lives with her parents (who immigrated from a Vietnamese refugee camp 25 years ago), an older brother, and a younger sister. You will find pain management a major aspect of your nursing interventions for Michelle, along with several cultural concerns.
- Donald is a 46-year-old male who is being treated for depression after the loss of his position as a loan banker because of his chronic absenteeism and poor job performance related to alcohol abuse. He has been drinking heavily recently and is suffering alcohol withdrawal since his admission. You will follow Donald through his other assessed healthcare needs of nutrition, coping, and changes in his role expectations.

These vignettes will provide many clinical examples throughout the text, offering a simulated practice environment and a touch of reality in planning the required continuity of client care.

Two suggested reading lists are included at the end of this first chapter to assist you in your journey of understanding the historical development of the nursing process and becoming knowledgeable about current publications describing these topics. Sometime during your busy program, take the time to read and reflect on these early authors' meaning and the language of nursing and the nursing process.

1. The ANA has defined nursing as: _____
_____
_____

2. My own definition of nursing is: _____
_____
_____

3. How has the information in this chapter affected your definition? _____
_____
_____

4. The ANA *Social Policy Statement* defines the phenomena of concern for nurses as: _____
_____
_____

5. The definition of *nursing process* is: _____
_____
_____

6. Name and define the five steps of the nursing process and provide an example of each step:

Step	Definition	Example
a. _____	_____	_____
b. _____	_____	_____
c. _____	_____	_____
d. _____	_____	_____
e. _____	_____	_____

7. List three advantages of using the nursing process:

   a. _____

   b. _____

   c. _____

8. List two of the fundamental philosophical beliefs that you believe are basic to decision making within the nursing process:

   a. _____

   b. _____

9. Identify the steps of the nursing process by placing the appropriate number of the activity in the space following the data presented in the following vignette: 1 = assessment; 2 = diagnosis; 3 = planning; 4 = implementation; 5 = evaluation.

VIGNETTE: Robert, a 72-year-old African-American male, is admitted with recurrent bilateral lower lobe pneumonia. _____

He reports this is his second episode in 6 months. _____

His temperature is 101°F, and his skin is hot and flushed. _____

He reports frequent hacking cough with moderate amount of thick, greenish mucus. _____

Auscultation of the chest reveals scattered rhonchi throughout. _____

His mucous membranes are pale, and his lips are dry and cracked. _____

He says that when he was sick last month, the doctor prescribed an antibiotic, which Robert discontinued after 6 days because he was feeling better. _____

You determine Robert has an airway clearance problem and a fluid volume deficit and is not managing his therapeutic regimen effectively, thus requiring teaching to promote adequate self-care and to prevent recurrence. _____

You establish the following outcomes:

• Expectorates secretions completely, with breath sounds clear and respirations noiseless _____
• Demonstrates adequate fluid balance with moist mucous membranes and loose respiratory secretions _____
• Verbalizes understanding of cause of condition and rationale for therapeutic regimen _____

You decide to set up a regular schedule for respiratory activities and fluid replacement. _____

You formulate a teaching plan to cover the identified concerns for self-care and illness prevention. _____

You provide a tube of petroleum jelly for Robert to use on his lips. _____

Every 2 hours, you visit Robert to encourage him to deep-breathe, cough, change his position, and drink a glass of fluid of his choice. _____

You discuss avoidance of crowds and individuals with upper respiratory infections and continuation of the treatment plan after discharge. _____

The following day, Robert's skin is no longer hot and flushed, temperature is 99°F, secretions are loose and readily expectorated, and breath sounds are clearing. _____

Robert's lips and oral mucous membranes are moist; he is able to explain in his own words how to care for himself and how to prevent pneumonia. _____

You decide that the current treatment plan is achieving the identified outcomes and to continue with the plan as written. _____

BIBLIOGRAPHY

American Nurses Association. (1980). *Nursing: A Social Policy Statement*. Kansas City, MO: Author.

American Nurses Association. (1995). *Nursing's Social Policy Statement*. Washington, DC: Author.

American Nurses Association. (2001). *Code of Ethics for Nurses*. Washington, DC: Author.

American Nurses Association. (2003). *Nursing's Social Policy Statement*. Washington, DC: Author.

American Nurses Association. (2004). *Nursing: Scope & Standards of Practice*. Washington, DC: Author.

Erickson, H. C., Tomlin, E. M., & Swain, M. A. P. (1983). *Modeling and Role-Modeling*. Englewood Cliffs, NJ: Prentice-Hall.

Johnson, M., Maas, M., & Moorhead, S. (2004). *Nursing Outcomes Classification (NOC)*, ed 3. St. Louis: Mosby.

King, L. (1971). *Toward a Theory for Nursing: General Concepts of Human Behavior*. New York: Wiley.

Martin, K. S. (2004). *The Omaha System: The Key to Practice, Documentation and Information Management*. Philadelphia: W. B. Saunders.

McCloskey, J. C., & Bulecheck, G. M. (2004). *Nursing Interventions Classification (NIC)*, ed 4. St. Louis: Mosby.

NANDA-I. (2007). *Nursing Diagnoses: Definitions & Classification*. Philadelphia: Author.

Nightingale, F. (1859). *Notes on Nursing: What It Is and What It Is Not* (facsimile edition). Philadelphia: J. B. Lippincott, 1946.

Peplau, H. E. (1952). *Interpersonal Relations in Nursing: A Conceptual Frame of Reference for Psychodynamic Nursing*. New York: Putnam.

Shore, L. S. (1988). *Nursing Diagnosis: What It Is and How to Do It, a Programmed Text*. Richmond, VA: Medical College of Virginia Hospitals.

Travelbee, J. (1971). *Interpersonal Aspects of Nursing*, ed 2. Philadelphia: F. A. Davis.

Yura, H., & Walsh, M. B. (1988). *The Nursing Process: Assessing, Planning, Implementing, Evaluating*, ed 5. Norwalk, CT: Appleton & Lange.

SUGGESTED READINGS

Classical Publications

American Nurses Association. (1973). *Standards of Nursing Practice*. Kansas City, MO: Author.

American Nurses Association. (1987). *The Scope of Nursing Practice*. Kansas City, MO: Author.

Aspinall, M. J., & Tanner, C. A. (1981). *Decision Making for Patient Care: Applying the Nursing Process*. New York: Appleton-Century-Crofts.

Bloch, D. (1974). Some crucial terms in nursing: What do they really mean? *Nursing Outlook, 22*(11):669–694.

Carlson, J. H., Craft, C. A., & McGuire, A. D. (1982). *Nursing Diagnosis*. Philadelphia: W. B. Saunders.

Carnevali, D. L. (1983). *Nursing Care Planning: Diagnosis and Management*, ed 3. Philadelphia: J. B. Lippincott.

Carnevali, D. L., & Thomas, M. D. (1993). *Diagnostic Reasoning and Treatment Decision Making in Nursing*. Philadelphia: J. B. Lippincott.

Hannah, K. J., Reimer, M., Mills, W. C., & Letourneau, S. (Eds.). (1988). *Clinical Judgment and Decision Making: The Future with Nursing Diagnosis*. New York: Wiley.

Orem, D. E. (1971). *Nursing: Concepts of Practice*. New York: McGraw-Hill.

Orlando, I. J. (1961). *The Dynamic Nurse-Patient Relationship: Function, Process, and Principles*. New York: Putnam.

Patterson, J. G., & Zderad, L. T. (1976). *Humanistic Nursing*. New York: Wiley.

U.S. Department of Health and Human Services. (1980). A classification scheme for client problems in community health nursing. DHHS Publication No. HRA 80-16.

Wiedenbach, E. (1964). *Clinical Nursing: A Helping Art*. New York: Springer.

Yura, H., & Walsh, M. B. (Eds.). (1967). *The Nursing Process*. Washington, DC: Catholic University of America Press.

Current Publications

Alfaro-Lefevre, R. (2005). *Applying Nursing Process: A Tool for Critical Thinking*, ed 6. Philadelphia: Lippincott Williams & Wilkins.

Carpenito-Moyet, L. J. (2007). *Nursing Diagnosis: Application to Clinical Practice*, ed 12. Philadelphia: Lippincott Williams & Wilkins.

Craft-Rosenberg, M. J., & Denehy, J. A. (Eds.). (2001). *Nursing Interventions for Infants and Children*. Thousand Oaks, CA: Sage Publications.

Erickson, H. L. (2007). *Modeling and Role-Modeling: A View from the Client's World*. Cedar Park, TX: Unicorns Unlimited.

Gordon, M. (2006). *Manual of Nursing Diagnosis*, ed 11. St. Louis: Mosby.

Hinz, M. D., et al. (2002). *Clinical Applications of Nursing Diagnosis: Adult, Child, Women's Psychiatric, Gerontic, and Home Health Considerations*, ed 4. Philadelphia: F. A. Davis.

Iowa Intervention Project. (1997). Nursing interventions classification (NIC): An overview. In M. J. Rantz & P. LeMone (Eds.). *Classification of Nursing Diagnoses: Proceedings of the Twelfth Conference, North American Nursing Diagnosis Association*. Glendale, CA: Cinahl Information Systems, pp 32–41.

Maas, M., Buckwalter, K. C., & Hardy, M. (1991). *Nursing Diagnosis and Interventions for the Elderly*. Menlo Park, CA: Addison-Wesley.

Maas, M. L. (1997). Nursing-sensitive outcomes classification (NOC): Completing the essential comprehensive languages of nursing. In M. J. Rantz & P. LeMone (Eds.). *Classification of Nursing Diagnoses: Proceedings of the Twelfth Conference, North American Nursing Diagnosis Association*. Glendale, CA: Cinahl Information Systems, pp 40–47.

Martin, K. S. (1997). The Omaha System. In M. J. Rantz & P. LeMone (Eds.). *Classification of Nursing Diagnoses: Proceedings of the Twelfth Conference, North American Nursing Diagnosis Association*. Glendale, CA: Cinahl Information Systems, pp 16–21.

Martin, K. S., & Scheet, N. J. (1992). *Omaha System: A Pocket Guide for Community Health Nursing*. Philadelphia: W. B. Saunders.

Chapter 2

The Assessment Step: Developing the Client Database

■ **ANA STANDARD 1:** Assessment: The registered nurse collects comprehensive data pertinent to the patient's health or the situation. (ANA, 2004)

The Client Database

The **ASSESSMENT** step of the nursing process is an organized dynamic process involving three basic activities:

- Gathering data systematically
- Sorting and organizing the data collected
- Documenting the data in a retrievable format

Using a number of techniques, you focus on eliciting a profile of the client that allows you to identify client problems or needs and corresponding nursing diagnoses, plan care, implement interventions, and evaluate outcomes. This profile is called the **CLIENT DATABASE,** and it serves as the fundamental pool of knowledge about the client from which all other steps of the nursing process proceed.

The client database supplies a sense of the client's overall health status, providing a picture of the client's physical, psychological, sociocultural, spiritual, cognitive, and developmental levels; economic status; functional abilities; and lifestyle. It is a combination of data gathered from the history-taking interview (a method of obtaining **SUBJECTIVE** information by talking with the client and/or significant other[s] and listening to their responses), the physical examination findings (a "hands-on" means of obtaining **OBJECTIVE** information), and information gathered from the laboratory/diagnostic studies. To be more specific, subjective data are what the client/significant others perceive, and objective data are what you observe.

Because consistency is important, the same data collection model should be used for both the client interview (history) and the physical examination, whether that model is a nursing framework, a systems approach, a head-to-toe review, or a combination defined by your own agency. Frequently, to enhance efficiency and effectiveness, these two activities are combined into one interactive process in which physical data are gathered while interview questions are asked.

FRAMEWORK FOR DATA COLLECTION

Several nursing models may be used to guide your data collection. Two of the most commonly used models are shown in Table 2–1: Doenges and Moorhouse's Diagnostic Divisions, and Gordon's Functional Health Patterns.

Using a nursing model as a framework for data collection (rather than a body systems approach, assessing the heart, moving on to the lungs, etc., or the commonly known head-to-toe approach) has the advantage of identifying and validating nursing diagnoses as opposed to **MEDICAL DIAGNOSIS.** An assessment model such as the General Assessment Tool in Appendix B limits repetitive collection of medical data and focuses data collection on the nurse's phenomena of concern—the human experience and response to birth, health, illness, and death. Such responses include self-care limitations; impaired functioning in areas such as sleep, rest, nutrition, elimination, and sexuality; pain; deficiencies in decision making; problematic relationships; or a desire simply to improve one's well-being (ANA, 1995). In addressing the client's responses across the lifespan, the nurse is also directed to consider the promotion of health and safety, the environment and prevention of disease, and the client's relationship with access to the healthcare system and quality of services (ANA, 2003).

TABLE 2–1. **Comparison of Nursing Models for Data Collection**	
Diagnostic Divisions (Doenges and Moorhouse, 2008)	**Functional Health Patterns (Gordon, 1994)**
Activity/Rest: Ability to engage in necessary/desired activities of life (work and leisure) and to obtain adequate sleep/rest.	**Health Perception/Health Management:** Client's perception of general health status and well-being. Adherence to preventive health practices.
Circulation: Ability to transport oxygen and nutrients necessary to meet cellular needs.	**Nutritional-Metabolic:** Patterns of food and fluid intake, fluid and electrolyte balance, general ability to heal.
Ego Integrity: Ability to develop and use skills and behaviors to integrate and manage life experiences.	**Elimination:** Patterns of excretory function (bowel, bladder, and skin), and client's perception.
Elimination: Ability to excrete waste products.	**Activity/Exercise:** Pattern of exercise, activity, leisure, recreation, and ADLs; factors that interfere with desired or expected individual pattern.
Food/Fluid: Ability to maintain intake of and use nutrients and liquids to meet physiological needs.	
Hygiene: Ability to perform basic ADLs.	**Cognitive-Perceptual:** Adequacy of sensory modes, such as vision, hearing, taste, touch, smell, pain perception, cognitive functional abilities.
Neurosensory: Ability to perceive, integrate, and respond to internal and external cues.	
Pain/Discomfort: Ability to control internal/external environment to maintain comfort.	**Sleep/Rest:** Patterns of sleep and rest-relaxation periods during 24-hour day as well as quality and quantity.
Respiration: Ability to provide and use oxygen to meet physiological needs.	**Self-perception/Self-concept:** Individual's attitudes about self, perception of abilities, body image, identity, general sense of worth, and emotional patterns.
Safety: Ability to provide safe, growth-promoting environment.	**Role/Relationship:** Client's perception of major roles and responsibilities in current life situation.
Sexuality: (Component of Ego Integrity and Social Interaction) Ability to meet requirements/characteristics of male/female role.	**Sexuality/Reproductive:** Client's perceived satisfaction or dissatisfaction with sexuality. Reproductive stage and pattern.
Social Interaction: Ability to establish and maintain relationships.	**Coping/Stress Tolerance:** General coping pattern, stress tolerance, support systems, and perceived ability to control and manage situations.
Teaching/Learning: Ability to incorporate and use information to achieve healthy lifestyle/optimal wellness.	**Value-Belief:** Values, goals, or beliefs that guide choices or decisions.

THE INTERVIEW PROCESS

Information in the client database is obtained primarily from the client (who is the most important source) and then from family members/significant others (secondary sources), as appropriate, through conversation and by observation during a structured interview. The nursing interview may take place over several contact sessions, but each contact should yield information, verify information already gathered, and/or

---

BOX 2–1

Subjective Data Compared With Objective Data

Subjective data are what the client/significant other(s) say, reflecting their own thoughts, feelings, and perceptions:

"My hip hurts."
"I'm worried about surgery."
"She didn't sleep well."
"I can't give my husband a shot."
"I haven't had a bowel
  movement for 3 days."

"I can't walk that far."
"I don't know what to do to
  lower my cholesterol level."
"His usual weight is 160 pounds."
"I don't think I'll ever get better."

Objective data are observable and measurable and include information gathered during the physical assessment and diagnostic studies:

Restless/agitated
Temperature 99.2°F
Old surgical scar
Flabby muscle tone
Hb 12.4

Cardiac murmur
Putrid odor
Bloody vomitus
Facial grimacing
Glucose 107

Remember:

- The better *prepared* you are for the interview, the better your chances of asking targeted questions that provide/elicit new insights about the client that, in turn, will help you to ask even more pertinent questions.
- The better the *listener* you are, the better your chances of hearing something meaningful in the client's responses.
- The more *perceptive* you are, the better your chances of seeing new relationships among the data collected.

clarify data. A well-conducted interview can be the first step in establishing a beneficial nurse-client relationship and the rapport needed for good communication.

However, the interview is not merely the routine completion of the items on a standardized form by whomever is available. Rather, it is a tool of communication that permits an interactive exchange of information: a process that produces a higher level of understanding than that which either person could achieve alone. The nursing interview has a specific purpose: collection of a set of specific data (information) from the client/significant other through conversation (subjective data) and observation (objective data). Box 2–1 provides examples that clarify the distinction between these two forms of data.

Clearly, the interview involves more than simply exchanging and processing data. Nonverbal communication is as important as the client's choice of words in providing the data. The ability to collect data that are meaningful to the client's health concerns depends heavily on your own knowledge base; the choice and sequence of questions; and the ability to give meaning to the client's responses, integrate the data gathered, and prioritize the resulting information. Your knowledge, understanding, and insight into the nature and behavior of the client are essential.

Read through Box 2–2, which identifies 10 key elements of a successful client interview. As you begin to understand and apply these interviewing techniques, you will see that they provide an opportunity for the client to use descriptive terms and to explain an answer fully. Keep these tips in mind as you complete the practice activities in this chapter.

BOX 2-2

Elements of a Successful Interview

A successful interview has 10 key elements: (1) a clear sense of the underlying purpose for conducting the interview, (2) preliminary or background research before the interview begins, (3) a formal request of the interviewee to conduct the interview, (4) sound interviewing strategy, (5) effective use of icebreakers, (6) smoothly addressing the business of the interview, (7) good rapport between nurse and client, (8) sensitivity to the client's needs during the interview process, (9) adequate time for recovery following discussion of sensitive areas, and (10) closure.

1. **Underlying purpose:** The information gathered during the interview will be used in formulating the plan of care. Knowing the underlying purpose provides guidance in asking and answering questions, especially when areas that appear to be unrelated to the current situation may need to be pursued.
2. **Preliminary research:** Investigate the client's and the family's current and previous situation. You can use resources such as records from the physician's office, receiving department (e.g., emergency department) or prior admissions, as well as other health-team members. Make notes to identify key points because research often generates questions that should be written down so they are not lost. This preparation will assist you when formulating questions in the interview. The end result of the interview depends on what is put into it.
3. **Request to conduct the interview:** Formally requesting the interview is courteous and can clearly promote a positive interaction. Identify yourself to the client, and explain precisely the purpose of collecting the data and how those data will be used. With the client, set a time for the interview, giving consideration to the needs and severity of the client's condition and the availability of significant others. Allow yourself as much time as possible to prepare. Your approach and attitude are important in helping the client be comfortable and understand the importance of the interview: "Mr. Jones, I would like to ask you some questions about yourself and your health status, so that together we may plan your care" is a more positive approach than "I need to know your history." The first approach not only sells the interview but also stimulates the client's thinking. The result is a more productive interview.
4. **Interview strategy:** Cover the details of the interview in accordance with the definition of its purpose with the client. Preparation and planning give a sense of security and a plan to fall back on if things go slowly or unexpectedly wrong. This also allows a comfortable departure from the plan when conversation takes an unexplored path into productive

Continued

Elements of a Successful Interview (*Continued*)

channels. A new twist and a refreshing insight are the gold nuggets of interviewing, leading to information that otherwise might not have been remembered or shared.

5. **Icebreakers:** Icebreakers are the words and phrases that can put the client at ease, set the stage, and promote a relaxed situation. They are the first bonds of human communication and trust in this new relationship. How the icebreakers are used during the first few minutes may determine how and if the interview proceeds, because the participants make important decisions concerning the future of this relationship. The client and/or significant others are making judgments about you (that you are sincere, trustworthy, sensitive, professionally competent, or not). Some examples of icebreakers that might be used are the acknowledgment of what you know and see: "You've been admitted for surgery." A simple comment about the weather may also put the client at ease. Offering something to drink, if allowed, and asking the client how he or she prefers to be addressed also serve to promote an atmosphere of relaxation. When you sit down and appear relaxed and interested, this goal is more readily achieved.

6. **Business:** Get to the business at hand. Ask your prepared questions, using terminology the client understands. Listen for answers and clues that will lead to other questions that you may not have anticipated. The relaxed informality that you have achieved needs to continue through this phase. Do not expect insights immediately; they usually come with time, increased comfort level, and trust.

7. **Rapport:** Call the participants by name, and monitor reactions to questions. Be careful not to bore or intimidate them with embarrassing questions. It is important to know when to shift gears, speed up, or slow down, or when to ask more challenging questions. Do not hurry the interview, and maintain eye contact as appropriate, based on cultural belief systems.

8. **Sensitivity:** It may be necessary to ask questions about issues that involve sensitive areas for the client. For example, questions about sexuality, lifestyle, or behaviors that put the person at risk for sexually transmitted diseases (STDs), including human immunodeficiency virus/acquired immunodeficiency syndrome (HIV/AIDS), may be perceived as threatening. Proceed cautiously being alert to verbal/nonverbal cues that may indicate that the area of discussion is particularly sensitive for the individual. Ceasing exploration at this point demonstrates respect for the individual's rights/privacy and can enhance the trust between participants. At a future point in the interview, the client's level of comfort may allow you to revisit the topic and gather necessary data.

9. **Recovery:** Recover any lost rapport. If the sensitive areas have been approached slowly, the recovery period should be fairly easy to accomplish. Warmth and caring evidenced by a smile and a touch of the hand are helpful.

10. **Closure:** Conclude the interview by summarizing the highlights of the interview, and encourage further communication by asking the client if he or she has anything else to add or any questions to ask of you.

The interview question is the major tool you will use to obtain information. How you phrase the question is a skill that is important in obtaining the desired results and getting the information necessary to arrive at accurate nursing diagnoses. Following are nine effective data collection questioning techniques:

- **Asking open-ended questions** allows the client maximum freedom to respond in his or her own way, impose no limitations on how the question may be answered, and may produce considerable information. For example, "How do you feel about your new medications?" or "Explain the injection technique to me."

- **Asking hypothetical questions** poses a situation and asks the client how it might be handled. You can learn whether the client has accurate information and can think about how a similar situation might be handled. For example, "What would you do if you felt dizzy?" These questions may be very useful in determining the extent to which the client has learned previously presented material.

- **Reflecting or "mirroring"** responses are useful techniques in getting at underlying meanings. By restating in the form of a question what the client has said, the client has the opportunity to continue to add detail to or clarify what he or she said. For example, the client might say, "Some days I'd like to throw this needle out the window." A mirror response would be, "So you'd like to throw your medication out the window?" Now the client is encouraged to verbalize what he or she is actually thinking or feeling. This response is nonevaluative and nonthreatening.

- **Focusing** shows the client that you are attending to what is being said and consists of eye contact (within cultural limits), body posture, and verbal responses. For example, "Tell me more about that."

- **Giving broad openings** encourages the client to take the initiative about what is to be talked about: for example, "Where would you like to begin?"

- **Offering general leads** encourages the client to continue: "...and then?"

- **Exploring** pursues a topic in more detail: "Would you describe it more fully?"

- **Verbalizing the implied** gives voice to what has been suggested; it is putting into words what the client has said indirectly. For instance, the client says, "It's no use taking this medicine anymore." You respond, "You're concerned that it isn't making a difference for you?"

- **Encouraging evaluation** helps the client to consider the quality of his or her own experience, such as: "How does that seem to you?"

However, even with a properly phrased question, there will be times when the answer you are seeking will not be given. The client has the right to refuse to answer any question at all, no matter how reasonably phrased. Some questioning strategies to be avoided because they are generally ineffective in eliciting information from clients include:

- **Asking closed-end questions** (such as "Why?") allow little or no freedom in choosing a response, such as, "Do you take your medicine?" (client responds "No") or "How long have you been taking insulin?" (client responds "3 years"). Typically, there are only one or two possible answers to a question. The interviewer remains in close control over the interview because of the rigid structure. Although the closed-end question may be useful in an emergency situation (when it is necessary to gather information in a short time), it is important to provide an opportunity for the client to explain the answers to questions in greater detail.
- **Leading questions** typically suggest the desired response, such as, "The infection seems to be getting better, don't you agree?" and thereby reduce the range of responses because the interviewee most commonly agrees with leading statements. Highly emotional questions, tone of voice, or inflection ("Where did you learn *that* injection technique?") may be interpreted as challenging, provoking the interviewee to "attack" or become defensive, thereby blocking communication.
- **Probing** is a persistent line of questioning—a demand for more information than is given willingly. "Now tell me about . . . ." creates an uneasy feeling in the client and may be interpreted as an invasion of privacy, resulting in a defensive response or withholding of information.
- **Agreeing/disagreeing** implies that the client is "right" or "wrong" ("I agree, that would be the thing to do" or "You didn't mean to do that, did you?") rather than promoting the client's idea as separate from your own. This can block exploration of an issue.

Complete Practice Activity 2–1.

PRACTICE ACTIVITY 2–1
Determining Types of Data

1. Identify subjective (S) versus objective (O) data:

Skin cool/damp
Sputum pale yellow
Allergic to eggs and sulfa
Pitting edema of feet and ankles
Usually voids three times per day
Chest pain lasting 15 minutes

2. Match the technique in Column A to the statements in Column B:

Column A	Column B
a. Open-ended question	"The next time this comes up, what would you do to handle it?"
b. Hypothetical question	"That feeling in your chest, can you describe it more fully?"
c. Reflection	"Do you use alcohol regularly?"
d. Closed-end question	"What would you like to talk about?"
e. Leading question	"You're feeling better today, aren't you?"

3. Rewrite the following, using effective data collection techniques:
a. "You felt like crying, didn't you?"
b. "You're in pain again?"
c. "Do you want to change occupations?"
d. "Since your physician has talked with you, you don't have any questions, do you?"
e. "Did you eat lunch?"

The Nursing Interview: Questioning and Listening

The client's medical diagnosis can provide a starting point for the nursing interview. Your knowledge about the anatomy and physiology of the disease/condition helps in choosing and prioritizing questions. When using a nursing model assessment tool, the results of the focused interview will point to the human responses to health, illness, and life processes and to the development of nursing (rather than medical) diagnoses. Let us visit our first client, Robert. Although you will ask Robert about the signs and symptoms associated with his pneumonia, your nursing focus is:

- How does his shortness of breath affect his ability to care for himself? (hygiene)
- Have the coughing episodes resulted in chest-wall pain or loss of sleep? (pain/discomfort, activity/rest)
- Has his appetite been affected by his frequent expectoration of purulent mucus? (food/fluid)
- How does he protect himself and others from transmission of infection? (safety, teaching/learning)

In addition, keep an open mind and pay attention to clues that may identify other human responses of concern requiring investigation.

THE CLIENT HISTORY

The history is more than simply recording information. You must review the data, organize and determine the relevance of each item (value the data), and document the facts. The quality of a history improves with your knowledge and experience with the history-taking process. Although such assessments are often lengthy and time-consuming in the beginning, more time is eventually saved by avoiding the necessity to retrace steps, correct misinformation, and undo actions. With practice, as you become skilled, the time required for this activity will decrease markedly.

GUIDELINES FOR HISTORY-TAKING

Listen Carefully

Be a good listener: Listen attentively to what the individual is saying. Listen for whole thoughts and ideas, not merely isolated facts. Facts may not be as important as the ideas that bind them together. For example, Robert tells you, "Sure, my doctor ordered some pills for me [antibiotics for pneumonia] last month." But Robert's tone of voice, facial expression, and body language communicate the idea that he may not be following his treatment regimen. Robert's nonverbal communication requires validation by asking either reflecting or open-ended questions, such as, "You seem to have a lack of enthusiasm as you tell me about your medication. What is that about?"

Active Listening

ACTIVE LISTENING: reflecting back what the other person has said to validate your understanding of the meaning. A restatement of the other person's total communication, including the words and the feelings.

Use skills of active listening, silence, and acceptance to provide ample time for the person to respond: Give your full attention to the interview and do not interrupt. Save your own comments until the speaker is completely finished. Finally, ask related questions to stimulate the individual's memory if blocks occur. Once again, "facts" may not be as important as the client's perception of reality. As you gain more experience in professional practice, you will begin to understand how important the client's perception is. This is especially true in your assessment, understanding, management, and treatment of your client's reported perception of pain.

Objectivity

Be as objective as possible: Identify only the client's and/or significant others' contributions to the history, and do not try to interpret the data at this point. Record subjective data from the client/significant others just as they were stated during the interview. Failure to do so may cause confusion and lead to inaccurate diagnoses. However, lengthy responses may need to be paraphrased.

Your initial responsibility is to observe, collect, and record data without drawing conclusions or making judgments and assumptions. Your self-awareness is a crucial factor in the interaction because perceptions, judgments, and assumptions can easily color the assessment findings unless they are recognized. Everyone has a responsibility to understand how biases affect conclusions drawn from data and not to be influenced by them. Review the beliefs cited in Chapter 1 and the Code for Nurses in Appendix A.

Manageable Detail

Keep the amount of detail manageable: The data collected about the client and/or significant others contain a vast amount of information, some of which may be repetitious. However, some of it will be valuable for eliciting information that was not recalled or volunteered previously.

Enough material needs to be noted in the history so that a complete picture is presented and yet not so much that the information will not be read or used. "Necessary" information includes all data (positive and negative) that are relevant to the situation. For example, Robert was admitted with the diagnosis of pneumonia. During the history, he reports, "I've been coughing a lot lately." Necessary information in this case is to clarify what Robert means by "coughing a lot lately." You need to know the frequency and time of coughing and factors that bring about or terminate an episode of coughing. Along with knowing there was a cough, you need to know whether the cough was productive. If productive, ascertain the descriptive characteristics of the mucus: what color was it? how much mucus does he expectorate? As you can see, the "necessary" information is that which clarifies and makes the communication of Robert's subjective data to other healthcare providers both useful and meaningful.

Sequence Information

Order is imperative: Develop and use a form that makes it easy to find information, identify problems, and choose nursing diagnoses. In addition, present the current health problems in chronological order, and include relevant events from the past. It is also useful to express topics in a uniform manner. For example, expressing the age at which events/illnesses/surgery occurred instead of just the year events occurred: "hysterectomy, age 35/1973."

Document Clearly

Unless you have computerized data collection, you must write legibly: This improves the communication and comprehension of your findings, thereby decreasing the chance of misunderstanding and saving time for you and other healthcare professionals who rely on your records.

Record Data in a Timely Way

Record the data during the interview, or write the history as soon as possible after gathering the information: This helps ensure greater accuracy of the data. The longer you wait to record, the more likely it is the data and specific details will fade and be more difficult to recall. Data not recorded are data lost.

Physical Examination: The Hands-On Phase

You perform the physical examination to gather objective information and also as a screening device. For the data collected during the physical examination to be meaningful, you need to know the normal physical and emotional characteristics of human beings sufficiently well to be able to recognize deviations.

FOCUS AND PREPARATION

To gain as much information as possible from the assessment procedure, approach the client with a positive, sincere attitude. Such an attitude conveys competence, interest, kindness, thoroughness, orderliness, and confidence. It may be frightening for the client if you give the impression that you do not know what you are doing or if you are awkward in performing assessment tasks. Give the client a clear explanation of the procedures you will be performing. Then, proceed with the examination according to the format you have chosen to gather and record the data: a nursing model (as suggested earlier), a systems approach (cardiovascular, respiratory, gastrointestinal, and so on), a head-to-toe review (head, neck, chest, and so on), or a combination of these. The same format should be used each time you perform a physical examination, to reduce the possibility of omissions and to increase your confidence and efficiency in completing the task.

However, the client's state of health/severity of condition may require you to place priority on specific portions of your assessment. This priority in data collection is based in part on the measurement criteria developed by the ANA. "[The nurse] prioritizes data collection activities based on the patient's immediate condition, or anticipated needs of the patient or situation" (ANA, 2003). For example, when examining a client with severe chest pain, you would probably choose to evaluate the pain and the cardiovascular system before addressing other areas. Likewise, the duration and specificity of any physical examination depend on circumstances such as the condition of the client and the urgency of the situation.

During the examination, emotional support and care should be offered as indicated. Use your professional judgment in selecting the steps and sequencing the assessment to provide emotional support as needed. The client with resolving chest pain may want to talk about his or her embarrassment of being perceived as "weak" during the episode of chest pain. Interrupting your examination to support and listen to your client is not only a correct intervention but also demonstrates the sensitive blending of the art and science of nursing. It is also important to provide the client with as much feedback as possible. While completing the examination process, you will find this is an excellent opportunity to provide education on associated procedures, assessment findings, and health teaching in general. Perceptual and observational skills are especially important in determining what your client needs.

ASSESSMENT METHODS

Four common methods used during the physical examination are inspection, palpation, percussion, and auscultation. These techniques incorporate the senses of sight, hearing, touch, and smell:

1. *Inspection* is a systematic process of observation that is not limited to vision; it also includes the senses of hearing and smell.

   Sight: Observing the skin for color, discolorations, lacerations; the lesion for drainage; the respiratory pattern for depth and symmetry; body language, movement, and posture; the use of extremities; the presence of physical limitations; the face for expressions.

   Hearing: Listening to the nature of a cough, the integrity of a joint, the tone of a voice, or content of interactions with others.

   Smell: Detecting significant odors.

2. *Palpation* is the touching or pressing of the external surface of the body with the fingers.

> *Touch:* Feeling a lump; noting temperature, amount of moistness, and texture of skin; or determining strength of uterine contraction.
>
> *Pressure:* Determining the character of a pulse, evaluating edema, noting position of the fetus, or pinching (tenting) to observe skin turgor.
>
> *Probing deeper:* Revealing muscle tone/tension or an abnormal pain response.

3. *Percussion* is the direct or indirect tapping of a specific body surface to ascertain information about underlying tissues or organs.

> *Using fingertips:* Tap the chest, and listen for the sound indicating the presence or absence of fluid, masses, or consolidation.
>
> *Using a percussion hammer:* Tap the knee, and observe the presence or absence of lower leg movement/reflexes.

4. *Auscultation* is listening for sounds within the body with the aid of a stethoscope and describing or interpreting them.

> *Hearing:* Listening at the antecubital space for blood pressure, the chest for heart/lung sounds, the abdomen for bowel sounds or fetal heart tones.

FOLLOW-UP CONSIDERATIONS

After completion of the physical examination, your client may require assistance. The client may need to be helped off the examination table for safety reasons or may require help with dressing. Consideration of these sometimes forgotten needs enhances the rapport and trust developed during the examination. Including these interventions personalizes the client-nurse interaction and makes the assessment process much more than just a gathering of required data.

You may need to verify or clarify communication associated with the physical examination. By repeating aloud what you have observed, you give the client the opportunity to validate the accuracy of the information obtained, and misunderstandings can be avoided; for example: observation—"I noticed that you flinched when I felt your abdomen"; response—"Yes, your hand was cold, and I'm ticklish."

Laboratory Tests and Diagnostic Procedures: Supporting Evidence

Laboratory and other diagnostic studies are a part of the information-gathering stage. They aid in the management, maintenance, and restoration of health. Some tests are used to diagnose disease, whereas others are useful in following the course of a disease or adjusting therapy. Your knowledge about the purpose, procedure, and results of various scans, x-rays, performance tests (e.g., treadmill electrocardiogram, pulmonary function), and numerous laboratory studies is necessary for the success of the study, promotion of timely nursing interventions, and a positive client outcome through proper preparation and education of the client about the prescribed studies.

In reviewing and interpreting laboratory tests, it is important to remember that the test material does not always correlate to an organ or body system. For example, a urine test might be done to detect the presence of bilirubin and urobilinogen, which could indicate liver disease, biliary obstruction, or hemolytic disease. In some cases, the relationship of the test to the pathology is clear, whereas in others, such as obtaining renal function studies in the presence of cardiac failure, it is not. This is a result of the interrelationships among the various organs and systems of the body. In a few cases, the results of a test are nonspecific because they indicate only that there is a disorder or abnormality and do not indicate the location of the cause of the problem. For example, an elevated erythrocyte sedimentation rate suggests the presence but not the location of an inflammatory process.

In evaluating laboratory tests, it is advisable to consider which drugs, over-the-counter medications, and herbal supplements are being administered to the client because they may have the potential to blur or falsify results, creating a misleading diagnostic picture.

FOR EXAMPLE:

- Heparin and aspirin products prolong blood clotting times.
- Oral iron preparations cause a false-positive result when the stool is tested for occult blood.
- Phenazopyridine (Pyridium) is a urinary tract analgesic that can color the urine red.
- Promethazine (Phenergan), an antiemetic, can cause a false-negative result in a pregnancy test.
- Ingestion of poppy seeds can provide a false-positive result for heroin; vitamin E can affect clotting times.

In some cases, it is necessary to note at what time medication was administered. Serum levels can be drawn to determine the varied concentrations of administered medications. Terms such as *peak* and *trough level* are used to determine the possible toxic effects and the therapeutic ranges of the medication.

There are also several mechanisms that may alter the laboratory results through the introduction of interfering materials.

FOR EXAMPLE:

- Foods that give a yellow color to blood serum (e.g., carrots, yams) alter a bilirubin test.
- Food may contribute to the presence of substances in body fluids/excretions, such as hemoglobin and myoglobin in meat, which may lead to a misdiagnosis of occult blood in the stool.
- Intramuscular injections can elevate creatine phosphokinase levels, which may be used to screen for acute myocardial infarction.

Organizing Information Elements

CLUSTERING THE COLLECTED DATA

Data gathered in the interview, from the physical examination, and from other records/sources are organized and recorded in a concise systematic way and clustered into similar categories. Various formats have been used to accomplish this, including a review of body systems. The body systems approach has been used by both medicine and nursing for many years but is actually more useful for the physician in making a medical diagnosis than for a nurse in identifying nursing diagnoses. Currently, nursing is developing and fine-tuning its own tools for recording and clustering data (e.g., Doenges, Moorhouse, & Murr 2008; Gordon, 1994; Guzzetta, et al., 1989). Organizing data using a nursing framework (Box 2–3) assists you in focusing your attention and in choosing specific nursing diagnosis labels to describe the data accurately. However, be aware of the advantages of each type of framework, and follow the approach recommended by your school or agency. Remember, consistency is the key. Before you meet Donald, read about Michelle in Box 2–4, and return to Table 2–1 to review the definitions of the 13 diagnostic divisions and the 11 functional health patterns.

BOX 2–3

Assessment Data for Robert Recorded in Doenges and Moorhouse Diagnostic Divisions Assessment Tool

Respiration
Reports (Subjective)
Dyspnea, related to: Climbing stairs/walking more than two blocks, close places/crowds
Cough/sputum: Thick, green, approximately 1/2 tsp, 6 to 10 times/day, especially with activity
History of:
Bronchitis: Diagnosed 2000
Asthma: No; **Tuberculosis:** No
Emphysema: Diagnosed 2000
Recurrent pneumonia: Yes; last admission approximately 6 months ago, recurrence 1 month ago
Exposure to noxious fumes: Not aware of past exposures (was a diesel trucker)
Smoker: Cigarettes (pack/day): 1 × 45 years, 1/2 × 8 years (since 2000)
Number of pack/years: 49
Use of respiratory aids: Inhaler and PO meds
Oxygen: No/"Doctor suggested I use oxygen at night, but I don't think I'm that bad."
Exhibits (Objective)
Respiratory: Rate: 28 at rest; **Depth:** Shallow
Symmetry: Increased AP diameter
Use of accessory muscles: Yes
Nasal flaring: None observed
Fremitus: Increased tactile; **Egophone:** Resonance increased
Percussion: Hyperresonate

Continued

*Assessment Data for Robert Recorded in Doenges
and Moorhouse Diagnostic Divisions Assessment Tool
(Continued)*

Breath sounds: Diminished, bronchovesicular, basilar inspiratory crackles bilateral, scattered rhonchi—limited clearing with cough
Cyanosis: Oral mucous membranes pale
Clubbing of fingers: Slight
Sputum characteristics: Green, tenacious, scant amount during assessment
Mentation/restlessness: Alert; responds to all questions; no restlessness
Other: Verbal responses slow; breathless—phrases four to five words long
Results chest x-ray: Bilateral lower lobe infiltrates
On reviewing the collected data for this client with pneumonia and noting cues (signs and symptoms) in the *Respiration* section of the database, you are referred to the *Respiration* section of the *Diagnostic Divisions*. Four possible labels are suggested: ineffective Airway Clearance, risk for Aspiration, ineffective Breathing Pattern, and impaired Gas Exchange.

BOX 2–4

*Organizing Assessment Data for Michelle Using a
Nursing Framework*

You obtain the following information for the client database during your assessment of Michelle (following her admission to the orthopedic unit, having had an external fixation device applied for multiple compound fractures of the right lower leg). The data have been clustered in two nursing frameworks by means of the identifying numbers for each data element.

Assessment Data

1. 14-year-old female
2. High-school student
3. Practicing Buddhist
4. Single
5. Living with parents, one older brother, one younger sister
6. Temperature 100°F
7. Sharp severe pain in right lower leg, "toes to knees," rated 9 on 0–10 scale, and right-sided headache rated 4
8. Hospitalized for tonsillectomy 4 years ago—2004/age 11
9. Alert and oriented, brief loss of consciousness at time of injury
10. Respirations 26, lungs clear, splinting with deep inspiration

11. Weight 98 pounds
12. Indwelling catheter in place; urine clear, amber
13. Independent in self-care
14. Usually sleeps 8 hours each night
15. Right lower leg—wound packed with sterile dressing; multiple puncture sites (external fixator in place)
16. Menarche at age 13
17. Manages stress by talking with friends, exercise (distance runner and mountain biking), meditation
18. States has no allergies
19. Concerned that injury will leave scars and affect participation in track activities
20. P 110, BP 100/78 (left arm/supine)

How you organize these data depends on the format you choose for recording. On occasion, data may be recorded in more than one section because the divisions/patterns are based on human responses instead of specific body systems. The above data could be recorded in two different nursing formats:

Doenges and Moorhouse: Diagnostic Divisions

Activity/Rest: 2, 9, 14, 17
Pain/Discomfort: 7
Circulation: 20   Respiration: 10
Ego Integrity: 3, 4, 17, 19   Safety: 6, 15, 18
Elimination: 12   Sexuality: 1, 4, 16
Food/Fluid: 11   Social Interaction: 4, 5
Hygiene: 13   Teaching/Learning: 2, 8
Neurosensory: 9

Gordon's: Functional Health Patterns

Health Perception/Health Management: 7, 8   Self-perception/
                                                   Self-concept: 19
Nutritional/Metabolic: 6, 10, 11, 15, 18, 20   Role/Relationship: 1, 2, 4, 5
                                                   Sexuality/Reproductive: 4, 16
Coping/Stress Tolerance: 17   Elimination: 12
Value/Belief: 3
Activity/Exercise: 10, 13, 17
Cognitive/Perceptual: 9   Sleep/Rest: 14

REVIEWING AND VALIDATING FINDINGS

VALIDATION is an ongoing process that occurs during the data collection phase and at its completion, when the data are reviewed and compared. You review the data to be sure that what has been recorded is factual and to identify errors of omission or inconsistencies that require additional investigation. Validation is particularly important when the data are conflicting, when the source of the data may not be reliable, or when serious harm to the client could result from any inaccuracies. Question the client or others to verify your impressions; for example, "tell me more about that" or "what I heard you say is ...." Validating the information gathered can prevent the possibility that wrong inferences are made or conclusions drawn that can lead to inaccurate nursing diagnoses, incorrect outcomes, and/or inappropriate nursing actions. Validating can be done by sharing your assumptions with the individuals involved and having them verify the accuracy of those conclusions. (Remember that data given in confidence should not be shared with other individuals unless the information is necessary for their evaluation of the client or for providing care. For example, information received in confidence regarding a client's sexual contacts should not be discussed with a parent or spouse without the client's consent, but it would be provided to public health officials in the presence of a reportable sexually transmitted disease.)

Data that are grossly abnormal are rechecked, and objective and subjective data are compared for congruencies and/or inconsistencies. For example, the client reports upper right abdominal pain, although musculature appears relaxed, and the client does not flinch on abdominal palpation. Additional investigation reveals that the pain is episodic and usually follows meal times. Temporary factors that may affect the data are also identified and noted. For example, you note the client's right hand is cool in comparison with the left hand. On questioning, you discover that the patient had been holding a glass of ice water in the right hand.

Finally, the client may remember something or may feel more comfortable in sharing information with you. As mentioned, although the data collected by any healthcare professional are confidential, it may be appropriate or necessary to share the information. For example, you may have a greater opportunity to observe interactions between family members during the assessment process, which could have an impact on the diagnostic process and/or the plan of care. Some of these findings may need to be brought to the attention of other healthcare professionals, such as the physician, dietitian, or physical therapist. Sharing these additional data aids in collaborative planning of care.

Summary

The assessment step of the nursing process emphasizes and should provide a holistic view of the client. The generalized assessment done during the overall gathering of data creates a profile of the client. A focused assessment may be done to obtain more information about a specific issue that needs expansion or clarification. Both types of assessment are important and complement each other. A successfully completed assessment provides data on the client's state of wellness, response to health problems, and risk factors.

To assist you in your assessment assignments and future applications of this first step of the nursing process, an extensive review of the current literature is provided. The Suggested Readings at the end of this chapter provide assessment references for adult health, the pediatric or geriatric client, telephone assessment, home health, and long-term care. Also included is a separate bibliography on genograms. A genogram is displayed in Practice Activity 2–2.

Donald has been admitted to the psychiatric hospital acute substance abuse unit for treatment of depression and withdrawal from alcohol.

Organize the data below according to diagnostic divisions and functional health patterns. Place the number of the listed data next to the category where you believe it fits (see Table 2–1).

1. 46-year-old male
2. Divorced, not currently involved in a relationship
3. Loan banker, laid off 5 months ago
4. Unsteady gait
5. Clothes rumpled, has not shaved for 2 days, dry skin
6. Eats 1 or 2 meals a day—donuts, sandwiches, meat and potatoes, no vegetables or fruits; coffee 4+cups/day
7. Stools have been loose, 3 to 4/day
8. BP 136/82 (right arm/sitting), radial pulse 92
9. Alert and oriented
10. Catholic, not practicing
11. Sleeps usually 3 to 4 hours a night, awakens around 5 a.m.
12. "I've been drinking a lot lately." (bourbon 1 fifth/day)
13. Worries about financial situation, unable to make child support payments
14. Congested nonproductive cough
15. Reports constant throbbing pain, left knee—old sports injury
16. Genogram

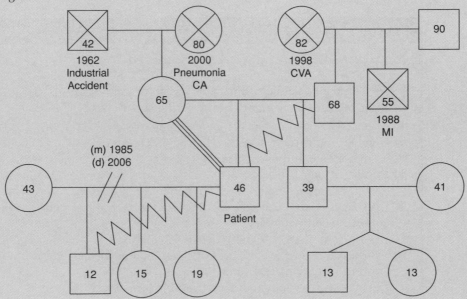

Continued

Organizing Data: Diagnostic Divisions and Functional Health Patterns (*Continued*)

Genogram: graphic representation of a family (may include several generations) reflecting medical data and relationships/roles.

Diagnostic Divisions	Functional Health Patterns
Activity/Rest:	Health Perception/Health Management:
Circulation:	Nutritional/Metabolic:
Ego Integrity:	Elimination:
Elimination:	Activity/Exercise:
Food/Fluid:	Cognitive/Perceptual:
Hygiene:	Sleep/Rest:
Neurosensory:	Self-perception/Self-concept:
Pain/Discomfort:	Role/Relationship:
Respiration:	Sexuality/Reproductive:
Safety:	Coping/Stress Tolerance:
Sexuality:	Value/Belief:
Social Interaction:	
Teaching/Learning:	

Return to the first ANA Standard of Practice, and review the measurement criteria necessary to achieve and ensure compliance with the standard. The knowledge and skills required to meet the criteria listed in Box 2–5 have been described in this chapter.

BOX 2–5

Measurement Criteria for ANA Standard 1

ANA Standard 1: Assessment: The registered nurse collects comprehensive data pertinent to the patient's health or the situation.

1. Collects data in a systematic and ongoing process.
2. Involves the patient, family, other healthcare providers, and environment, as appropriate, in holistic data collection.
3. Prioritizes data collection activities based on the patient's immediate condition, or anticipated needs of the patient or situation.
4. Uses appropriate evidence-based assessment techniques and instruments in collecting pertinent data.
5. Uses analytical models and problem-solving tools.
6. Synthesizes available data, information, and knowledge relevant to the situation to identify patterns and variances.
7. Documents relevant data in a retrievable format.

(ANA, 2004)

1. Rewrite the following questions so that they are open-ended:

    a. You're feeling better after the respiratory treatment, aren't you?

    _____

    b. Have you taken your medicine today?

    _____

    c. Do you understand these directions?

    _____

2. Using the interview techniques described in this chapter, write a question to clarify these client statements:

    a. Do you think I should tell my doctor about my concern?

    Reflecting/mirroring: _____

    b. I got into a fight with my roommate.

    Exploring: _____

    c. I don't think I can go on without my husband.

    Verbalize the implied: _____

    d. I feel like running out the door.

    General lead: _____

3. When might a closed-ended question be helpful?

    _____

4. Describe the three components of the client database:

    a. _____

    b. _____

    c. _____

5. The four activities involved in the physical assessment are:

    a. _____ b. _____ c. _____ d. _____

6. The client database is important to the provision of client care because:

    _____

7. For assessment purposes, the difference between subjective data and objective data is:

    _____

8. Underline the subjective data, and circle the objective data in the following vignette:

> **VIGNETTE:** Sally comes to the obstetric department for evaluation of her stage of labor. Back pains began about 3 hours ago (8 p.m.) while she was on her job as a respiratory therapist. Contractions are 5 minutes apart, lasting 30 seconds for the past 45 minutes. BP 146/84 (left arm/lying), P 110, respirations 24. Weight 155 pounds (up 4 pounds this week). Cervix dilated 4 cm, membranes intact. Fetal head engaged, heart tones slightly muffled in right lower quadrant, rate 132. Nauseated since a dinner of fried chicken 4 hours ago. Appears anxious and seems irritated that her physician is not present. Voided 1 hour ago; has not had a bowel movement for 2 days. Stopped smoking 8 months ago. Lungs clear. No allergies. Married, husband plans to attend the birth. Two children are in the care of their grandmother tonight. Appears well groomed with a well-fitting maternity uniform and low-heeled shoes. Requests to leave contacts in to observe the birth. Last physical examination 1 week ago. Gestation 37 weeks, with due date 3 weeks off—3/11/08.

9. An important benefit of doing "research" or reviewing available information before an interview is:

_____

10. An interview should be "requested" because:

_____

11. Check the information resources that can be useful in helping the nurse to prepare for the interview:

Family/significant other   Physician notes

Old medical records   Textbooks/reference journals

Diagnostic studies   Other nurses/healthcare providers

12. Sensitivity of the nurse is important during the interview process to:

_____

13. List three abilities of the nurse that are necessary in order to collect a relevant client database:

a. _____

b. _____

c. _____

14. In the following vignette, cluster and record the assessment data (following the numbers) into the appropriate diagnostic divisions listed below. Refer to Table 2–1 as needed for the type of data included in the specific divisions to assist you in clustering the data.

VIGNETTE: Robert, a 72-year-old (1) African-American male admitted to the medical unit at 1 p.m. for (2) bilateral lower lobe pneumonia. (3) Has had liquids only by mouth for several days. (4) Last BM—2 days ago, brown/formed stool, (5) voided at 1:20 p.m.—clear, dark amber. He reports (6) "my chest hurts," as he splints chest while coughing. (7) Small amount thick, green sputum expectorated with cough. (8) Appears anxious, fidgeting with sheets, face tense, watching nurse intently. (9) Tympanic temperature 101°F, (10) BP 178/102 (left arm/lying), P 100/regular, (11) respirations 28/shallow. (12) Skin warm, moist; color pale. (13) Has difficulty hearing questions, left hearing aid (R ear) at home. (14) Reports "This is the second episode in a month." (15) Doctor prescribed antibiotic (drug unknown) a month ago; client did not complete treatment. (16) States he lives alone (widower) and is (17) responsible for meeting his own needs. In reviewing diagnostic studies, you note that the (18) chest x-ray reveals infiltrates in both lower lobes, and a (19) Gram stain of the sputum reveals Gram-negative bacteria.

Diagnostic Divisions

Activity/Rest: _____   Hygiene: _____   Sexuality: _____

Circulation: _____   Neurosensory: _____   Social Interaction: _____

Ego Integrity: _____   Pain/Discomfort: _____   Teaching/Learning: _____

Elimination: _____   Respiration: _____

Food/Fluid: _____   Safety: _____

The next chapter presents the second step of the nursing process-diagnosis. In this chapter, the diagnostic reasoning process is used to analyze/synthesize the information obtained from the client database and to identify the client healthcare needs or nursing diagnoses that form the basis for the development of the plan of care.

BIBLIOGRAPHY

American Nurses Association. (1995). *Nursing's Social Policy Statement*. Washington, DC: Author.

American Nurses Association. (2003). *Nursing's Social Policy Statement*, ed 2. Washington, DC: Author.

American Nurses Association. (2004). *Nursing: Scope & Standards of Practice*. Washington, DC: Author.

Doenges, M. E., Moorhouse, M. F., & Murr, A. C. (2008). *Nurse's Pocket Guide: Diagnoses, Interventions, and Rationales*, ed 11. Philadelphia: F. A. Davis.

Gordon, M. (1994). *Nursing Diagnosis: Process and Application*, ed 3. St. Louis: Mosby.

Guzzetta, C. E., Bunton, S. D., Prinkey, L. A., & Sherer, A. (1989). *Clinical Assessment Tools for Use With Nursing Diagnoses*. St. Louis: Mosby.

SUGGESTED READINGS

Allen, J. E. (1997). *Long-Term Care Facility Resident Assessment Instrument User's Manual: For Use With Version 2.0 of HCFA: Minimum Data Set Resident Assessment Protocols and Utilization Guidelines, October 1995, Plus HCFA's 249 Questions and Answers, August 1996*. New York: Springer.

Barkauskas, V. H., Baumann, L. C., & Darling-Fisher, C. (2002). *Health & Physical Assessment*, ed 3. St. Louis: Mosby.

Bates, B. (2002). *Visual Guide to Physical Examination: Head-to-Toe Adult Assessment*. Philadelphia: Lippincott Williams & Wilkins.

Cole, S. A., & Bird, J. (2000). *The Medical Interview: The Three-Function Approach*, ed 2. St. Louis: Mosby.

Coulehan, J. L., & Block, M. R. (2001). *The Medical Interview: Mastering Skills for Clinical Practice*, ed 4. Philadelphia: F. A. Davis.

D'Avanzo, C. (2008). *Pocket Guide to Cultural Health Assessment*, ed 4. St. Louis: Mosby.

Dillon, P. M. (2007). *Nursing Health Assessment: Student Applications*, ed 2, Philadelphia: F. A. Davis.

Engel, K. (2002). *Pocket Guide to Pediatric Assessment*, ed 3. St. Louis: Mosby.

Expert 10-Minute Physical Examinations, ed 2. (2005). St. Louis: Mosby.

Fuller, J., & Schaller-Ayers, J. (2000). *Health Assessment: A Nursing Approach*, ed 3. Philadelphia: Lippincott.

Giger, J. N., & Davidhizar, R. E. (Eds.). (2008). *Transcultural Nursing: Assessment and Intervention*, ed 5. St. Louis: Mosby.

Hogstel, M. O., & Curry, L. C. (2005). *Health Assessment: Through the Lifespan*, ed 4. Philadelphia: F. A. Davis.

Leasia, M. S., & Monahan, F. D. (2002). *A Practical Guide to Health Assessment*, ed 2. Philadelphia: W. B. Saunders.

Nursing Assessment and Older People. (2004). London: Royal College of Nursing. Accessed 2007 at http://www.rcn.org.uk/members/downloads/nursingassessmentolder.pdf

Pesut, D. F., & Herman, J. (1999). *Clinical Reasoning: The Art and Science of Critical and Creative Thinking*. Albany, NY: Delmar.

Seidel, H. M., Ball, J. W., Dains, J. E., & Benedict, G. W. (2006). *Mosby's Guide to Physical Examination*, ed 6. St. Louis: Mosby.

Simonsen, S. M. (2001). *Telephone Health Assessment: Guidelines for Practice*, ed 2. St. Louis: Mosby.

Springhouse. *Assessment: A 2-in-1 Reference for Nurses*. (2004). Philadelphia: Lippincott Williams & Wilkins.

Thompson, J. M., & Wilson, S. F. (2000). *Health Assessment for Nursing Practice*, ed 2. St. Louis: Mosby.

Weber, J. (2007). *Nurses' Handbook of Health Assessment*, ed 6. Philadelphia: Lippincott Williams & Wilkins.

Zimbrzuski, C. (2001). *Clinical Companion for Assessment of the Older Adult*. Cengage Delmar.

Genogram References

Beauchesne, M., Kelley, B., & Gauthier, M. A. (1997). News, notes & tips. The genogram: A health assessment tool. *Nurse Educator, 2*(3):9, 16.

Beck, R. (1987). The genogram as process. *American Journal of Family Therapy, 15*:343–351.

Engelman, S. R. (1988). Use of the family genogram technique with spinal cord injured patients. *Clinical Rehabilitation, 2*:7–15.

Friedman, H., Rohrbaugh, M., & Krakauer, S. (1988). The time-line genogram: Highlighting temporal aspects of family relationships. *Family Process, 27*(3):293–303.

Herth, K. A. (1989). The root of it all: Genograms as a nursing assessment tool. *Journal of Gerontological Nursing, 15*:32–37.

Hurley, P. M. (1982). Family assessment: Systems theory and the genogram. *Children's Health Care, 10*:76–82.

Like, R. C., Rogers, J., & McGoldrick, M. (1988). Reading and interpreting genograms: A systematic approach. *Journal of Family Practice*, (4):407–412.

Marinelli, R. D. (1995). The genogram in health education. *Journal of Health Education, 26*(4):243–244.

McGoldrick, M., Gerson, B., & Petry, S. (2008). *Genograms: Assessment & Intervention*, ed 3. New York: W. W. Norton.

Puskar, K., & Nerone, M. (1996). Genogram: A useful tool for nurse practitioners. *Journal of Psychiatric and Mental Health Nursing, 3*(1):55–60.

Richards, W. R., Burgess, D. E., Petersen, F. R., & McCarthy, D. L. (1993). Genograms: A psychosocial assessment tool for hospice. *Hospice Journal: Physical, Psychosocial, and Pastoral Care of the Dying, 9*(1):1–12.

Rogers, J. C., & Rohrbaugh, M. (1991). The SAGE-PAGE trial: Do family genograms make a difference? *Journal American Board of Family Practice, 4*(5):319–326.

Rogers, J. C., Rohrbaugh, M., & McGoldrick, M. (1992). Can experts predict health risk from family genograms? *Family Medicine, 24*(3):209–215.

Shore, W. B., Wilkie, H. A., & Croughan-Minihane, M. (1994). Family of origin genograms: Evaluation of a teaching program for medical students. *Family Medicine, 26*(4):238–243.

Visscher, E. M., & Clore, E. R. (1992). The genogram: A strategy for assessment. *Journal of Pediatric Health Care, 6*(6):361–367.

Waters, I., Watson, W., & Wetzel, W. (1994). Genograms: Practical tools for family physicians. *Canadian Family Physician, 40*:282–287.

Chapter 3

The Diagnosis Step: Analyzing the Data

■ **ANA STANDARD 2:** Diagnosis: The registered nurse analyzes the assessment data to determine the diagnoses or issues. (ANA, 2004)

The second step of the nursing process is often referred to as **ANALYSIS**, as well as **need (or problem) identification or nursing diagnosis**. Although all these terms may be used interchangeably, the purpose of this step of the nursing process is to draw conclusions regarding a client's specific needs or human responses of concern so that effective care can be planned and delivered. We have chosen to label this step of the nursing process **DIAGNOSIS**. To be more specific, this is a process of data analysis using diagnostic reasoning (a form of clinical judgment) in which judgments, decisions, and conclusions are made about the meaning of the data collected to determine whether nursing intervention is indicated.

The diagnosis of client needs has been determined by nurses on an informal basis since the beginning of the profession. The term came into formal use in the nursing literature during the 1950s (Fry, 1953), although its meaning continued to be seen in the context of medical diagnosis. A group of interested nursing leaders met and held a national conference in 1973 (Gebbie & Lavin, 1975). Their purpose

ANALYSIS: the process of examining and categorizing information to reach a conclusion about a client's needs.

DIAGNOSIS: the second step of the nursing process, in which the data collected are analyzed and, through the process of diagnostic reasoning, specific client diagnostic statements are created.

was to identify the client needs that fall within the scope of nursing, label them, and develop a classification system that could be used by nurses throughout the world. This group called these labels **NURSING DIAGNOSES**. Regional, national, and international workshops and conferences continue to be held since that first conference. NANDA International (NANDA-I) (formerly the North American Nursing Diagnosis Association) meets every 2 years to review its work on the development and classification of nursing diagnoses as well as the work of other nursing groups worldwide, representing varied clinical specialties and healthcare settings.

The American Nurses Association (ANA) standards of practice were first developed in 1973. With the acceptance of the ANA *Social Policy Statement* in 1980, which defined nursing as the "diagnosis and treatment of human responses to actual or potential health problems," and the 1995 update description as the "diagnosis and treatment of human responses to health and illness" (ANA, 1995), the movement for broad use of a common language was enhanced. The system developed by NANDA-I provides a standard terminology that is accepted by ANA and various specialty groups and is being used across the United States and in many countries around the world. NANDA-I has established a liaison with the International Council of Nursing to support and contribute to the global effort to standardize the language of health care, with the goal that NANDA-I labels will be included in the International Classification of Diseases (ICD-11). In the meantime, NANDA-I nursing diagnoses are included in the U.S. version of International Classification of Diseases–Clinical Modifications (ICD-10-CM). The NANDA, Nursing Interventions Classification (NIC), and Nursing Outcomes Classification (NOC) classifications have been coded into the Systematized Nomenclature of Medicine (SNOMED). (Inclusion in an international coded terminology is essential if nursing's contribution to health care is to be recognized. Indexing of the entire medical record supports disease management activities, research, and analysis of outcomes for quality improvement for all healthcare disciplines. Coding also supports telehealth, the use of telecommunications technology to provide medical information and healthcare services over distance, and facilitates access to healthcare data across care settings and different computer systems.)

The use of the nursing process and NANDA-I diagnoses is rapidly becoming an integral part of an effective system of nursing practice. It is a system that can be used within existing conceptual frameworks, because it is a generic approach adaptable to all academic and clinical settings. In addition, as mentioned in the first chapter, organizing schemata of nursing problems other than NANDA-I are used within the profession. Additional schemata, such as the Omaha System, the Patient Care Data Set, the Clinical Care Classification (formerly Home Health Care Classification), and the Perioperative Nursing Data Set (see individual bibliographies for each of these), have been approved for use. This edition introduces you to the Omaha System by presenting associated Omaha System problems with the NANDA-I diagnoses in the case studies.

Defining Nursing Diagnosis

The term *nursing diagnosis* has been used as both a verb and a noun. This may result in confusion. Nursing diagnosis is used as a noun in reference to the work of NANDA-I. For the purposes of this text, *nursing diagnosis* refers to the NANDA-I list of nursing diagnosis labels (Table 3–1) that form the stem of the client diagnostic statement.

TABLE 3–1. Nursing Diagnoses (Accepted for Use and Research [2007])

Activity Intolerance [specify level]	Coping, compromised family
Activity Intolerance, risk for	Coping, defensive
Airway Clearance, ineffective	Coping, disabled family
Allergy Response, latex	Coping, ineffective
Allergy Response, risk for latex	Coping, ineffective community
Anxiety [specify level]	Coping, readiness for enhanced
Anxiety, death	Coping, readiness for enhanced community
Aspiration, risk for	Coping, readiness for enhanced family
Attachment, risk for impaired parent/child	
Autonomic Dysreflexia	Death Syndrome, risk for sudden infant
Autonomic Dysreflexia, risk for	Decision Making, readiness for enhanced
	Denial, ineffective
Behavior, risk-prone health	Dentition, impaired
Body Image, disturbed	Development, risk for delayed
Body Temperature, risk for imbalanced	Diarrhea
Bowel Incontinence	Dignity, risk for compromised human
Breastfeeding, effective	Distress, moral
Breastfeeding, ineffective	Disuse Syndrome, risk for
Breastfeeding, interrupted	Diversional Activity, deficient
Breathing Pattern, ineffective	
	Energy Field, disturbed
Cardiac Output, decreased	Environmental Interpretation Syndrome, impaired
Caregiver Role Strain	
Caregiver Role Strain, risk for	Failure to Thrive, adult
Comfort, readiness for enhanced	Falls, risk for
Communication, impaired verbal	Family Processes: alcoholism, dysfunctional
Communication, readiness for enhanced	Family Processes, interrupted
Conflict, decisional (specify)	Family Processes, readiness for enhanced
Conflict, parental role	Fatigue
Confusion, acute	Fear
Confusion, chronic	Fluid Balance, readiness for enhanced
Confusion, risk for acute	[Fluid Volume, deficient (hyper/hypotonic)]
Constipation	Fluid Volume, deficient [isotonic]
Constipation, perceived	Fluid Volume, excess
Constipation, risk for	Fluid Volume, risk for deficient
Contamination	Fluid Volume, risk for imbalanced
Contamination, risk for	

Continued

CLIENT DIAGNOSTIC STATEMENT: the outcome of the diagnostic reasoning process; a three-part statement identifying the client's need, the cause of the need (or human response of concern), and the associated signs/ symptoms.

Distinguishing between Medical and Nursing Diagnoses....

- **Medical diagnoses** are illnesses/ conditions, such as diabetes, heart failure, hepatitis, cancer, and pneumonia, that reflect alteration of the structure or function of organs/ systems and are verified by medical diagnostic studies. The medical diagnosis usually does not change.
- **Nursing diagnoses** address human responses to actual and potential health concerns/ life processes, (e.g., ineffective Airway Clearance, ineffective Health Maintenance, Grieving, readiness for enhanced Hope) and change as the client's situation or perspective changes/resolves.

TABLE 3–1. Nursing Diagnoses (Accepted for Use and Research [2007]) (Continued)

Gas Exchange, impaired
Glucose, risk for unstable blood
Grieving
Grieving, complicated
Grieving, risk for complicated
Growth & Development, delayed
Growth, risk for disproportionate

Health Maintenance, ineffective
Health-Seeking Behaviors [specify]
Home Maintenance, impaired
Hope, readiness for enhanced
Hopelessness
Hyperthermia
Hypothermia

Identity, disturbed personal
Immunization Status, readiness for enhanced
Infant Behavior, disorganized
Infant Behavior, readiness for enhanced organized
Infant Behavior, risk for disorganized
Infant Feeding Pattern, ineffective
Infection, risk for
Injury, risk for
Injury, risk for perioperative-positioning
Insomnia
Intracranial Adaptive Capacity, decreased

Knowledge, deficient [Learning Need] [specify]
Knowledge, readiness for enhanced

Lifestyle, sedentary
Liver Function, risk for impaired
Loneliness, risk for

Memory, impaired
Mobility, impaired bed
Mobility, impaired physical
Mobility, impaired wheelchair

Nausea
Neglect, unilateral

Noncompliance [Adherence, ineffective] [specify]
Nutrition: less than body requirements, imbalanced
Nutrition: more than body requirements, imbalanced
Nutrition, readiness for enhanced
Nutrition: more than body requirements, risk for imbalanced

Oral Mucous Membrane, impaired

Pain, acute
Pain, chronic
Parenting, readiness for enhanced
Parenting, impaired
Parenting, risk for impaired
Peripheral Neurovascular Dysfunction, risk for
Poisoning, risk for
Post-Trauma Syndrome
Post-Trauma Syndrome, risk for
Power, readiness for enhanced
Powerlessness
Powerlessness, risk for
Protection, ineffective

Rape-Trauma Syndrome
Rape-Trauma Syndrome: compound reaction
Rape-Trauma Syndrome: silent reaction
Religiosity, impaired
Religiosity, readiness for enhanced
Religiosity, risk for impaired
Relocation Stress Syndrome
Relocation Stress Syndrome, risk for
Role Performance, ineffective

Self-Care, readiness for enhanced
Self-Care Deficit, bathing/hygiene
Self-Care Deficit, dressing/grooming
Self-Care Deficit, feeding
Self-Care Deficit, toileting

Self-Concept, readiness for enhanced

Self-Esteem, chronic low

Self-Esteem, risk for situational low

Self-Esteem, situational low

Self-Mutilation

Self-Mutilation, risk for

Sensory Perception, disturbed (specify: visual, auditory, kinesthetic, gustatory, tactile, olfactory)

Sexual Dysfunction

Sexuality Pattern, ineffective

Skin Integrity, impaired

Skin Integrity, risk for impaired

Sleep Deprivation

Sleep, readiness for enhanced

Social Interaction, impaired

Social Isolation

Sorrow, chronic

Spiritual Distress

Spiritual Distress, risk for

Spiritual Well-being, readiness for enhanced

Stress Overload

Suffocation, risk for

Suicide, risk for

Surgical Recovery, delayed

Swallowing, impaired

Therapeutic Regimen Management, effective

Therapeutic Regimen Management, ineffective

Therapeutic Regimen Management, ineffective community

Therapeutic Regimen Management, ineffective family

Therapeutic Regimen Management, readiness for enhanced

Thermoregulation, ineffective

Thought Processes, disturbed

Tissue Integrity, impaired

Tissue Perfusion, ineffective (specify type: renal, cerebral, cardiopulmonary, gastrointestinal, peripheral)

Transfer Ability, impaired

Trauma, risk for

Urinary Elimination, impaired

Urinary Elimination, readiness for enhanced

Urinary Incontinence, functional

Urinary Incontinence, overflow

Urinary Incontinence, reflex

Urinary Incontinence, stress

Urinary Incontinence, total

Urinary Incontinence, risk for urge

Urinary Incontinence, urge

Urinary Retention [acute/chronic]

Ventilation, impaired spontaneous

Ventilatory Weaning Response, dysfunctional

Violence [actual/]risk for other-directed

Violence [actual/]risk for self-directed

Walking, impaired

Wandering [specify sporadic or continual]

Information that appears in brackets has been added by the authors to clarify and facilitate the use of nursing diagnoses.

Although nurses work within the nursing, medical, and psychosocial domains, nursing's phenomena of concern are patterns of human response, not disease processes. Therefore, nursing diagnoses do not parallel medical/psychiatric diagnoses; they involve independent nursing activities as well as collaborative roles and actions.

The nursing diagnosis is a conclusion, drawn from data collected about a client, that serves as a means of describing a health need amenable to treatment by nurses. A uniform or standardized way of identifying, focusing on, and labeling specific phenomena allows the nurse to deal effectively with individual client responses.

Although there are different definitions of the term *nursing diagnosis*, NANDA -I has accepted the following: Nursing diagnosis is a clinical judgment about individual, family, or community responses to actual or potential health problems/life processes. Nursing diagnoses provide the basis for selection of nursing interventions to achieve outcomes for which the nurse is accountable.

The nursing diagnosis is as correct as the current data allow because it is supported by these data. It says what the client's situation is at the present time and reflects changes in the client's condition as they occur. Each decision the nurse makes is time-dependent; with additional information gathered later, decisions may change. Unlike medical diagnoses, nursing diagnoses change as the client progresses through various stages of illness/maladaptation to resolution of the need for nursing intervention or to the conclusion of the condition. For example, for a client undergoing cardiac surgery, initial needs may be acute Pain; decreased Cardiac Output; ineffective Airway Clearance; and risk for Infection. As the client progresses, needs may shift to risk for Activity Intolerance; deficient Knowledge (Learning Need) (specify); and ineffective Role Performance.

THE USE OF NURSING DIAGNOSES

Although not yet comprehensive, the current NANDA-I list of diagnostic labels defines/refines professional nursing activity. The continued growth of nursing diagnoses is dependent upon nurses using the proposed diagnoses on a daily basis, becoming familiar with the parameters of each individual diagnosis and identifying its strengths and weaknesses, thus promoting research and further development.

Frequently asked questions are "Why should we use a nursing diagnosis? What is its value to the nursing profession?" The use of a nursing diagnosis can provide many benefits. The accurate choice of a nursing diagnosis to label a client need:

- **Gives nurses a common language:** Promotes improved communication among nurses, other healthcare providers, and alternate care settings.

  FOR EXAMPLE: Using the nursing diagnosis ineffective Airway Clearance instead of noting "difficulty breathing" conveys a distinct image. With the former, a clear picture begins to develop in your mind as your thoughts focus on the musculature of the upper airway, mucus production, and cough effort. With the second label, you do not have a clear idea as to what is happening with this client, and you question whether the client is experiencing an airway maintenance problem, impaired movement of the chest, or decreased perfusion to the lungs.

SIGN: objective or observable evidence or manifestation of a health need.

This improved communication may result in improved quality and continuity of the care provided to the client.

SYMPTOM: subjectively perceptible change in the body or its functions that indicates disease or the kind or phases of disease.

- **Promotes identification of appropriate goals:** Aids in the choice of correct nursing interventions to alleviate the identified need and provides guidance for evaluation. Whereas nursing actions were once based on variables such as **SIGNS** and **SYMPTOMS**, test results, or a medical diagnosis, nursing diagnosis is a uniform way of identifying, focusing on, and dealing with specific client responses to health and illness (i.e., the phenomena of concern for nurses).

FOR EXAMPLE: "Risk for Infection" compared with "presence of urinary catheter": the risk or potential threat of an infection brings to mind specific goals/outcomes and interventions to protect the client, but what is your concern, if any, with the urinary catheter?

- **Provides acuity information:** Ranks the amount of work that involves nursing care and can serve as a basis for client classification systems. This method of ranking can be used to determine individual staffing needs. It can also serve as documentation to provide justification for third-party reimbursement.

FOR EXAMPLE: Nursing diagnoses can be given different, weighted values according to the amount of nursing involvement required. For example, impaired Gas Exchange may require a considerable amount of skilled nursing time to promote adequate ventilation, to provide oxygen and respiratory treatments, and to monitor laboratory studies; acute Urinary Retention may require a much shorter period for inserting a catheter into the bladder and periodically measuring the urine output. In addition, some third-party payers (such as Medicare and other insurance companies) include nursing diagnoses when considering extended length of stay or delayed discharge.

- **Can create a standard for nursing practice:** Provides a foundation for quality improvement programs, a means for evaluating nursing practice, and a mechanism for costing delivery of nursing care.

FOR EXAMPLE: Did the nursing interventions address and resolve the need? Did the client experience the desired result (e.g., alleviation of pain)? Were the goals met, or is there documentation of the reasons why they were not met? Were the expected outcomes revised to meet changing client needs?

- **Provides a quality improvement base:** Clinicians, administrators, educators, and researchers can document, validate, or alter the process of care delivery, which then improves the profession.

FOR EXAMPLE: The use of universally understood labels enhances retrieval of specific data for review to determine accuracy, to validate and/or change nursing actions related to specific nursing diagnoses, and to evaluate an individual nurse's performance.

Identifying Client Needs

During the assessment step, the collection, clustering, and validation of client data flow directly into the diagnosis step of the nursing process, in which you sense needs or problems and choose nursing diagnoses.

DIAGNOSTIC REASONING: ANALYZING THE CLIENT DATABASE

Identifying client needs and then selecting a nursing diagnosis label involves the use of your experience, expertise, and intuition. There are six steps in need identification, which constitute the activities of diagnostic reasoning. The result

REMEMBER: nursing diagnoses may represent a physical, sociological, or psychological finding.

PHYSICAL NURSING DIAGNOSES include those that pertain to circulation (e.g., ineffective peripheral Tissue Perfusion), ventilation (e.g., ineffective Airway Clearance), elimination (e.g., Constipation), and so on.

PSYCHOSOCIAL NURSING DIAGNOSES include those that pertain to the mind (e.g., disturbed Thought Processes), emotion (e.g., Anxiety [specify level]), or lifestyle/relationships (e.g., ineffective Sexuality Patterns; Social Isolation).

PES: format for combining a nursing diagnosis label, client-specific cause, and signs/symptoms to create an individualized diagnostic statement.

CUE: signal that indicates a possible need/direction for care.

is a client diagnostic statement that identifies the client need, suggests its potential cause or etiology, and notes its signs and symptoms. This is known as the **PES** format, reflecting Problem, Etiology, and Signs/Symptoms (Gordon, 1976).

Step 1: Problem Sensing

Data are reviewed and analyzed to identify **CUES** (signs and symptoms) suggesting client needs that can be described by nursing diagnosis labels. If the data have been recorded in a nursing format (e.g., diagnostic divisions or functional health patterns), the nurse is automatically guided to specific groups of nursing diagnoses when certain cues from the data are identified (Box 3–1). This helps to focus attention on appropriate diagnoses. Reviewing the NANDA-I definitions of specific diagnoses (see Appendix I) can be of further assistance in deciding between two or more similar diagnostic labels; for instance, there are seven different diagnoses for urinary incontinence (see step 4).

BOX 3–1

Nursing Diagnoses Organized According to Diagnostic Divisions

After data have been collected and areas of concern/need have been identified, consult the Diagnostic Divisions framework to review the list of nursing diagnoses that fall within the individual categories. This will assist with the choice of specific diagnostic labels to accurately describe data from the client database. Then, with the addition of etiology (when known) and signs and symptoms, the client diagnostic statement emerges.

Diagnostic Division: Activity/Rest
Ability to engage in necessary/desired activities of life (work and leisure) and to obtain adequate sleep/rest

Diagnoses

Activity Intolerance [specify level]	Lifestyle, sedentary
	Mobility, impaired bed
Activity Intolerance, risk for	Mobility, impaired wheelchair
Disuse Syndrome, risk for	Sleep, readiness for enhanced
Diversional Activity, deficient	Sleep Deprivation
Fatigue	Transfer Ability, impaired
Insomnia	Walking, impaired

Diagnostic Division: Circulation
Ability to transport oxygen and nutrients necessary to meet cellular needs

Diagnoses

Autonomic Dysreflexia
Autonomic Dysrefexia, risk for
Cardiac Output, decreased
Intracranial Adaptive Capacity,
  decreased

Tissue Perfusion,
  ineffective (specify type:
  cerebral, cardiopulmonary,
  renal, gastrointestinal,
  peripheral)

Diagnostic Division: Ego Integrity

Ability to develop and use skills and behaviors to integrate and manage life experiences

Diagnoses

Anxiety [specify level]
Anxiety, death
Behavior, risk-prone health
Body Image, disturbed
Conflict, decisional (specify)
Coping, defensive
Coping, ineffective
Coping, readiness for enhanced
Decision Making, readiness for
  enhanced
Denial, ineffective
Dignity, readiness for enhanced
Distress, moral
Energy Field, disturbed
Fear
Grieving
Grieving, complicated
Grieving, risk for complicated
Hope, readiness for enhanced
Hopelessness
Personal Identity, disturbed
Post-Trauma Syndrome
Post-Trauma Syndrome, risk for

Power, readiness for enhanced
Powerlessness
Powerlessness, risk for
Rape-Trauma Syndrome
Rape-Trauma Syndrome:
  compound reaction
Rape-Trauma Syndrome: silent
  reaction
Religiosity, impaired
Religiosity, ready for enhanced
Religiosity, risk for impaired
Relocation Stress Syndrome
Relocation Stress Syndrome, risk for
Self-Concept, readiness for
  enhanced
Self-Esteem, chronic low
Self-Esteem, risk for situational low
Self-Esteem, situational low
Sorrow, chronic
Spiritual Distress
Spiritual Distress, risk for
Spiritual Well-being, readiness for
  enhanced

Diagnostic Division: Elimination

Ability to excrete waste products

Diagnoses

Bowel Incontinence
Constipation

Constipation, perceived
Constipation, risk for

Continued

Nursing Diagnoses Organized According to Diagnostic Divisions (Continued)

Diarrhea
Urinary Elimination, impaired
Urinary Elimination, readiness
  for enhanced
Urinary Incontinence, functional
Urinary Incontinence, overflow
Urinary Incontinence, reflex

Urinary Incontinence, risk for
  urge
Urinary Incontinence, stress
Urinary Incontinence, total
Urinary Incontinence, urge
Urinary Retention [acute/
  chronic]

Diagnostic Division: Food/Fluid

Ability to maintain intake of and use nutrients and liquids to meet physiological needs

Diagnoses

Breastfeeding, effective
Breastfeeding, ineffective
Breastfeeding, interrupted
Dentition, impaired
Failure to Thrive, adult
Fluid Balance, readiness for
  enhanced
[Fluid Volume, deficient hyper/
  hypotonic]
Fluid Volume, deficient [isotonic]
Fluid Volume, excess
Fluid Volume, risk for deficient
Fluid Volume, risk for imbalanced

Glucose, risk for unstable blood
Infant Feeding Pattern,
  ineffective
Nausea
Nutrition: less than body
  requirements, imbalanced
Nutrition: more than body
  requirements, imbalanced
Nutrition: risk for more than body
  requirements, imbalanced
Nutrition, readiness for enhanced
Oral Mucous Membrane, impaired
Swallowing, impaired

Diagnostic Division: Hygiene

Ability to perform basic activities of daily living

Diagnoses

Self-Care, readiness for
  enhanced
Self-Care Deficit, bathing/
  hygiene

Self-Care Deficit, dressing/
  grooming
Self-Care Deficit, feeding
Self-Care Deficit, toileting

Diagnostic Division: Neurosensory

Ability to perceive, integrate, and respond to internal and external cues

Diagnoses

Confusion, acute
Confusion, chronic

Confusion, risk for acute
Infant Behavior, disorganized

Infant Behavior, readiness for
   enhanced organized
Infant Behavior, risk for disorganized
Memory, impaired
Neglect, unilateral
Peripheral Neurovascular
   Dysfunction, risk for

Sensory Perception, disturbed
   (specify: visual, auditory,
   kinesthetic, gustatory, tactile,
   olfactory)
Stress Overload
Thought Processes,
   disturbed

Diagnostic Division: Pain/Discomfort

Ability to control internal/external environment to maintain comfort

Diagnoses

Comfort, readiness for enhanced
Pain, acute
Pain, chronic

Diagnostic Division: Respiration

Ability to provide and use oxygen to meet physiological needs

Diagnoses

Airway Clearance, ineffective
Aspiration, risk for
Breathing Pattern, ineffective
Gas Exchange, impaired

Ventilation, impaired
   spontaneous
Ventilatory Weaning Response,
   dysfunctional

Diagnostic Division: Safety

Ability to provide safe, growth-promoting environment

Diagnoses

Allergy Response, latex
Allergy Response, risk for
   latex
Body Temperature, risk for
   imbalanced
Contamination
Contamination, risk for
Death Syndrome, risk for
   sudden infant
Environmental Interpretation
   Syndrome, impaired
Falls, risk for

Health Maintenance,
   ineffective
Home Maintenance, impaired
Hyperthermia
Hypothermia
Immunization Status, readiness
   for enhanced
Infection, risk for
Injury, risk for
Injury, risk for perioperative
   positioning
Mobility, impaired physical

Continued

Nursing Diagnoses Organized According to Diagnostic Divisions (Continued)

Poisoning, risk for
Protection, ineffective
Self-Mutilation
Self-Mutilation, risk for
Skin Integrity, impaired
Skin Integrity, risk for impaired
Suffocation, risk for
Suicide, risk for
Surgical Recovery, delayed

Thermoregulation, ineffective
Tissue Integrity, impaired
Trauma, risk for
Violence, [actual/]risk for other-directed
Violence, [actual/]risk for self-directed
Wandering [specify sporadic or continual]

Diagnostic Division: Sexuality

(Component of Ego Integrity and Social Interaction) Ability to meet requirements/characteristics of male/female role

Diagnoses

Sexual Dysfunction
Sexuality Pattern, ineffective

Diagnostic Division: Social Interaction

Ability to establish and maintain relationships

Diagnoses

Attachment, risk for impaired parent/child
Caregiver Role Strain
Caregiver Role Strain, risk for
Communication, impaired verbal
Communication, readiness for enhanced
Conflict, parental role
Coping, compromised family
Coping, disabled family
Coping, ineffective community

Coping, readiness for enhanced community
Coping, readiness for enhanced
Family Processes: alcoholism, dysfunctional
Family Processes, interrupted
Loneliness, risk for
Parenting, impaired
Parenting, risk for impaired
Role Performance, ineffective
Social Interaction, impaired
Social Isolation

Diagnostic Division: Teaching/Learning

Ability to incorporate and use information to achieve healthy lifestyle/optimal wellness

Diagnoses

Development, risk for delayed
Growth, risk for disporportionate
Growth and Development, delayed
Health-Seeking Behaviors [specify]
Knowledge, deficient [Learning Need] [specify]
Knowledge (specify), readiness for enhanced
Noncompliance [Adherence, ineffective] [specify]

Therapeutic Regimen Management, effective
Therapeutic Regimen Management, ineffective
Therapeutic Regimen Management: ineffective community
Therapeutic Regimen Management: ineffective family
Therapeutic Regimen Management, readiness for emhanced

FOR EXAMPLE: When the Diagnostic Divisions format is used, body temperature is recorded in the Safety section. When the client's temperature rises, the nurse reviews the diagnostic labels under Safety to find a possible fit, such as Hyperthermia or risk for Infection. At the same time, cues are noted in other sections of the database that may be combined with fever or may be totally unrelated. In fact, cues may have relevance in more than one section, as you can see in Box 3–2.

BOX 3–2

Walking Through the Use of Diagnostic Divisions

During the Assessment phase, the following data were obtained from Robert:

Activity/Rest
Reports (Subjective)
Occupation: Retired truck driver
Usual Activities/Hobbies: Used to like to hunt and fish
Leisure Time Activities: Mostly watches baseball on TV, takes short walks—one to two blocks
Feelings of Boredom/Dissatisfaction: "Wish I could do more; just getting too old"
Limitations Imposed by Condition: "I get short of breath; stay at home mostly"
Sleep: Hours: 5; **Naps:** After lunch—2 hr; **Aids:** None
Insomnia: Only if short of breath (1 or 2 ×/wk) or needs to void (1 ×/night)

Continued

Walking Through the Use of Diagnostic Divisions (Continued)

Rested on Awakening: Not always; "feel weak most of the time"
Other: "Sometimes, it feels like there isn't enough air"
Exhibits (Objective)
Observed Response to Activity: Cardiovascular: BP 178/102, P 100 after walking half-length of corridor from floor scale **Respiratory:** 32, rapid, leaning forward ("to catch breath")
Mental Status (i.e., withdrawn/lethargic): Alert, responding to all questions
Neuromuscular Assessment: Muscle mass/tone: Decreased/bilaterally equal/ diminished; Posture: Leans forward to breathe
Tremors: No; **ROM:** Movement in all extremities; **Strength:** Moderate
Deformity: No
Having previously noted respiratory cues of dyspnea with activity when you reviewed the respiratory data in Box 2–3, you return to the Activity/Rest section of the Diagnostic Divisions, where the effects/limitations of this condition on both activity and sleep would also be considered. You are referred to the following nursing diagnoses: Activity Intolerance [specify level]; risk for Activity Intolerance; risk for Disuse Syndrome; deficient Diversional Activity; Fatigue; Insomnia; sedentary Lifestyle; impaired bed Mobility; impaired wheelchair Mobility; readiness for enhanced Sleep; Sleep Deprivation; impaired Transfer Ability; and impaired Walking, as possible choices to describe or label Robert's needs.

Step 2: Rule-Out Process

Alternative explanations are considered for the identified cues to determine which nursing diagnosis label may be the most appropriate. This step is crucial in establishing an adequate list of diagnostic statements. As you compare and contrast the relationships among and between data, etiological factors are identified within or between categories based on an understanding of the biological, physical, and behavioral sciences.

> **FOR EXAMPLE:** Although Hyperthermia or risk for Infection was suggested during the first step of diagnostic reasoning, another consideration might be deficient Fluid Volume. In another example, cues of increased tension, restlessness, elevated pulse rate, and reported apprehension may initially be thought to indicate Anxiety (specify level). However, a similar diagnosis of Fear should be considered as well as the possibility that these cues may be physiologically based, thus requiring medical treatment and nursing interventions related to education and monitoring.

If you encounter difficulty in choosing a nursing diagnosis label, asking yourself the following questions may provide additional guidance:

1. What are my concerns about this client?
2. Can I do something about it?
3. Can the overall risk be reduced by nursing intervention?

For example, in the teenaged client with bulimia, electrolyte imbalance may occur. Questions to ask might be:

- What is a major concern about electrolyte imbalance?
  - The client may develop a cardiac dysrhythmia or even arrest.
- Can I do something about it?
  - Yes, you can monitor signs of imbalance, encourage foods/fluids rich in necessary eletrolytes, administer supplements, and educate client regarding nutritional needs.
- Can the overall risk be reduced by nursing interventions?
  - Yes, the risk of cardiac dysrhythmias can be reduced if electrolyte balance is maintained/restored.

Conclusion: The nursing diagnosis would be risk for decreased Cardiac Output, and the client diagnostic statement would be risk for decreased Cardiac Output, risk factor of decreased potassium intake/excessive loss.

Step 3: Synthesizing the Data

Considering the data as a whole (including information collected by other members of the healthcare team) can provide a comprehensive picture of the client in relation to past, present, and future health status. This is called **SYNTHESIZING** the data. The suggested nursing diagnosis label is combined with the identified **RELATED FACTOR(S)** and cues to create a hypothesis.

> **FOR EXAMPLE:** Sally had a period of bleeding during delivery of the placenta following the unexpected delivery of twins. Blood loss was estimated to be approximately 600 mL. In addition, she experienced several episodes of vomiting before delivery and reduced oral intake because of nausea. The nursing diagnosis label: deficient [isotonic] Fluid Volume related factors of hemorrhage, vomiting, poor oral intake; cues of dark urine, dry mouth/lips, low blood pressure.

Step 4: Evaluating or Confirming the Hypothesis

Test the hypothesis for appropriate fit; that is, review the NANDA-I nursing diagnosis and definition. Then, compare the assessed possible **ETIOLOGY** with NANDA-I's related factors or **RISK FACTORS**. Next, compare the assessed client cues with NANDA-I's Defining Characteristics, which are used to support and provide an increased level of confidence in your selected nursing diagnosis. Appendix I provides a complete listing of NANDA-I nursing diagnostic labels, definitions, defining characteristics, and related factors. This listing will be helpful as you work through the practice activities and work pages contained in each chapter. Review Box 3–3: the information provides a beginning effort in assessing the appropriateness of a specific nursing diagnosis label.

SYNTHESIZING: reviewing all data as a whole to obtain a comprehensive picture of the client.

ETIOLOGY: identified causes and/or contributing factors responsible for the presence of a specific client need.

RELATED FACTOR: conditions/ circumstances that contribute to the development/ maintenance of a nursing diagnosis; forms the "related to" component of the client diagnostic statement.

RISK FACTOR: environmental factors and physiological, psychological, genetic, or chemical elements that increase the vulnerability of an individual, family, or community to an unhealthy event.

BOX 3–3

Elements of NANDA-I Nursing Diagnostic Labels

Appendix I supplies a complete listing of NANDA-I nursing diagnosis labels, which will be helpful to you as you work through the exercises in this chapter and throughout the book. It is important to become familiar with this list so that you can find information quickly in the clinical setting. Identify the key elements of the diagnostic label "deficient Fluid Volume" as excerpted below.

deficient [isotonic] Fluid Volume

Definition: Decreased intravascular, interstitial, and/or intracellular fluid. This refers to dehydration, water loss alone without change in sodium.

Related Factors: Active fluid volume loss, failure of regulatory mechanisms.

Defining Characteristics: Decreased urine output; increased urine concentration; weakness; sudden weight loss (except in third spacing); decreased venous filling; increased body temperature; change in mental state; elevated hematocrit; decreased skin/tongue turgor; dry skin/mucous membranes; thirst; increased pulse rate; decreased blood pressure; decreased pulse volume/pressure.

Lunney (1989, 1990) addressed the self-monitoring task of accuracy determination, defining the characteristics of accuracy and providing an ordinal scale for measurement. The scale ranges from the highest assigned accuracy point value, which describes a diagnosis that is consistent with all the cues, to the lowest point value, which describes a diagnosis indicated by more than one cue but recommended for rejection based on the presence of at least two disconfirming cues (see Appendix C). Additionally, Appendix D, Self-Monitoring of Accuracy Using the Integrated Model: A Guide (taken from Lunney), is an excellent self-evaluation of your progress in diagnostic efforts. (Also, a separate section in the Suggested Readings is dedicated to the topic of accuracy of nursing diagnoses.) The completed evaluation provides feedback regarding your diagnostic abilities. Reflection and self-monitoring are tools to assist you in developing your critical thinking skills. The attention you give to measuring the accuracy of your suggested nursing diagnosis is time well spent. Comparing the subjective and objective data gathered from the client with the defining characteristics of the possible nursing diagnoses that are listed not only helps ensure the accuracy of your statement but also stresses the importance of objectivity in this diagnostic process.

Return to Box 3–2. In reviewing Robert's database, you sense that he may have a problem with activity. After reviewing the NANDA-I nursing diagnosis labels and definitions relevant to the Activity/Rest Diagnostic Division, you choose risk for Activity Intolerance. To confirm your hypothesis, compare the cues from the database with the related factors and defining characteristics noted in Appendix I. Practice Activity 3–1 presents an Interactive Care Plan Worksheet for the client problem of Activity Intolerance, on which you can document the identified cues.

PRACTICE ACTIVITY 3–1
Interactive Care Plan Worksheet

In the appropriate spaces on this worksheet, record the cues from Box 3–2 that are relevant to the problem of Activity Intolerance identified for Robert.

INTERACTIVE CARE PLAN WORKSHEET	Student Name:	
ACTIVITY INTOLERANCE	Client's Medical Diagnosis:	
DEFINITION:	Insufficient physiological or psychological energy to endure or complete required or desired daily activities.	
DEFINITION: CHARACTERISTICS:	Verbal report of fatigue or weakness; abnormal heart rate or blood pressure response to activity; exertional discomfort or dyspnea; ECG changes reflecting dysrhythmias or ischemia.	
RELATED FACTORS:	Bedrest and/or immobility; generalized weakness; sedentary lifestyle; imbalance between oxygen supply and/or demand.	
STUDENT INSTRUCTIONS:	In the space below, enter the subjective and objective data gathered during your client assessment.	

A S S E S S M E N T	**Subjective Data Entry**	**Objective Data Entry**

	TIME OUT!	**Student Instructions:** To be sure your client diagnostic statement written below is accurate you need to review the defining characteristics and related factors associated with the nursing diagnosis and see how your client data match. Do you have an accurate match or are additional data required, or does another nursing diagnosis need to be investigated?
D I A G N O S I S	**CLIENT DIAGNOSTIC STATEMENT:**	Nursing Diagnosis (specify) _____ _____ Related to _____ _____ _____

Step 5: List the Client's Needs

Based on the data obtained from steps 3 and 4, the accurate nursing diagnosis label is combined with the assessed etiology and signs/symptoms, if present, to finalize the client diagnostic statement.

> **FOR EXAMPLE:** Sally is diagnosed with deficient [isotonic] Fluid Volume related to hemorrhage, vomiting, reduced intake as evidenced by dark urine, dry mucous membranes, hypotension, and hemoconcentration. This individualized

---

BOX 3–4

Components of the Client Diagnostic Statement: Problem (Need), Etiology, and Signs and Symptoms (PES)

P = Problem (Need) is the name or diagnostic label identified from the NANDA-I list. The key to making an accurate nursing diagnosis is identifying the label that focuses attention on a current or potential physical or behavioral response to health/illness or a life process that may affect the client's quality of life. The label addresses concerns of the client/significant other(s) and the nurse that require or will benefit from nursing intervention and management.

    E = Etiology is the suspected cause or reason for the response that has been identified from the assessment (client database). The nurse makes inferences based on knowledge and expertise, such as understanding pathophysiology and situational or developmental factors. The etiology is stated as "related to." *Note:* One problem or need may have several suspected causes, such as chronic low Self-Esteem related to feelings of abandonment by SO (significant other), ineffective social functioning.

    S = Signs and Symptoms are the manifestations (or cues) identified in the assessment that substantiate the nursing diagnosis. They are stated as "evidenced by," followed by a list of subjective and objective data. It is important to note that risk diagnoses are not accompanied by signs and symptoms because the need has not yet actually occurred. In this instance, the "S" component of the diagnostic statement is omitted, and the "E" component would be replaced by an itemization of the identified risk factors that suggest that the diagnosis could occur (e.g., risk for Infection: risk factors of trauma, malnutrition, and invasive procedures).

---

diagnosis reflects the PES format for a three-part diagnostic statement, as described in Box 3–4. A diagnostic statement is required for each client need or problem you identify. Complete Practice Activity 3–2.

Step 6: Re-evaluate the Client Problem List

Be sure all areas of concern are noted. Once all nursing diagnoses are identified, list them according to priority, and classify them according to status: an actual need; a risk need; or a resolved need.

ACTUAL DIAGNOSIS: existing in fact or reality, existing at the present time (NANDA-I 2007).

- **Actual diagnoses:** Describe human responses to health conditions/life processes that currently exist in an individual, family, or community. They are supported by defining characteristics (manifestations/signs and symptoms) that cluster in patterns of related cues or inferences (NANDA-I, 2007). They are expressed by the use of a three-part PES statement.

Identifying the PES Components of the Client Diagnostic Statement

Questions 1–5: Identify the PES components of each of these diagnostic statements:

1. severe Anxiety related to changes in health status of fetus/self and threat of death as evidenced by restlessness, tremors, focus on self/fetus.

   P =_____ E =_____ S =_____

2. disturbed Thought Processes related to pharmacological stimulation of the nervous system as evidenced by altered attention span, disorientation, and hallucinations.

   P =_____ E =_____ S =_____

3. ineffective Coping related to maturational crisis as evidenced by inability to meet role expectations and alcohol abuse.

   P =_____ E =_____ S =_____

4. Hyperthermia related to increased metabolic rate and dehydration as evidenced by elevated temperature, flushed skin, tachycardia, and tachypnea.

   P =_____ E =_____ S =_____

5. acute Pain related to tissue distention and edema as evidenced by verbal reports, guarding behavior, and changes in vital signs.

   P =_____ E =_____ S =_____

6. Explain the difference between actual and risk diagnoses:

   _____

7. Give an example of an actual and a risk need for a client with second-degree burns of the hand.

   _____

FOR EXAMPLE: A client is admitted for a medical workup because of difficulties with bladder function related to her diagnosis of multiple sclerosis. An actual diagnosis might be Urinary Retention.

- **Health promotion diagnoses:** Describe a clinical judgment of an individual, family, or community regarding motivation and desire to increase well-being and actualize human health potential as expressed in their readiness to enhance specific health behaviors (NANDA-I, 2007). With this actual diagnosis the client can be in any state of health.

HEALTH PROMOTION DIAGNOSIS: behavior motivated by the desire to increase well-being and actualize human health potential.

FOR EXAMPLE: An individual's desire to improve his or her diet could be labeled readiness for enhanced Nutrition as evidenced by following the American Diabetic Association guidelines for intake and expressed willingness to enhance nutrition. A community may desire to increase the immunization rate for children above the acceptable level of 80%. A health promotion diagnosis of readiness for enhanced Immunization Status would be appropriate.

WELLNESS DIAGNOSIS:
quality or state of
being healthy.

- **Wellness diagnoses:** Provide another form of an actual diagnosis describing human responses to levels of wellness in an individial, family, or community that have a readiness for enhancement (NANDA-I, 2007). In such cases, the client has an assessed opportunity to improve an aspect of his or her health or well-being. (*Note:* See section on Wellness and Health Promotion in Suggested Readings.) The diagnostic statement is written as readiness for enhanced....

FOR EXAMPLE: A client's need to improve his or her sense of harmony with others (i.e., family members) could be labeled readiness for enhanced Spiritual Well-being. The family of a client with multiple sclerosis (MS) has been supportive during periods of exacerbated symptoms; however, the family wants to learn how to optimize the client's health status, thereby improving and enriching the client's lifestyle. Therefore, a wellness diagnosis of readiness for enhanced family Coping is appropriate.

RISK DIAGNOSIS:
vulnerability,
especially as a result
of exposure to factors
that increase the
chance of injury or
loss.

- **Risk diagnoses:** Refer to human responses to health conditions/life processes that may develop in a vulnerable individual, family, or community. They are supported by risk factors that contribute to increased vulnerability (NANDA-I, 2007). They represent a need that you believe could develop, but because it has not yet occurred there are no signs or symptoms—only "risk factors"—so it would be written as a two-part statement.

FOR EXAMPLE: The client's MS has been in remission; however, the client has had difficulty in the past with physical mobility. This past problem must be considered when planning this client's care to minimize the possibility of recurrence. A potential problem would then be identified as risk for impaired physical Mobility.

- **Resolved Diagnoses:** Those that no longer require intervention. Because the need no longer exists, no diagnostic statement is needed.

FOR EXAMPLE: Your client formerly suffered a decubitus ulcer (impaired Skin Integrity); however, she has learned techniques to prevent recurrence of this problem, and her skin is in good condition. Therefore, as long as she is able to participate in or direct her own care, this is of no significant concern to you at this time.

DIAGNOSTIC ERROR: a
mistaken assumption
leading to a wrong
conclusion.

Finally, validate the diagnostic conclusions/impressions with the client and/or a colleague. This helps reduce the possibility of **DIAGNOSTIC ERRORS** and/or omissions as discussed in Box 3–5. Inclusion of the client/significant others promotes understanding and participation in the planning of individualized care.

BOX 3–5

Potential Errors in Choosing a Nursing Diagnosis

* Overlooking cues results in a missed diagnosis: leads to worsening of the problem.

FOR EXAMPLE: A client reports discomfort at the insertion site of an intravenous catheter. You notice that the area is slightly reddened but fail to consider the risk for infection. As a result, the client develops sepsis or a blood infection, requiring emergency intervention and longer hospital stay.

* **Making a diagnosis with an insufficient database:** Can lead in the wrong direction, wasting valuable time and resources.

FOR EXAMPLE: The client displays signs of anxiety. Without additional assessment, you administer a mild antianxiolytic agent in the belief that the signs and symptoms are psychologically based. Later, when checking the client, you find signs of cyanosis, suggesting inadequate oxygenation. Thus, the anxiety was probably at least in part physiological and needed other nursing interventions.

* **Stereotyping:** Leads to treatment of all clients in the same way and negates individualization.

FOR EXAMPLE: In a medical-surgical setting, the assumption is often made that a client with a psychiatric diagnosis is apt to become violent.

The process of identifying client needs is more complex than simply attaching a label. In reviewing the definition of nursing, it can be seen that "the human responses to health and illness" are complex, and the process of accurately diagnosing these human responses attests to the complexity of nursing.

OTHER CONSIDERATIONS FOR NEED/PROBLEM IDENTIFICATION

The medical/psychiatric diagnosis can provide a starting point for identifying associated client needs (problem sensing). Review Box 3–6 for several medical/psychiatric diagnoses with examples of associated nursing diagnoses. Although the presence of a medical/psychiatric diagnosis can suggest several nursing diagnoses, these nursing diagnoses must be supported by cues in the client database.

> **FOR EXAMPLE:** In experiencing a myocardial infarction, the client often suffers pain, anxiety, and activity intolerance and requires teaching activities. In addition, the client may be at risk for decreased Cardiac Output, ineffective Tissue Perfusion, and excess Fluid Volume. These needs do not necessarily occur in each client with this condition. One client may actually be pain-free, whereas another could demonstrate a sleep disturbance or report spiritual distress. Therefore, a medical diagnosis can provide an initial point for problem sensing, but the validity of a nursing diagnosis depends on the presence of individually appropriate supporting data.

BOX 3–6

Applicable Nursing Diagnoses Associated With Selected Medical/Psychiatric Disorders

Certain nursing diagnoses may be linked to specific health problems (e.g., medical disorders). This linkage is often presented as choices in a diagnostic database, in various types of clinical pocket manuals, or on preprinted or computerized care planning forms. The purposes are to assist the clinician in rapidly identifying other applicable nursing diagnoses, based on the changing needs of the client, and to develop a decisive plan of care.

Because the nursing process is cyclical and ongoing, other nursing diagnoses may become appropriate as the individual client situation changes. Therefore, you must continually assess, identify, and validate new needs and evaluate the effectiveness of subsequent care. Keep in mind that the client may have needs unrelated to the medical diagnosis.

AIDS

risk for Infection [progression to sepsis/opportunistic overgrowth]: risk factors may include depressed immune system, inadequate primary defenses, use of antimicrobial agents, broken skin, malnutrition, and chronic disease processes.
risk for Deficient Fluid Volume: risk factors may include excessive losses (copious diarrhea, profuse sweating, vomiting, hypermetabolic state, and fever) and impaired intake (nausea, anorexia, lethargy).
Fatigue may be related to disease state, malnutrition, anemia, negative life events, stress/anxiety possibly evidenced by inability to maintain usual routines, decreased performance, lethargy/listlessness, and disinterest in surroundings.

Labor Stage I (Active Phase)

acute Pain/[Discomfort] may be related to contraction-related hypoxia, dilation of tissues, and pressure on adjacent structures combined with stimulation of both parasympathetic and sympathetic nerve endings, possibly evidenced by verbal reports, guarding/distraction behaviors (restlessness), increased muscle tension, and narrowed focus.
impaired Urinary Elimination may be related to retention of fluid in the prenatal period, increased glomerular filtration rate, decreased adrenal stimulation, dehydration, pressure of the presenting part, and regional anesthesia, possibly evidenced by frequency, urgency/incontinence, or retention.
risk for ineffective Coping [Individual/Couple]: risk factors may include stressors accompanying labor, inadequate level of confidence in ability to cope, inadequate level of perception of control.

Fractures

acute Pain may be related to movement of bone fragments, muscle spasms, tissue trauma/edema, traction/immobility device, stress, and anxiety, possibly evidenced by verbal reports, distraction behaviors, self-focusing/narrowed focus, facial mask of pain, guarding/protective behavior, alteration in muscle tone, and autonomic responses (changes in vital signs).

deficient Knowledge [Learning Need] regarding healing process, therapy requirements, potential complications, and self-care needs; may be related to lack of information, possibly evidenced by verbalizations, inappropriate behaviors—apathy and inaccurate follow-through of instructions.

impaired physical Mobility may be related to loss of integrity of bone structures, pain/discomfort, prescribed movement restrictions (bed rest, extremity immobilization), and reluctance to initiate movement, possibly evidenced by difficulty turning, limited range of motion, and uncoordinated movements.

Depressive Disorders (Mood Disorders)

Major Depression/Dysthymia

risk for self- /other-directed Violence: risk factors may include depressed mood, feelings of worthlessness/hopelessness, and history of substance abuse.*

[moderate to severe] Anxiety/disturbed Thought Processes may be related to unmet needs, unconscious conflict about essential values/goals of life, threat to self-concept, interpersonal transmission/contagion, sleep deprivation, possibly evidenced by reports of apprehension or fearfulness, feelings of inadequacy, irritability, restlessness, jittery, difficulty concentrating/impaired attention, diminished ability to problem solve, focusing on physiological symptoms, ideas of reference, hallucinations/delusions.

Insomnia may be related to depression (biochemical alterations—decreased serotonin levels), unresolved anxieties, and decreased activity, possibly evidenced by difficulty falling/staying asleep, waking up early, reports of nonrestorative sleep, lack of energy.

*A risk diagnosis is not evidenced by signs and symptoms as the problem has not occurred; rather, nursing interventions are directed at prevention.

Adapted from Doenges, M. E., Moorhouse, M. F., & Murr, A. C. (2008). *Nurse's Pocket Guide, Nursing Diagnoses with Interventions*, ed 11. Philadelphia: F.A. Davis.

The client's or family member's understanding of normal body function, individual expectations (including cultural), or mistaken perceptions may result in the belief that a need exists, even in the absence of diagnostically appropriate supporting data. Even though the need seems to exist only in the mind of the client/significant other, it needs to be addressed and resolved in order to promote optimal wellness and allow the client to focus on the supported needs.

FOR EXAMPLE:

1. The parent of a child with cancer may believe that the child is incapable of self-care activities, even though the child's level of function and development indicates otherwise. This is not a client problem with self-care but rather the parent's problem—possibly, compromised family Coping.

2. A female client may believe that sexual desire normally disappears after menopause/hysterectomy, and the fact that it does not indicates to her that something is wrong. Although sexual dysfunction may have occurred, the assessment reveals inadequate information and misconceptions. Therefore, the nursing diagnosis is deficient Knowledge of normal sexual functioning.

3. An elderly, confused client with a diagnosis of Alzheimer's disease is found wandering in the day room. She has soiled herself and is smearing feces on the walls and couch. The problem is not one of bowel elimination but of disturbed Thought Processes. Interventions should be addressed to behavioral management rather than only to bowel control.

As noted in the previous examples, it is important to reduce the need to its basic component in order to focus interventions on the roots of the human response. It is also important to take the related factors and the defining characteristics to the lowest "denominator" possible so the client and nurse are better able to formulate individually specific goals/outcomes and identify appropriate interventions/actions to be taken to correct or alleviate the need.

> **FOR EXAMPLE:** impaired Social Interaction related to neurological impairment and the resulting sequelae (i.e., cognitive, behavioral, and emotional changes) is better stated as "related to skill deficit about ways to enhance mutuality, communication barriers, limited physical mobility as evidenced by family report of change in pattern of interacting, dysfunctional interactions with peers and family, observed discomfort in social situations." This simplifies care and increases the likelihood of a timely and satisfactory resolution.

Neurological impairment is a broad label that reflects general pathophysiology and lacks the specificity that is necessary to guide nursing actions/interventions. By identifying specific responses, you focus attention directly on issues that can be corrected or altered by nursing interventions.

For beginners, it is advisable to use the NANDA-I list in Appendix I when choosing a diagnostic label. Because the list is still evolving, "holes" may exist. With practice and experience, you may very well identify a need that is treatable with nursing interventions but for which there is no appropriate NANDA-I label. In this situation, the diagnosis should be stated clearly using the PES format and then reviewed with other nursing colleagues to verify that the meaning and intent are communicated accurately. Finally, the work should be documented and submitted to NANDA-I for consideration.

Nursing knowledge is both objective and subjective, and it is the combination of intuition and analysis that guides nursing's methodology. Experienced nurses may use **INTUITION** to arrive at a conclusion as an integral part of critical thinking. This skill is difficult to teach, and it may not develop in all nurses; however, it needs to be respected, valued, and encouraged. Intuition is grounded in knowledge, skill, and experience. It is the recognition of previously experienced patterns and the detection of subclinical changes (Benner & Tanner, 1987).

Paying attention to your feelings or sense of something for which there are no data can add an important dimension to the diagnostic reasoning process. Intuition,

INTUITION: a sense of something that is not clearly evidenced by known facts.

applied responsibly by checking, rechecking, and validating impressions (to avoid errors in judgment), can lead to insights not available in any other way.

Finally, identification of a client's needs may be assisted by entering the client database into a computer. On-line diagnostic software programs are available that contain lists of frequently used nursing diagnoses correlated to specific medical diagnoses. Other programs may suggest possible nursing diagnoses based on cues that the program identifies in the client database. Such programs are support tools and do not eliminate your need to use the diagnostic reasoning process to identify and formulate appropriate client diagnostic statements *independently* of computer recommendations.

Writing a Client Diagnostic Statement: Using PES Format

As NANDA-I's list of nursing diagnosis labels has increased, issues of **WELLNESS** are being addressed. The focus of a nursing diagnosis is no longer limited solely to problems but may also include the client's needs and strength areas for potential enhancement. For this reason, although this textbook uses the PES format, we have chosen to identify the outcome of the diagnostic reasoning process as the *Client Diagnostic Statement* instead of the commonly used term *Client Problem*.

WELLNESS: a state of optimal health, physical and psychosocial.

According to the PES format, the problem (need), etiology, and signs and symptoms (or risk factors) are combined into a neutral statement that avoids value-laden or judgmental language. The use of ambiguous or judgmental terms, such as "too often," "uncooperative," or "manipulative," can lead to misunderstanding on the part of the reader. Clients may become defensive, or readers may be influenced to make an inaccurate or biased decision, resulting in a negative treatment outcome.

The *need* and *etiology* sections of the diagnostic statement are joined by the phrase "related to." Phrases such as "due to" or "caused by" indicate a specific/limited causal link that should therefore be avoided. "Related to" suggests a connection between the nursing diagnosis and the identified factors, leaving open the possibility that there may be other contributing factors not yet recognized.

When writing a diagnostic statement, remember to include qualifiers or quantifiers as appropriate. NANDA-I has provided for some flexibility of the nursing language by creating a multi-axial taxonomy. An *axis* is defined as a dimension of the human response that is considered in the diagnostic process. The first axis is the diagnostic concept. The other six axes (subject of the diagnosis, judgment, location, age, time, and status of the diagnosis) can be used to modify the diagnostic concept (see Appendix G). Some modifiers are already included in the label.

> **FOR EXAMPLE:** ineffective community Coping. Coping (diagnostic concept) is the principal element or human response of concern. It has been modified by a judgment (ineffective) and the subject of the diagnosis (community). In adult Failure to Thrive, "adult" reflects an age modifier.

If the term "specify" is noted with a diagnostic label, it is important that the correct information for the individual client be provided to make the communication clear.

FOR EXAMPLE: In ineffective Tissue Perfusion (specify), the modifier to be specified is from the location axis (e.g., cerebral, renal). However, in the diagnostic label deficient Knowledge (specify), the modifier is actually the area or topic for which the client has deficient knowledge, such as *regarding care of the newborn.* In the case of decisional Conflict (specify), the modifier is the subject of the conflict or life crisis. The client diagnostic statement might read "decisional Conflict regarding divorce related to perceived threat to value system as evidenced by vacillation between alternative choices, increased muscle tension, and reports of distress."

By definition, nursing diagnoses identify client needs that can be positively affected, or possibly prevented, by nursing actions. Some diagnoses permit greater independent function, whereas others are more collaborative. This may be visualized as a continuum without a fixed midpoint differentiating independent from dependent actions (Fig. 3–1). Furthermore, the extent of independent function is influenced by the individual nurse's experience, level of expertise, and work setting and the presence of established **PROTOCOLS**, or standards of care. For this reason, the authors recommend that nurses identify the nursing component and appropriate interventions for any client need instead of labeling independent versus **COLLABORATIVE PROBLEMS** or potential complications.

FOR EXAMPLE:

- During and following Sally's bleeding episode, the nursing component would be deficient [isotonic] Fluid Volume, and the nurse would not only monitor the problem but also take action to control/prevent further blood loss (e.g., fundal massage), increase fluid intake (oral, intravenous [IV], or both), administer prescribed antiemetic, and provide assurance to the client.

PROTOCOL: written guidelines of steps to be taken for providing client care in a particular situation/ condition.

COLLABORATIVE PROBLEM: a need, identified by another discipline, that contains a nursing component requiring nursing intervention and/or monitoring and therefore is an element of the interdisciplinary plan of care.

FIGURE 3–1. Representative comparison of the amount of independent nursing function in two nursing diagnoses. Nursing diagnoses have varying amounts of independent function, and nursing actions can be identified for any client situation. As shown in this diagram, the nursing diagnosis *Anxiety* has a high degree of independent nursing action, whereas *Cardiac Output* has a lower degree.

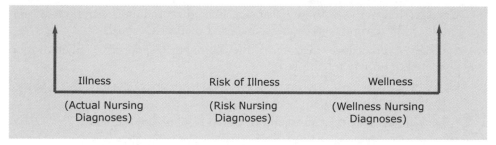

FIGURE 3–2. Trifocal model for client assessment. Adapted from Kelly, Frisch, & Avant, 1995.

- A low-serum potassium level may result in dysrhythmias that can be addressed in risk for decreased Cardiac Output, requiring electrocardiographic (ECG) interpretation, possible limiting of activities, provision of potassium-containing foods/fluids as appropriate and, possibly, other interventions based on protocols.

- Michelle has a subclavian IV catheter. You might be concerned with risk for Infection, with implications for sterile dressing changes, observation of the site, and monitoring of vital signs.

Debate concerning the amount of independent function associated with nursing diagnoses and the interpretation of the definition of nursing diagnoses has been ongoing. These debates attest to the perceived and actual importance that nursing diagnoses have had and continue to have in the structuring of both the education and the practice of nursing. A bifocal model of nursing diagnosis and collaborative problems has existed for many years (Carpenito, 1997; Wallace & Ivey, 1989). Also, a trifocal model of nursing diagnosis (Kelly et al., 1995) that reinforces the wellness diagnoses has been developed (Fig. 3–2).

In creating a diagnostic statement, it is important to be aware of common errors that can result in an incorrect nursing diagnosis. An incorrect nursing diagnosis or misstatement of needs can lead to incorrect goals/outcomes and inappropriate nursing interventions. This can result in inappropriate/inadequate treatment of the client that may not resolve the need and that may occasionally place the nurse at risk for legal liability.

- **Using the medical diagnosis:** Self-Care Deficit related to stroke.

  Correct: Self-Care Deficit related to neuromuscular impairment as evidenced by inability to manipulate clothing and dress self.

- **Relating the problem to an unchangeable situation:** risk for Injury related to blindness.

  Correct: risk for Injury: risk factors of unfamiliarity with surroundings.

- **Confusing the etiology or signs/symptoms with the need:** Postoperative lung congestion related to ineffective cough.

Correct: Ineffective Airway Clearance related to retained secretions as evidenced by adventitious breath sounds and ineffective cough .

- **Using a procedure instead of the "human response":** Catheterization related to urinary retention.

Correct: Urinary Retention related to blockage/perineal swelling as evidenced by bladder distention.

- **Lacking Specificity:** Constipation related to nutritional intake.

Correct: Constipation related to poor eating habits, insufficient fiber and fluid intake as evidenced by hard/formed stool.

- **Combining two nursing diagnoses:** Anxiety and Fear related to separation from parents.

Correct: Fear related to separation from parents, or moderate Anxiety related to change in environment and unmet needs as evidenced by voice quivering, irritability, distress.

- **Relating one nursing diagnosis to another:** Ineffective Coping related to anxiety.

Correct: severe Anxiety related to change in role function and threat to economic status as evidenced by uncertainty, feelings of inadequacy, diminished ability to problem solve.

- **Using judgmental/value-laden language:** chronic Pain related to secondary/ monetary gain.

Correct: chronic Pain related to physical disability/recurrent muscle spasms and psychosocial disability as evidenced by verbal report, self-focusing, reduced interaction with people. **Note:** The client's report is valid, but the issue of secondary gain may require additional assessment to reveal other appropriate nursing diagnoses and interventions.

- **Making assumptions:** risk for impaired Parenting: risk factors of inexperience (new mother).

Correct: deficient Knowledge regarding child-care issues related to lack of previous experience, unfamiliarity with resources as evidenced by verbalization of problem, and inaccurate follow-through of instruction. **Note:** The label "deficient Knowledge" can have negative connotations for the client and may result in defensive responses. The authors support the use of a substitute label "Learning Need."

- **Writing a legally inadvisable statement:** impaired Skin Integrity related to not being turned every 2 hours.

Correct: impaired Skin Integrity related to prolonged pressure and impaired circulation as evidenced by destruction of skin layers. **Note:** If a client complication occurs as a result of poor care/failure to meet standards of care, an incident/occurrence report would be completed to document what happened.

With this in mind, review In a Nutshell before proceeding to Practice Activity 3–3.

In a Nutshell

How to Write a Client Diagnostic Statement

1. Using physical assessment and history-taking interview techniques, collect subjective and objective data from the client, significant other, family members, other healthcare providers, and/or client records as appropriate. A nursing framework is recommended, such as Diagnostic Divisions (Doenges and Moorhouse) or Functional Health Patterns (Gordon).

2. Organize the collected data using a nursing framework (see item 1, above), a body systems approach (cardiovascular, gastrointestinal, and so on), a head-to-toe review (head, neck, thorax, and so on), or a combination of these. Your institution may use its own clustering model. If you have used a nursing framework, however, you will discover that information in the client database is already conveniently structured for ease in identifying applicable nursing diagnoses.

3. Using diagnostic reasoning skills, review and analyze the database to identify cues (signs and symptoms) suggesting needs that can be described by nursing diagnostic labels. Check the NANDA-I definitions of specific diagnoses for further assistance in distinguishing between two or more potentially applicable labels (see Appendix I).

4. Consider alternative rationales for the identified cues by comparing and contrasting the relationships among and between data and isolating etiological factors. This will allow you to determine which nursing diagnostic labels may be most appropriate and rule out those that are not.

5. Test your selection of nursing diagnostic label(s) and associated etiology(ies) for appropriateness by:

Confirming the NANDA-I nursing diagnosis and definition for your choice of diagnostic label (P)

Comparing your proposed etiology with the NANDA-I Related Factors or Risk Factors associated with that particular diagnosis (E)

Comparing your identified signs and symptoms (cues) with the NANDA-I Defining Characteristics for the selected diagnosis (S)

6. Re-evaluate your list of selected diagnoses to be sure that all client needs are considered. Then, order your list according to a needs priority model (the Maslow or Kalish model is usually used) with validation from the client, and classify each diagnosis as actual (signs and symptoms supporting it are already present), risk for (risk factors are present, but the problem has not yet occurred), readiness for enhanced (there is a desire to move to a higher state), or resolved (need no longer requires nursing action).

7. Write the client diagnostic statement for each diagnosis on your list. A three-part statement using the PES format is indicated for actual or wellness

Continued

In a Nutshell (Continued)

diagnoses, and an adaptation of the PES format is used to create the two-part statement for risk diagnoses. Resolved diagnoses do not require diagnostic statements.

Three-Part Client Diagnostic Statement

Combine (1) the confirmed nursing diagnosis label (P), (2) related factors (E), and (3) defining characteristics (S). These elements are linked by the phrases "related to" and "as evidenced by":

NEED (PROBLEM): [nursing diagnostic label]
ETIOLOGY: Related to [etiological factors]
SIGNS AND SYMPTOMS: As evidenced by [defining characteristics]

Two-Part Client Diagnostic Statement

Combine (1) the confirmed risk nursing diagnosis label (P) and (2) the associated risk factors (E). These elements are linked by the phrase "risk factors of."

NEED (PROBLEM): [risk nursing diagnosis label]
ETIOLOGY: Risk factors of [associated risk factors]

PRACTICE ACTIVITY 3–3
Identifying Correct and Incorrect Client Diagnostic Statements

Label each client diagnostic statement as correct or incorrect. Identify why a statement is incorrect.

1. ineffective Airway Clearance related to increased pulmonary secretions and bronchospasm, evidenced by wheezing, tachypnea, and ineffective cough.
2. impaired Thought Processes related to delusional thinking or reality base, evidenced by persecutory thoughts of "I am victim" and interference with ability to think clearly and logically.
3. impaired Gas Exchange related to bronchitis, evidenced by rhonchi, dyspnea, and cyanosis.
4. deficient Knowledge regarding diabetic care, related to inaccurate follow-through of instructions, evidenced by information misinterpretation and lack of recall.
5. acute Pain related to tissue distention and edema, evidenced by reports of severe colicky pain in right flank, elevated pulse and respirations, and restlessness.

Finally, although the PES format is a commonly recognized way of structuring the client diagnostic statement, other formats may be appropriate when a different standardized language is used. For example, the Omaha System identifies four levels of a diagnostic statement: Level 1—Domain, Level 2—Problem Classification, Level 3—Modifier, and Level 4—Signs/Symptoms (Box 3–7).

BOX 3–7

Omaha System Example

In Box 3–2, Robert is assessed using the Activity/Rest Diagnostic Division, revealing a range of possible NANDA-I nursing diagnosis labels including:

Activity Intolerance
risk for Disuse Syndrome
deficient Diversional Activity
Fatigue
Insomnia
Sleep Deprivation
Impaired Walking

These lead to a client diagnostic statement of: Activity Intolerance related to imbalance between oxygen supply/demand as evidenced by dyspnea and tachycardia with exertion, weakness, and limitation of desired activities.

   If we apply the Omaha System to the assessment data for Robert's level of physical activity, his problem would be documented as:

Level 1—Domain IV, Health-Related Behaviors
Level 2—Problem Classification, No. 37. Physical Activity
Level 3—Modifier, Individual Impairment
Level 4—Signs/Symptoms, No. 3. Inappropriate Type/Physical Condition

You are encouraged to read the articles and texts included in the Omaha System section of the Suggested Readings at the end of this chapter.

Summary

Identification of an accurate nursing diagnosis requires time to analyze the gathered data and to validate the diagnosis. This process is critical because it is the pivotal part of the nursing process. The time you take to formulate an accurate client diagnostic statement and to plan the required care results in increased nursing efficiency, better use of time for all nursing staff, and the delivery of appropriate client care—with the end result of better client outcomes.

   Some nurses still organize care around medical diagnoses, spending most of their time following medical orders. Medical diagnoses have a narrower focus than nursing diagnoses because they are based on pathology, whereas a nursing diagnosis takes into account the psychological, social, spiritual, and physiological responses of the client, family, or community. NANDA-I diagnostic labels listed in Appendix I are used in formulating diagnostic statements that are structured in a three-part Problem (Need), Etiology, and Signs/Symptoms (PES) format. Two-part statements may be used for risk diagnoses.

   At times, something that appears easy to do in theory may seem difficult to achieve in practice. As you work with and become more familiar with nursing diagnoses, the client goals, related outcomes, and nursing interventions for attaining these goals and outcomes become more readily apparent. An accurate and complete nursing diagnosis serves as the basis for the activities of the planning step of the nursing process, discussed in Chapter 4.

Before continuing, return to the second ANA Standard of Practice, and review the measurement criteria necessary to achieve and ensure compliance with the standard as discussed in this chapter (Box 3–8).

BOX 3–8

Measurement Criteria for ANA Standard 2

ANA Standard 2: Diagnosis: The registered nurse analyzes the assessment data to determine the diagnoses or issues.

1. Derives the diagnoses or issues based on assessment data.
2. Validates the diagnoses or issues with the patient, family, and other health-care providers when possible and appropriate.
3. Documents diagnoses or issues in a manner that facilitates the determination of the expected outcomes and plan.

1. What is the definition of Diagnosis?

   _____

2. What two factors influenced the development and acceptance of nursing diagnosis as the language of nursing?

   _____

3. List three reasons for using nursing diagnosis.

   a. _____

   b. _____

   c. _____

4. List the six steps of diagnostic reasoning.

   a. _____

   b. _____

   c. _____

   d. _____

   e. _____

   f. _____

5. Name the components of the Client Diagnostic Statement.

   a. _____

   b. _____

   c. _____

6. If a risk diagnosis is identified, how is the Client Diagnostic Statement altered?

   _____

7. What is the difference between a medical and a nursing diagnosis?

   _____

8. Which of these client diagnostic statements are stated correctly? Indicate by placing a C before correct or an I before incorrect statements. Then, differentiate actual (A) from risk (R) needs by placing an A or R by each statement.

   a. deficient Knowledge regarding drug therapy, related to misinterpretation and unfamiliarity with resources as evidenced by request for information and inaccurate follow-through of instruction.

   b. risk for Infection: risk factors of decreased ciliary action, decreased hemoglobin, and invasive procedures.

   c. impaired Urinary Elimination, related to indwelling catheter evidenced by inability to void.

   d. moderate Anxiety related to change in health status, role function, and economic status evidenced by apprehension, insomnia, and feelings of inadequacy.

9. Underline the cues in the following client database that indicate that a need may exist, and write a Client Diagnostic Statement based on your findings.

VIGNETTE: Sally is 2 days post-delivery. She reports that her bowels have not moved but says she has been drinking plenty of fluids, including fruit juices, and has been eating a balanced diet.

Elimination (Excerpt From the Client Database)

Subjective
Usual bowel patterns: Every morning
Laxative use: Rare/MOM p.m.
Character of stool: Brown, formed
Last BM: 4 days ago
History of bleeding: No
Hemorrhoids: Past 5 weeks
Constipation: Currently
Diarrhea: No
Usual voiding pattern: 3–4 ×/day
Character of urine: Yellow
Incontinence: No
Urgency: No
Pain/burning/difficulty voiding: No
History of kidney/bladder disease: Several bladder infections, last one 6 years ago
Associated concerns: Pain with stool, nausea, "I just can't go no matter what I do."

Objective
Abdomen tender: Yes
Soft/firm: Somewhat firm
Palpable mass: No
Size/girth: Enlarged/postpartal
Bowel sounds: Present all four quadrants, hypoactive every 1 to 2 minutes
Hemorrhoids: Visual examination not done

Write the Client Diagnostic Statement. Refer to the listing of nursing diagnoses in Appendix I to compare diagnostic labels addressing bowel elimination.

BIBLIOGRAPHY

American Nurses Association. (1980). *Nursing: A Social Policy Statement.* Kansas City, MO: Author.
American Nurses Association. (1995). *Nursing's Social Policy Statement.* Washington, DC: Author.
American Nurses Association. (2004). *Nursing: Scope & Standards of Practice.* Washington, DC: Author.
Benner, P., & Tanner, C. A. (1987). How expert nurses use intuition. *American Journal of Nursing, 87*(1): 23–31.

Carpenito, L. J. (1997). *Nursing Diagnosis: Application to Clinical Practice*, ed 7. Philadelphia: J. B. Lippincott.

Fry, V. S. (1953). The creative approach to nursing. *American Journal of Nursing*, 53:301–302.

Gebbie, K. M., & Lavin, M. A. (1975). *Classification of Nursing Diagnoses: Proceedings From the First National Conference*. St. Louis: Mosby.

Gordon, M. (1976). Nursing diagnosis and the diagnostic process. *American Journal of Nursing*, 76(8):1298–1300.

Kelly, J., Frisch, N., & Avant, K. (1995). A trifocal model of nursing diagnosis: Wellness reinforced. *Nursing Diagnosis*, 6(3):123–128.

Lunney, M. (1989). Self-monitoring of accuracy using an integrated model of diagnostic process. *Journal of Advanced Medical Surgical Nursing*, 1(3):43–52.

Lunney, M. (1990). Accuracy of nursing diagnosis: Concept development. *Nursing Diagnosis*, 1(1):12–17.

NANDA International. (2007). *Nursing Diagnoses: Definition & Classification*. Philadelphia: Author.

Wallace, D., & Ivey, J. (1989). The bifocal clinical nursing model: Descriptions and applications to patients receiving thrombolytic or anticoagulant therapy. *Journal of Cardiovascular Nursing*, 4(1): 33–45.

SUGGESTED READINGS

Nursing Language, Classification, Theory, and Taxonomy

Advant, K. C. (1990). The art and science in nursing diagnosis development. *Nursing Diagnosis*, 1(1):51–56.

Dobryzn, J. (1995). Components of written nursing diagnostic statements. *Nursing Diagnosis*, 6(1):29–38.

Kerr, M. (1991). Validation of taxonomy. In R. M. Carroll-Johnson (Ed.). *Classification of Nursing Diagnoses: Proceedings of the Ninth Conference North American Nursing Diagnosis Association*. Philadelphia: J. B. Lippincott.

Kerr, M., et al. (1992). Development of definitions for taxonomy II. *Nursing Diagnosis*, 3(2):65–71.

Kerr, M., et al. (1993). Taxonomic validation: An overview. *Nursing Diagnosis*, 4(1):6–14.

Loomis, M. E., & Conco, D. (1991). Patients' perception of health, chronic illness, and nursing diagnosis. *Nursing Diagnosis*, 2(4):162–170.

Miers, L. J. (1991). NANDA's definition of nursing diagnosis: A plea for conceptual clarity. *Nursing Diagnosis*, 2(1):9–18.

Mills, W. C. (1991). Nursing diagnosis: The importance of a definition. *Nursing Diagnosis*, 2(1):3–8.

Shoemaker, J. (1984). Essential features of a nursing diagnosis. In M. Kim, G. K. McFarland, & A. M. McLane (Eds.). *Classification of Nursing Diagnoses: Proceedings of the Fifth Conference, North American Nursing Diagnosis Association*. St. Louis: Mosby.

Spackman, K. (2000). SNOMED RT and SNOMED CT: The promise of an international clinical terminology. *MD Computing*, 17(6):29.

Warren, J. J., & Hoskins, L. M. (1990). The development of NANDA's nursing diagnosis taxonomy. *Nursing Diagnosis*, 1(4):162–168.

Whitley, G. G., & Gulanick, M. (1995). Barriers to use of nursing diagnosis in clinical settings. *Nursing Diagnosis*, (5):25–32.

Texts

Carmona, E. V., & de Moraes Lopes, M. H. B. (2006). Content validation of parental role conflict in the neonatal intensive care unit. *International Journal of Nursing Terminologies and Classifications*, 17(1):3–9.

Carpenito-Moyet, L. J. (2007). *Nursing Diagnosis: Application to Clinical Practice*, ed 12. Philadelphia: Lippincott Williams & Wilkins.

Doenges, M. E., Moorhouse, M. F., & Murr, A. C. (2006). *Nursing Care Plans: Guidelines for Individualizing Client Care Across the Life Span*, ed 7. Philadelphia: F. A. Davis.

Leuner, J. D., Manton, A. K., Kelliher, D., Sullivan, S. D., & Doherty, M. (1990). *Mastering the Nursing Process: A Case Study Approach*. Philadelphia: F. A. Davis.

Maas, M., Buckwalter, K. C., & Hardy, M. (1991). *Nursing Diagnosis and Interventions for the Elderly*. Menlo Park, CA: Addison-Wesley.

Newfield, S., et al. (2007). *Cox's Clinical Applications of Nursing Diagnosis: Adult, Child, Women's, Mental Health, Gerontic, and Home Health Considerations*, ed 5. Philadelphia: F. A. Davis.

Validation of Nursing Diagnoses

Brukwitzki, G., Holmgen, C., & Maibusch, R. M. (1996). Validation of the defining characteristics of the nursing diagnosis ineffective airway clearance. *Nursing Diagnosis, 7*:63–69.

Chiang, L., Ku, N., & Lo, C. K. (1994). Clinical validation of the etiologies and defining characteristics of altered nutrition: Less than body requirements in patients with cancer. In R. M. Carroll-Johnson & M. Paquette (Eds.). *Classification of Nursing Diagnoses: Proceedings of the Tenth Conference, North American Nursing Diagnosis Association.* Philadelphia: J. B. Lippincott.

Chung, L. (1997). The clinical validation of defining characteristics and related factors of fatigue in hemodialysis patients. In M. J. Rantz & P. Lemone (Eds.). *Classification of Nursing Diagnoses: Proceedings of the Twelfth Conference, North American Nursing Diagnosis Association.* Glendale, CA: Cinahl.

Dougherty, C. (1997). Reconceptualization of the nursing diagnosis decreased cardiac output. *Nursing Diagnosis: The Journal of Nursing Language and Classification, 8*:29–36.

Ennen, K. A., Komorita, N. I., & Pogue, N. (1997). Validation of defining characteristics of the nursing diagnosis: Fluid volume excess. In M. J. Rantz, P. Guirao-Goris, & G. Duarte-Climents. (2007). The expert nurse profile and diagnostic content validity of sedentary lifestyle: The Spanish validation. *International Journal of Nursing Terminologies and Classifications, 18*(3):84–92.

Fowler, S. B. (1997). Impaired verbal communication: During short-term oral intubation. *Nursing Diagnosis: The Journal of Nursing Language and Classification, 8*:93–98.

Hensley, L. D. (1994). Spiritual distress: A validation study. In R. M. Carroll-Johnson & M. Paquette (Eds.). *Classification of Nursing Diagnoses: Proceedings of the Tenth Conference, North American Nursing Diagnosis Association.* Philadelphia: J. B. Lippincott.

Kerr, M., et al. (1993). Development of definitions for taxonomy II. *Nursing Diagnosis, 3*(2):65–71.

Kraft, L. A., Maas, M., & Hardy, M. A. (1994). Diagnostic content validity of impaired physical mobility in the older adult. In R. M. Carroll-Johnson & M. Paquette (Eds.). *Classification of Nursing Diagnoses: Proceedings of the Tenth Conference, North American Nursing Diagnosis Association.* Philadelphia: J. B. Lippincott.

Lee, E., & Lee, M. (2006). Comparison of nursing interventions performed by medical-surgical nurses in Korea and the United States. *International Journal of Nursing Terminologies and Classifications, 17*(2): 110–117.

Lemone, P. (1993). Validation of the defining characteristics of altered sexuality. *Nursing Diagnosis, 4*(2): 56–62.

Lemone, P., & James, D. (1997). Nursing assessment of altered sexuality: A review of salient factors and objective measures. *Nursing Diagnosis: The Journal of Nursing Language and Classification, 8*:120–128.

Lemone, P., & Weber, J. (1995). Validating gender-specific defining characteristics. *Nursing Diagnosis, 6*(2):64–72.

Levin, R. F., Krainovich, B. C., Bahrenburg, E., & Mitchell, C. A. (1988). Diagnostic content validity of nursing diagnosis. *Image: The Journal of Nursing Scholarship, 21*(1):40–44.

Morton, N. (1997). Validation of the nursing diagnosis decreased cardiac output in a population without cardiac disease. In M. J. Rantz & P. Lemone (Eds.). *Classification of Nursing Diagnoses: Proceedings of the Twelfth Conference, North American Nursing Diagnosis Association.* Glendale, CA: Cinahl.

Rantz, M. J. & Lemone, P. (Eds.). *Classification of Nursing Diagnoses: Proceedings of the Twelfth Conference, North American Nursing Diagnosis Association.* Glendale, CA: Cinahl.

Sidani, S., & Woodtli, M. A. (1994). Testing and validating an instrument to assess the defining characteristics of stress and urge incontinence. In R. M. Carroll-Johnson & M. Paquette (Eds.). *Classification of Nursing Diagnoses: Proceedings of the Tenth Conference, North American Nursing Diagnosis Association.* Philadelphia: J. B. Lippincott.

Simon, J., Baumann, M. A., & Nolan, L. (1995). Differential diagnostic validation: Acute and chronic pain. *Nursing Diagnosis, 6*(2):73–79.

Smith, J. E., et al. (1997). Risk for suicide and risk for violence: A case study approach for separating the current violence diagnoses. *Nursing Diagnosis: The Journal of Nursing Language and Classification, 8*:67–77.

Tiesinga, L. J., Dassen, T. W. N., & Halfens, R. J. G. (1997). Validation of the nursing diagnosis fatigue among patients with chronic heart failure. In M. J. Rantz & P. Lemone (Eds.). *Classification of Nursing Diagnoses: Proceedings of the Twelfth Conference, North American Nursing Diagnosis Association.* Glendale, CA: Cinahl.

Wall, B., Howard, J., & Perry-Phillips, J. (1995). Validation of two nursing diagnoses: Increased intracranial pressure and high risk for increased intracranial pressure. In M. J. Rantz & P. Lemone (Eds.). *Classification of Nursing Diagnoses: Proceedings of the Eleventh Conference, North American Nursing Diagnosis Association.* Glendale, CA: Cinahl.

Whitley, G. G. (1992). Concept analysis of anxiety. *Nursing Diagnosis, 3*(3):107–116.
Whitley, G. G. (1992). Concept analysis of fear. *Nursing Diagnosis, 3*(4):155–161.

Specific Nursing Diagnoses

Bakker, R. H., Kastermans, M.C., & Dassen, T. W. N. (1995). An analysis of the nursing diagnosis ineffective management of therapeutic regimen compared to noncompliance and Orem's self-care deficit theory. *Nursing Diagnosis,* 6:161–168.
Bakker, R. H., Kastermans, M. C., & Dassen, T. W. N. (1997). Noncompliance and ineffective management of therapeutic regimen: Use in practice and theoretical implications. In M. J. Rantz & P. Lemone (Eds.). *Classification of Nursing Diagnoses: Proceedings of the Twelfth Conference, North American Nursing Diagnosis Association.* Glendale, CA: Cinahl.
Harness-DoGloria, D., & Pye, C. G. (1995). Risk for impaired skin integrity: Incorporation of the risk factors from AHCPR guidelines. In M. J. Rantz & P. Lemone (Eds.). *Classification of Nursing Diagnoses: Proceedings of the Eleventh Conference, North American Nursing Diagnosis Association.* Glendale, CA: Cinahl.
Heliker, D. (1992). Reevaluation of the nursing diagnosis: Spiritual distress. *Nurs Forum, 27*(4):15–20.
Lunney, M. (2006). Stress overload: A new nursing diagnosis. *International Journal of Nursing Terminologies and Classifications, 17*(4):165–175.
Mahon, S. M. (1994). Concept analysis of pain: Implications related to nursing diagnoses. *Nursing Diagnosis, 1*(5):15–25.
Minton, J. A., & Creason, N. S. (1991). Evaluation of admission nursing diagnoses. *Nursing Diagnosis, 2*(1):119–125.
Schmelz, J. O. (1997). Ineffective airway clearance: State of the science. In M. J. Rantz & P. Lemone (Eds.). *Classification of Nursing Diagnoses: Proceedings of the Twelfth Conference, North American Nursing Diagnosis Association.* Glendale, CA: Cinahl.
Smucker, C. (1995). A phenomenological description of the experience of spiritual distress. In M. J. Rantz & P. Lemone (Eds.). *Classification of Nursing Diagnoses: Proceedings of the Eleventh Conference, North American Nursing Diagnosis Association.* Glendale, CA: Cinahl.
Tiesinga, L. J., Dassen, T. W. N., & Halfens, R. J. G. (1995). Fatigue: A summary of definitions, dimensions, and indicators. *Nursing Diagnosis,* 7:51–62.
Whitley, G. G. (1997). A comparison of two methods of clinical validation of nursing diagnosis. In M. J. Rantz & P. Lemone (Eds.). *Classification of Nursing Diagnoses: Proceedings of the Twelfth Conference, North American Nursing Diagnosis Association.* Glendale, CA: Cinahl.
Whitley, G. G., & Tousman, S. A. (1996). A multivariate approach for the validation of anxiety and fear. *Nursing Diagnosis,* 7:116–124.
Woodtli, A. (1995). Stress incontinence: Clinical identification and validation of defining characteristics. *Nursing Diagnosis,* 6:115–122.
Woodtli, M. A., & Yocum, K. (1994). Urge incontinence: Identification and clinical validation of defining characteristics. In R. M. Carroll-Johnson and M. Paquette (Eds.). *Classification of Nursing Diagnoses: Proceedings of the Tenth Conference, North American Nursing Diagnosis Association.* Philadelphia: J. B. Lippincott.
Woolridge, J., et al. (1998). A validation study using the case-control method of the nursing diagnosis risk for aspiration. *Nursing Diagnosis: The Journal of Nursing Language and Classification,* 9:5–14.

Accuracy of Nursing Diagnoses

Levin, R. F., Lunney, M., & Krainovich-Miller, B. (2004). Improving diagnostic accuracy using an evidence-based nursing model. *International Journal of Nursing Language and Classification, 15*(4):114-122.
Lunney, M. (1992). Divergent productive thinking factors and accuracy of nursing diagnoses. *Research in Nursing and Health, 15*(3):303–311.
Lunney, M. (1994). Measurement of accuracy of nursing diagnosis. In R. M. Carroll-Johnson & M. Paquette (Eds.). *Classification of Nursing Diagnoses: Proceedings of the Tenth Conference, North American Nursing Diagnosis Association.* Philadelphia: J. B. Lippincott.
Lunney, M., Karlik, B. A., Kiss, M., & Murphy, P. (1995). Accuracy of nursing diagnosis in clinical settings. In M. J. Rantz & P. Lemone (Eds.). *Classification of Nursing Diagnoses: Proceedings of the Eleventh Conference, North American Nursing Diagnosis Association.* Glendale, CA: Cinahl.

Lunney, M., Karlik, B. A., Kiss, M., & Murphy, P. (1997). Accuracy of nursing diagnosis of psychosocial responses. *Nursing Diagnosis: The Journal of Nursing Language and Classification*, 8:157–166.

Lunney, M., & Paradiso, C. (1995). Accuracy of interpreting human responses. *Nursing Management*, 26(10):48H–48K.

Wellness (Health Promotion)

Allen, C. (1989). Incorporating a wellness perspective for nursing diagnosis in practice. In R. M. Carroll-Johnson (Ed.). *Classification of Nursing Diagnoses: Proceedings of the Eighth Conference, North American Nursing Diagnosis Association*. Philadelphia: J. B. Lippincott.

Appling, S. E. (1997). Wellness issues: Sleep: Linking research to improved outcomes. *MEDSURG Nursing*, 6(3):159–161.

Armentrout, G. (1993). A comparison of the medical model and the wellness model: The importance of knowing the difference. *Holistic Nursing Practice*, 7(4):57–62.

Carpenito-Moyet, L. J. (2007). *Nursing Diagnosis: Application to Clinical Practice*, ed 12. Philadelphia: Lippincott Williams & Wilkins.

Fleury, J. (1991). Empowering potential: A theory of wellness motivation. *Nursing Research*, 40:286–291.

Fleury, J. (1991). Wellness motivation in cardiac rehabilitation. *Heart & Lung: Journal of Critical Care*, 20(1):3–8.

Fleury, J. (1996). Wellness motivation theory: An exploration of theoretical relevance. *Nursing Research*, 45:277–283.

Kelly, J., Frisch, N., & Avant, K. (1995). A trifocal model of nursing diagnosis: Wellness reinforced. *Nursing Diagnosis*, 6(3):123–128.

Moch, S. (1989). Health within illness: Conceptual evolution and practice possibilities. *Advances in Nursing Science*, 11:230–231.

Murdaugh, C. L., & Vanderboom, C. (1997). Individual and community models for promoting wellness. *Journal of Cardiovascular Nursing*, 11(3):1–14.

Pender, N. J., Murdaugh, C. L., & Parsons, M. A. (2005). *Health Promotion in Nursing Practice*, ed 5. Upper Saddle River, NJ: Prentice Hall.

Popkess-Vawter, S. (1991). Wellness nursing diagnoses: To be or not to be? *Nursing Diagnosis*, 2(1):19–25.

Ryan, J. P. (1993). Wellness and health promotion of the elderly. *Nursing Outlook*, 41(3):143.

Stolte, K. M. (1994). Health-oriented nursing diagnoses: Development and use. In R. M. Carroll-Johnson & M. Paquette (Eds.). *Classification of Nursing Diagnoses: Proceedings of the Tenth Conference, North American Nursing Diagnosis Association*. Philadelphia: J. B. Lippincott.

Stolte, K. M. (1996). *Wellness Nursing Diagnosis for Health Promotion*. Philadelphia: Lippincott Williams & Wilkins.

Omaha System

Barrera, C., Machanga, M., Connolly, P. M., & Yoder, M. (2003). Nursing care makes a difference: Application of the Omaha System. *Outcomes Management*, 7(4):181–185.

Bednarz, P. K. (1998). The Omaha system: A model for describing school nurse case management. *Journal of School Nursing*, 4(3):24–30.

Bowles, K. H. (1999). The Omaha system: Bridging hospital and home care. On-line *Journal of Nursing Informatics*, 3(1):7–11. Accessed Sept 2007 at http://www.eaa-knowledge.com/ojni/ni/dm/ojni.html

Bowles, K. H. (2000). Application of the Omaha system in acute care. *Research in Nursing and Health*, 23(2): 93–105.

Elfrink, V. (1999). The Omaha system: Bridging nursing education and information technology. *On-line Journal of Nursing Informatics*, 3(1): 15–19. Accessed Sept 2007 at http://www.eaa-knowledge.com/ojni/ni/dm/ojni.html

Elfrink, V. L., & Martin, K. S. (1996). Educating for community nursing practice: Point of care technology. *Healthcare Information Management*, 10(2):81–89.

Erdogan, S., & Esin N. M. (2006). The Turkish version of the Omaha System: Its use in practice-based family nursing education. *Nurse Education Today*. Accessed Sept 2007 at http://dx.doi.org/10.1016/j.nedt.2005.11.009

Lang, N., et al. (1997). *Nursing Practice and Outcomes Measurement*. Oakbrook Terrace, IL: Joint Commission on Accreditation of Healthcare Organizations, pp 17–34.

Martin, K. S. (1989). The Omaha system and NANDA: A review of similarities and differences: In R. M. Carroll-Johnson (Ed.). *Classification of Nursing Diagnoses: Proceedings of the Eighth Conference, North American Nursing Diagnosis Association.* Philadelphia: J. B. Lippincott, pp 171–172.

Martin, K. S. (1997). The Omaha System. In M. J. Rantz & P. Lemone (Eds.). *Classification of Nursing Diagnoses: Proceedings of the Twelfth Conference, North American Nursing Diagnosis Association.* Glendale, CA: Cinahl, pp 16–21.

Martin, K. S. (2005). *The Omaha System: A Key to Practice, Documentation, and Information Management,* ed 2. St. Louis: Elsevier.

Martin, K. S., Leak, G. K., & Aden, C. A. (1992). The Omaha System: A research-based model for decision making. *Journal of Nursing Administration, 22:*44–52.

Martin, K. S., & Martin, D. L. (1997). How can the quality of nursing practice be measured? In J. C. McCloskey & H. K. Grace (Eds.). *Current Issues in Nursing,* ed 5. St. Louis: Mosby, pp 315–321.

Martin, K. S., & Norris, J. (1996). The Omaha System: A model for describing practice. *Holistic Nursing Practice, 11*(1):75–83.

Martin, K. S., & Scheet, N. J. (1992). *The Omaha System: A Pocket Guide for Community Health Nursing.* Philadelphia: W. B. Saunders.

Martin, K. S., & Scheet, N. J. (1992). *The Omaha System: Applications for Community Health Nursing.* Philadelphia: W. B. Saunders.

Martin, K. S., Scheet, N. J., & Stegman, M. R. (1993). Home health care clients: Characteristics, outcomes of care, and nursing interventions. *Am Journal of Public Health* 83:1730–1734.

Merrill, A. S., Hiebert, V., Moran, M., & Weatherby, F. (1998). Curriculum restructuring using the practice-based Omaha System. *Nurse Educator, 23*(3):41–44.

Plowfield, L. A., Hayes, E. R., & Hall-Long, B. (2005). Using the Omaha system to document the wellness needs of the elderly. *Nursing Clinics of North America, 40*(4): 817–829.

Sloan, H. L., & Delahoussaye, C. P. (2003). Clinical application of the Omaha system with the Nightingale tracker. *Nurse Educator, 28*(1):15–17.

Westra, B. (1995). Implementing nursing diagnoses in community settings. In M. J. Rantz & P. Lemone (Eds.). *Classification of Nursing Diagnoses: Proceedings of the Eleventh Conference, North American Nursing Diagnosis Association.* Glendale, CA: Cinahl, pp 47–51.

Westra B. L. (2005). National Health Information Infrastructure (NHII) and nursing: Implementing the Omaha system in community-based practice. Accessed Sept 2007 at http://www.himss.org/content/files/ImplementationNursingTerminologyCommunity.pdf

Clinical Care Classification (Home Healthcare Classification)

Saba, V. K. (1992). Home health care classification. *Caring, 11*(5):58–60.

Saba, V. K. (1992). The classification of home health care nursing: Diagnoses and interventions. *Caring, 11*(3):5–57.

Saba, V. K. (1994). *Home Health Care Classification (HHCC) of Nursing Diagnoses and Interventions (Revised).* Washington, DC: Author.

Saba, V. K. (1997). An innovative Home Health Care Classification (HHCC) System. In M. J. Rantz & P. Lemone (Eds.). *Classification of Nursing Diagnoses: Proceedings of the Twelfth Conference, North American Nursing Diagnosis Association.* Glendale, CA: Cinahl.

Saba, V. K. (1999). Home Health Care Classification: Written testimony for National Committee on Vital and Health Statistics—Work Group on Computer-based Patient Record. Accessed 2007 at http://www.ncvhs.hhs.gov/990517t7.htm

Saba, V. K. (2007). *Clinical Care Classification (CCC) System Manual: A Guide to Nursing Documentation.* New York City: Springer.

Saba, V. K., & Zucherman, A. E. (1992). A new home health care classification method. *Caring, 11*(10):27–34.

Patient Care Data Set

Ozbolt, J. G. (1997). From minimum data to maximum impact: Using clinical data to strengthen patient care. *MD Computing, 14:*295–301. [Note: Adapted from *Advanced Practice Nursing Quarterly* (1996:1:62–69).]

Ozbolt, J. G. (1997). Multiple attributes for patient care data: Toward a multiaxial, combinatorial vocabulary. Accessed Sept 2007 at http://www.amia.org/pubs/symposia/D004400.pdf

Ozbolt, J. G. (1999). The patient care data set: Profile. Accessed Sept 2007 at http://www.ncvhs.hhs.gov/990518t3.pdf

Ozbolt, J. G., Fruchtnicht, J. N., & Hayden, J. R. (1994). Toward data standards for clinical nursing information. *Journal of the American Medical Information Association* 1:175–185.

Ozbolt, J. G., Russo, M., & Schultz, M. P. (1995). Validity and reliability of standard terms and codes for patient care data. In R. M. Gardner (Ed.). *Proceedings of the Nineteenth Annual Symposium on Computer Applications in Medical Care,* pp 37–41. Philadelphia: Hanley & Belfus.

Perioperative Nursing Data Set

Beyea, S. C. (2001). Data fields for intraoperative records using the perioperative nursing data set. *AORN Journal, 73*(5):952, 954.

Beyea, S. C. (2002). *Perioperative Nursing Data Set (PNDS),* ed. 2. Denver: AORN.

Dawes, B. S. (2001). Communicating nursing care and crossing language barriers. *AORN Journal, 73*(5):892, 894.

Junttilla, K., Lauri, S., Salantera, S., & Hupli, M. (2002). Initial validation of the perioperative nursing data set in Finland. *International Journal of Nursing Language and Classification, 13*(2):41–52.

Kleinbeck, S. (2007). PNDS—*Perioperative Nursing Data Set,* ed 2. Denver, CO: AORN.

Kleinbeck, S., & Dopp, A. (2005). The PNDS—a new language for documenting care. *AORN Journal, 82* (1):50–57. Accessed Sept 2007 at http://findarticles.com/p/articles/mi_m0FSL/is_1_82/ai_n15394472/pg_1

Chapter 4

The Planning Step: Creating the Plan of Care

■ **ANA STANDARD 3:** Outcomes identification: The registered nurse identifies expected outcomes for a plan individualized to the patient or situation.

■ **ANA STANDARD 4:** Planning: The registered nurse develops a plan that prescribes strategies and alternatives to attain expected outcomes. (American Nurses Association, 2004)

PLANNING: third step of the nursing process, during which goals/outcomes are determined and interventions chosen.

Once the etiology, signs, and symptoms previously identified are incorporated into a client diagnostic statement, proceed to the **PLANNING** step of the nursing process. Attention is now focused on the actions that are most appropriate to addressing the client's

PLAN OF CARE: written evidence of the second and third steps of the nursing process that identifies the client's needs, goals/ outcomes of care, and interventions for treating the need and achieving the outcomes.

needs. Begin to set priorities, establish goals, identify desired outcomes, and determine specific nursing interventions. These actions are documented as the **PLAN OF CARE**, which serves to guide the activities of all healthcare workers who are involved in the client's care. It is a priority that clients and/or significant others be included in the process of planning so they can contribute to, participate in, and take responsibility for their own care and the achievement of the desired outcomes and goals.

Setting Priorities for Client Care

Generally, the starting point for planning care is ranking the client's needs so that the nurse's attention and subsequent actions are properly focused. Although there are many ways of prioritizing client needs, a useful framework is one developed by Abraham Maslow (Fig. 4–1). In 1943 Maslow theorized that human behavior is motivated by a hierarchy arranged from basic to progressively higher-level needs (Maslow, 1970). According to Maslow, physiological needs are generally considered baseline survival needs because they must be met in order for life to continue. When these base-level needs (such as food, fluid, and oxygen) are not satisfied, it is difficult or impossible to focus on or attempt to meet higher-level needs (such as love, belonging, and self-esteem). Keep in mind that some clients with chronic problems may achieve higher-level needs even though baseline survival needs may be compromised. This is possible because as clients learn to function within physiological limitations, they may be able to refocus some energy on other needs.

Richard Kalish (1983) expanded and further subdivided the structure of Maslow's hierarchy, resulting in a more comprehensive description of the specific need categories. This expanded hierarchy can help you, as a nurse, to identify and prioritize client needs more effectively and to plan desired outcomes and the associated nursing interventions (Fig. 4–2). Failure to meet human needs at any level can significantly interfere with a client's overall progress. Clearly, it is difficult to use active listening techniques (meeting a higher-level client need for self-esteem) to explain

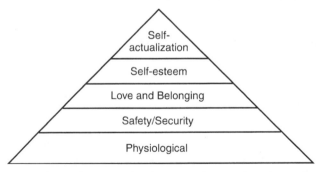

FIGURE 4–1. Maslow's hierarchy of needs. The pyramid of Maslow's hierarchy is a model that provides a view of human behavior in a structured way to determine physiological and psychological needs. Physiological needs appear at the bottom, or base, of the pyramid. Maslow's theory indicates that these lower-level needs must be met before higher-level needs (such as self-esteem) can be addressed. Knowledge of needs that must be met first can help the nurse determine the priorities of client care.

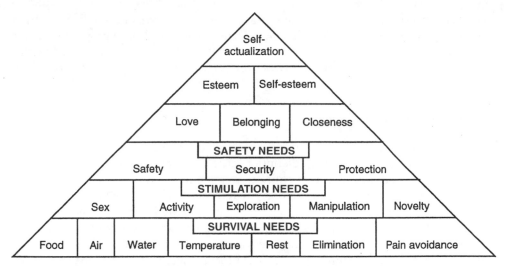

FIGURE 4–2. Kalish's expanded hierarchy. In an expansion of Maslow's model, Kalish restructured the first two levels of Maslow's pyramid (physiological and safety/security needs) into three levels and identified more specific subcategories. The base level is labeled survival, the second level stimulation, and the third level safety. The refinement of these subcategories can further assist the nurse in identifying the priorities for planning client care.

the importance of maintaining a patent airway to a client who is choking (a basic need of survival).

Once you have determined the priorities of care, the client's care needs can also be ranked according to a system (such as Maslow's hierarchy; see Appendix H) that can help you identify basic to higher-level actions/interventions. This is necessary because it is usually difficult to plan and provide care effectively when more than three to five nursing diagnoses exist at one time, depending on their complexity. By ranking the client's needs, you can proceed in a logical way to facilitate your client's recovery.

FOR EXAMPLE:

- Basic survival needs (i.e., air, water, and food) must be met before other needs can be considered. Sample diagnostic labels involving basic survival needs include ineffective Airway Clearance and imbalanced Nutrition: less than body requirements.
- Safety needs are next in order of importance. Nursing diagnostic labels relating to safety needs include risk for self-directed Violence, risk for Injury, and impaired Home Maintenance.
- Once these categories of needs are met, concerns regarding needs in the social, self-esteem, and self-actualization categories can be considered. Examples of nursing diagnostic labels related to these categories include impaired Social Interaction (a need for relationships with others), Self-Esteem [specify] (the need to feel good about oneself), and readiness for enhanced family Coping (a need for family and belonging).

GOALS: broad guidelines, divided into long-term and short-term goals, indicating the overall direction for movement as a result of the interventions of the healthcare team.

Setting priorities for client care is a complex and dynamic challenge. What you may perceive today as the number one client care need or appropriate nursing intervention could change tomorrow or, for that matter, within minutes. Practice Activity 4–1 gives you some experience in prioritizing client concerns based on levels of need.

ESTABLISHING CLIENT GOALS

Once you have prioritized client needs, establish the goals for treatment/discharge. The client care goal is a broad description of the general direction in which your client is expected to progress in response to treatment.

LONG-TERM GOALS: those goals that may not be achieved before discharge from care and that may require continued attention by client and/or others.

Goals may be either long-term or short-term. **LONG-TERM GOALS** indicate the overall direction or end result of care and may very well not be achieved before discharge from care. Examples of long-term goals are "Maintains control of blood glucose level" or "Uses resources/supports to prevent rehospitalization." **SHORT-TERM GOALS** are more specific guides for care and must usually be met before discharge or transfer to a less acute level of care, supervision, or support. Short-term goals may be building blocks for attaining long-term goals. Nursing care can be planned more accurately when the focus is directed on short-term goals. Depending on the client's anticipated length of stay, a short-term goal may be evaluated within a few hours or over the period of several therapeutic sessions. This period may be as long as several calendar weeks if the client is seen for counseling/therapy on a weekly or

SHORT-TERM GOALS: those goals that usually must be met before discharge or movement to a less acute level of care.

PRACTICE ACTIVITY 4–1
Prioritizing Nursing Diagnoses

Instructions: Prioritize the nursing diagnoses listed in each separate set by using the Maslow or Kalish model. Rank the four diagnoses by using 1 to designate the most basic or more immediate client need, and continue to 4, which designates the highest-level need (but least in priority). Review Appendix I as needed to compare definitions of these nursing diagnoses.

a. stress Urinary Incontinence
ineffective Sexuality Pattern
ineffective Airway Clearance
risk for impaired Skin Integrity

b. impaired Gas Exchange
deficient Knowledge
Hypothermia
risk for Infection

c. acute Pain
chronic low Self-Esteem
impaired physical Mobility
Social Isolation

monthly basis. Examples of short-term goals are "Learns to use blood glucose monitoring system" or "Uses two support agencies within the community to meet needs."

If the short-term goal is to be met within the nursing shift or visit during which it is identified, it is not necessary to write the goal on the plan of care; it can be noted in the progress note. If the goal is not accomplished by the end of the shift/visit, it is added to the plan of care with a new time frame so that those involved in the client's care can continue to work toward it.

IDENTIFYING DESIRED OUTCOMES

The next step in developing the plan of care is to determine specific **OUTCOMES**, which are defined as client responses that are achievable and desired by the client and that can be attained within a defined period, given the present situation and resources. Planned outcomes are the desired results of actions taken to achieve the broader goal; they are the measurable steps toward achieving the treatment/discharge criteria that were established earlier. They are also useful in monitoring nursing practice, advancing standards of care, and documenting nursing's contributions to healthcare.

OUTCOMES: measurable steps to achieve the goals of treatment and to meet discharge criteria; outcomes are results of actions undertaken to achieve a broader goal.

Because outcomes must be measurable, outcome statements need to:

- Be specific
- Be realistic
- Consider the client's circumstances and desires
- Indicate a definite time frame
- Provide measurable evaluation criteria for determining success or failure

Desired outcomes are written by listing items/behaviors that can be observed and monitored to determine whether a positive/acceptable outcome has been achieved within the indicated time frame (for example, "Verbalizes understanding of disease process and potential complications...."). A broad goal for a client with chronic obstructive pulmonary disease might be "Ventilation/oxygenation adequate to allow a functional lifestyle"; the integral outcomes needed for this goal to be achieved could include:

NURSING-SENSITIVE OUTCOMES: an individual, family, or community state, behavior, or perception that is measured along a continuum in response to a nursing intervention (Moorhead, Johnson, & Maas, 2004).

- Maintains patent airway with breath sounds clear....
- Demonstrates techniques to improve airway clearance with use of pursed-lip breathing, liquefying secretions, and/or nebulizer therapy....
- Initiates necessary lifestyle changes and participates in treatment regimen....

This itemized listing of outcomes serves as the evaluation tool, which is discussed more fully in Chapter 6.

Measurable action verbs are used to describe outcomes. Some examples of this type of verb include *discusses, states, identifies, administers, explains,* and *reports.* For instance, "Client will: Ambulate with use of cane." (Refer to Box 4–1 for additional examples.) Passive words are generally avoided. Specific time elements in outcome statements also provide measurable criteria, such as: "Client will: Ambulate with cane without assistance within 3 days." Some outcomes may be ongoing because they do not include a specific time frame other than discharge from care. Examples of these ongoing outcomes are statements such as "Client will: Maintain a patent airway" or "Client will: Be free of skin breakdown." It is your job to monitor each of these

BOX 4-1

Action Verbs Useful in Writing Measurable Outcomes

Using active rather than passive verbs provides a clearer method for determining client progress. The following are examples of action verbs that can be measured or observed:

List, Record, Name, State
Describe, Explain, Identify
Demonstrate, Use, Schedule
Differentiate, Compare, Relate
Design, Prepare, Formulate, Calculate
Select, Choose, Compare
Increase/Decrease, Stand, Walk, Participate

FOR EXAMPLE: The client will: *List* three things he understands about his diagnosis. The client will: *Walk* to the end of the hall and back three times today.

Below are a few samples of passive verbs. Notice that the actions described by the verbs are not measurable:

Understand, Feel, Learn, Know, Accept

FOR EXAMPLE: The client will: *Understand* his treatment plan. How will the nurse measure achievement and *know* that the client understands?

situations and document regularly any client findings. However, the situation may not be resolved until the client's condition/status changes or discharge has occurred.

When outcomes are written properly, they provide direction for planning and validating the choice of appropriate nursing interventions.

FOR EXAMPLE:

- Client will: Identify individual nutritional needs within two visits.
- Client will: Formulate a dietary plan based on these needs within three visits.

From these desired outcomes, the client's level of dietary knowledge should be assessed and individual client needs identified; in addition, client teaching information should be presented to provide the client with the tools necessary to formulate a dietary plan.

Interventions can be wide-ranging. The outcome statement "Client will: Verbalize acceptance of actual body image within 2 weeks" may call for interventions ranging from learning to recognize and express feelings about body changes, to developing a program of diet and exercise to promote weight loss, to instruction in the use of makeup, hairstyles, and ways of dressing that maximize figure assets/minimize perceived faults.

All outcomes should tell the reader specifically what the client is working on or doing. If the outcome does not seem to relate logically to the goals for treatment/discharge, it should be questioned. Is the outcome, in fact, a valid component of the plan of care? There is a simple and straightforward method of determining whether an outcome is written correctly: ask yourself if you could *observe* the client in the performance of the behavior indicated. If the answer is no, the desired, measurable outcome you have written should be modified. Below are several pairs of correctly and incorrectly written outcomes with notations to identify the desired elements. When you have finished looking them over, work through the exercises in Practice Activity 4–2.

1. **Incorrect:** "Understands insulin therapy within 48 hours."
   Rationale: This client outcome states a clear time line, but can you measure a client's "understanding"? This outcome needs a measurable action verb.
   Correct: "Demonstrates correct insulin administration techniques within 48 hours."
   or
   "Explains reasons for the steps of insulin administration within 48 hours."
   Rationale: These are well-written outcomes that are observable, measurable, and time-limited.

2. **Incorrect:** "Requires no reminders from staff regarding dietary restrictions within 3 days."
   Rationale: This outcome tells what the staff will do, not what the client will do.
   Correct: "Lists individual dietary restrictions and makes appropriate choices from daily menu within 3 days."
   Rationale: This outcome is observable and easy to document.

3. **Incorrect:** "Receives fewer restrictions for defying staff instructions during the next 2 weeks."
   Rationale: What is the definition of "fewer"? A specific number is clearer. What constitutes "defiance," and what is the client doing? According to this outcome, the client "receives" fewer restrictions, which places the client in an essentially passive role. Good measurable outcomes state what the client actively does.
   Correct: "Adheres to unit rules with decrease of infractions from the current rate of one per day to no more than two per week within 7 days."
   Rationale: Incidents of violation of unit rules are events that are observable, well documented, and easy to track. This outcome is also time-limited.

PRACTICE ACTIVITY 4–2
Identifying Correctly Stated Outcomes

Instructions: Identify which of the following outcome statements is written correctly or, if written incorrectly, state why it is incorrect. Modify those statements that are not correct.

1. Client will: List individual risk factors and appropriate interventions.
2. Client will: Identify four adaptive/protective measures for individual situation by discharge.
3. Client will: Understand behaviors, lifestyle changes necessary to promote physical safety within 72 hours.
4. Airway patent, aspiration prevented, ongoing.
5. Client will: Assume responsibility for own learning by participating in group discussions twice a day no later than 10/29/08.

As mentioned in Chapter 1, a classification of outcomes associated with both nursing diagnoses and nursing interventions has been researched and developed. The Nursing Outcomes Classification (NOC) was developed by a research team at the University of Iowa's College of Nursing. The current work, including the 330 nursing outcomes, is entitled *Iowa Outcomes Project: Nursing Outcomes Classification (NOC)*. A sample of NOC labels includes Abuse Cessation, Bone Healing, Cardiac Pump Effectiveness, Child Adaptation to Hospitalization, Dignified Life Closure, Hope, Leisure Participation, Oral Hygiene, Quality of Life, Social Support, and Will to Live.

NOC is designed to describe the client state following the implementation of nursing interventions. Whereas the nursing diagnosis Activity Intolerance is defined by NANDA-I as "Insufficient physiological or psychological energy to endure or complete required or desired daily activities," the nursing outcome of "Endurance: Capacity to sustain activity" describes the state (or status) the client would achieve after the implementation of selected nursing interventions (Box 4–2).

Each outcome has an associated list of indicators that are measured by a variety of specific 5-point Likert scales. Thus, the outcome is a variable state, with indicators used to measure the client response to the care provided by measuring the client's status before and after implementing the plan of care to provide a comparitive baseline. For example, Robert, with questioned Insomnia as possibly diagnosed in the last chapter, can have an outcome state of "Sleep," and indicators of "sleep quality" and "hours of sleep," which, measured on a 1–5 scale of *severely compromised* to *not compromised* and the indicator of inappropriate napping measured on a 1–5 scale of *severe* to *none*, reveal the extent of compromise. It is important to note that these are subjective measures because, for example, there is no specific definition for *severe* in relation to inappropriate napping.

BOX 4–2

Pairing NANDA-I With NOC Outcomes

In the preceding chapter, Robert had the possible nursing diagnosis of either Activity Intolerance or Insomnia. Possible nursing outcomes identified in NOC associated with these diagnoses include:

Nursing Diagnosis:	Activity Intolerance
Outcomes:	Endurance
	Mobility
	Pain: Disruptive Effects
Nursing Diagnosis:	Insomnia
Outcomes:	Comfort Level
	Rest
	Sleep

Moorhead, S., Johnson, M., & Maas, M. (Eds.). (2004). *Iowa Outcomes Project: Nursing Outcomes Classification (NOC)*, ed 3. St. Louis: Mosby.

Now revisit Robert, and review how another language of nursing, the Omaha System, assists in goal development. See Box 4–3 for the application of the Omaha System to Robert's NANDA-I Activity Intolerance nursing diagnosis and the Omaha System Problem: No. 37, Physical Activity.

BOX 4–3

Application of the Omaha System: Goal Development—Part I

NANDA-I Nursing Diagnosis: Activity Intolerance
Omaha System Problem: No. 37, Physical Activity
The Omaha System has a Problem Rating Scale for Outcomes. This scale rates three conceptual components: knowledge, behavior, and status. Each scale has a 5-point Likert scale. As with NOC, each concept has an associated scale. For example, Robert's knowledge of his level of physical activity can range in the following:

1. No knowledge
2. Minimal knowledge
3. Basic knowledge
4. Adequate knowledge
5. Superior knowledge

When Robert is questioned about his current medical condition and its effect on cardiac activity, you may find that Robert's knowledge of his physical activity is 1, No knowledge.

Robert's behavior is also rated using the following:

1. Not appropriate
2. Rarely appropriate
3. Inconsistently appropriate
4. Usually appropriate
5. Consistently appropriate

Robert's behavior toward physical activity is assessed at 3, inconsistently appropriate. The assessed data indicate that Robert does try to complete some activities, but data do not confirm that he participates in a routine exercise program.

Robert's status is rated using:

1. Extreme signs/symptoms
2. Severe signs/symptoms
3. Moderate signs/symptoms
4. Minimal signs/symptoms
5. No signs/symptoms

Further assessment data would be required to assess his level of independence. For this example, however, you could assign a rating of 3, moderate signs/symptoms, based on the decrease in physical activity due to current medical condition and past health history of limited physical activity and no routine exercise program.

Selecting Appropriate Nursing Interventions

NURSING INTERVENTIONS: any treatment based upon clinical judgment and knowledge, that a nurse performs to enhance patient/client outcomes. (McCloskey Dochterman & Bulechek, 2004, p 3).

NURSING INTERVENTIONS are prescriptions for behaviors, treatments, activities, or actions that assist the client in achieving the expected outcomes. Nursing interventions, like nursing diagnoses, are key elements of the knowledge of nursing; the scientific body of knowledge of nursing interventions, like that of nursing diagnoses, continues to grow as research supports the connection between actions and outcomes (McCloskey & Bulechek, 1994). In Chapter 3, the need to select the right nursing diagnosis was discussed. Selecting the appropriate nursing intervention so that your client can achieve the desired outcomes is as important as accuracy in diagnosing. It also is another method of individualizing your client's care. The Nursing Interventions Classification (NIC) (McCloskey Dochterman & Bulechek, 2004) contains a diverse list of 514 independent and collaborative intervention labels that nurses do on behalf of clients to provide both direct and indirect care such as Abuse Protection Support, Infant Care, Organ Procurement, Blood Products Administration, and Code Management.

Naturally your expectation is that the interventions you select will benefit the client and/or family/significant other in a predictable way. For optimum success, base your nursing interventions on the client's nursing diagnosis; the established goals and desired outcomes; your ability to successfully implement the intervention; the ability and willingness of the client to undergo the intervention; and the appropriateness of the intervention. In addition, interventions need to be age-/situation-appropriate and must promote identified client strengths, when possible.

FOR EXAMPLE:

- Discussion of fears may help to reduce the adult client's level of anxiety, whereas an infant may respond more positively to holding and cuddling.
- Although a walk down the hall to take a shower or bath may be desired by many new mothers, cultural beliefs may dictate that the new mother remain on bedrest for 7 days or refrain from a full shower for 2 to 4 weeks.
- Orange juice is a good choice for fluid replacement unless the client has open lesions on the oral mucosa, in which case mild fruit nectars would be preferred because acidic juices cause pain.
- Visualization to assist with stress or pain management may be the appropriate intervention for the client assessed as having creative abilities, but it may not be successful in clients who are concrete thinkers or have developmental delays.

You are accountable for being current and accurate in identifying nursing interventions. Therefore, you must be familiar with the body of scientific knowledge (rationale) that supports these interventions in addition to respecting your client's personal preferences and cultural/religious beliefs.

NURSING STANDARD: identified criterion against which nursing care is compared and evaluated; generally reflects the minimum level of nursing care.

NURSING STANDARDS and agency policy must also be considered in choosing specific interventions. For example, one nursing standard describes the minimum level for nursing care related to urinary catheterization. The standard also contains the policies and procedures required to meet that standard. The policy identifies the level of educational preparation that is required for the nurse to perform the procedure, and the procedural section lists the needed equipment, suggested method of performing the procedure, and documentation requirements.

The interventions you choose must be deliberate and purposeful; they must include information on independent nursing activities (such as frequency of monitoring activities/focused assessments, whether counseling and/or teaching will be provided, the need to suction an airway) as well as any collaborative activities necessary for the nurse to carry out orders from other healthcare providers (including consultation by and referral to other providers).

To be communicated accurately, nursing interventions, like nursing diagnoses and client care goals and outcomes, must be developed in the correct format, and they must be written specifically and clearly. The following items must be included when creating and documenting the intervention in the client's plan of care:

- The date when the intervention is written
- An action verb describing the activity to be performed
- Qualifiers of how, when (time/frequency), where, and amount
- Signature and/or initials of originating nurse

FOR EXAMPLE:

- 1/27 Assist as needed with self-care activities each a.m. AG
- 6/12 Record respiratory and pulse rates before, during, and after activity. BB
- 3/13 Inspect wound during each dressing change. MR
- 10/12 Measure intake and output hourly. SP

Note: Depending on agency policy, when the original plan of care is written or developed, a single date and signature are sufficient. As subsequent interventions are added, the entries should be dated and initialed or signed individually. Now, take a moment to complete Practice Activity 4–3 before proceeding to Box 4–4, which walks you through the first three steps of the nursing process. Client data are presented, and a client need is identified. Then a goal, outcomes, and appropriate interventions are chosen to address the need.

Having completed that activity, consider how you would identify appropriate interventions using the Omaha System. In Robert's case, the Omaha System first presented a problem based on the assessed signs/symptoms. When the planning of care was begun for Robert, the Outcome Rating Scales were used to assess knowledge, behavior, and status. The next portion of the Omaha System, the Intervention Scheme, is used to complete the plan of care (Box 4–5).

The three standardized nursing languages—NANDA-I, NIC, and NOC—have been combined into the NNN Alliance for a comprehensive classification of nursing. Having chosen the NANDA-I diagnosis of Activity Intolerance and the NOC of Endurance for Robert, determine the appropriate nursing intervention (NIC) to address Robert's problem (Box 4–6).

The Client Plan of Care

Planning care can save valuable time when the goals of care, client outcomes, and nursing interventions to achieve them are clearly identified and recorded for all to see. The documentation of the planning process is provided in the client's plan of care, which some nurses refer to as the "care plan." This plan of care is written to:

PRACTICE ACTIVITY 4–3
Identifying Correctly Stated Interventions

Instructions: Identify which of the following interventions are correctly stated, and rewrite those that are not.

1. Walk length of hall 2 ×/day with assistance from two staff members.

2. Force fluids.

3. Pericare after each BM.

4. Encourage deep-breathing exercises and cough q2h.

5. Reduce environmental stimuli.

6. Provide written handout for side effects of medications before discharge.

BOX 4–4

Application of the Nursing Process Through the Planning Step

Step I: Assessment

On 6/11/08 at 5:30 p.m., Michelle, a 14-year-old female (DOB 3/2/94), is admitted with compound multiple fractures of the right tibia and fibula and a mild concussion following a mountain-bike accident.

Assessment Data

Pain/Discomfort:
Subjective
Location: R lower leg, as well as general muscle aches, multiple skin abrasions, and right-sided headache.
Intensity (0–10): 9
Frequency: Since accident
Quality: Sharp stabbing and aching R leg (headache dull, throbs)
Duration: Constant
Radiation: Toes to knee

Precipitating factors: Movement
How relieved: Morphine sulfate in ED
Associated symptoms: Muscle spasms
Objective
Facial grimacing: Yes
Guarding affected area: Yes
Emotional response: Tearful
Narrowed focus: Yes

Step II: Need Identification

Based on this assessment (and additional data recorded in other sections of the Assessment Tool), using the diagnostic reasoning process and working with Appendix I, you choose the nursing diagnosis label acute Pain and write the plan of care.

6/11/08 6 p.m.

Client Diagnostic Statement: acute Pain related to movement of bone fragments R lower leg, soft tissue injury/edema, and use of external fixator as evidenced by verbal reports, guarding, muscle tension, narrowed focus, and tachycardia.

Step III: Planning

Goal: Pain-free or controlled
Outcomes:
Client will:

- Verbalize relief of pain within 5 minutes of IV bolus/45 minutes of PO administration of medication
- Use relaxation skills to reduce level of pain by 6/12, 9 a.m.
- Identify methods that provide relief by 6/12, 4 p.m.

Interventions:

- Maintain limb rest of R leg × 24 hours (6/12, 6 p.m.)
- Elevate lower leg with folded blanket
- Apply ice to area 20 minutes on/20 minutes off, as tolerated × 48 hours (6/13, 6 p.m.)
- Place cradle over foot of bed
- Document reports and characteristics of pain
- Medicate with morphine sulfate-PCA and bolus per peds protocol, advance to Vicodin 5 mg PO q4h, prn.
- Demonstrate/encourage use of progressive relaxation techniques, deep-breathing exercises, and visualization.
- Provide alternate comfort measures, position change, backrub. *BB*

(*Note:* Michelle has reported a dull headache associated with the concussion, but it is not a major concern for her at this time; some of the interventions noted previously will be effective in relieving this pain as well.)

BOX 4–5

Application of the Omaha System: Goal Development—Part II

NANDA-I Nursing Diagnosis: Activity Intolerance
Omaha System Problem: No. 37, Physical Activity
Knowledge Rating Scale =1
Behavior Rating Scale =3
Status Rating Scale =3
The Omaha System also has an Intervention Scheme. The scheme has 62 specific targets or objects of nursing actions. For example, Behavioral Modification No. 2 may be selected to assist Robert in his lack of an exercise program.
The scheme has four categories of intervention application:

1. Health teaching, guidance, and counseling
2. Treatments and procedures
3. Case management
4. Surveillance

Based on the assessed data and the outcome ratings on Robert's physical activity, the selection of the category Health teaching, Guidance, and Counseling is appropriate. The actual target for the nursing actions could be No. 2, Behavioral Modification, or No. 19, Exercises.

    Authors' Note: This is just an example of one possible application of the Omaha System. The Omaha System is a comprehensive nursing language system, and different problems, ratings, intervention categories, and targets can apply to Robert's case and would attest to your critical thinking skills.

BOX 4–6

Pairing NANDA-I With NIC Interventions

To continue the process of planning care for Robert, you have chosen the NANDA-I diagnosis of Activity Intolerance and the NOC (outcome) of Endurance, with the following indicators as measured by the 1–5 scale of "extremely compromised" to "not compromised."

1. Performance of usual routine
2. Activity
3. Blood oxygen level
and on the 1–5 scale of "severe" to "none"
4. Exhaustion

After reviewing NIC, you might choose Activity Therapy (*Definition:* Prescription of and assistance with specific physical, cognitive, social, and spiritual activities to increase the range, frequency, or duration of an individual's activity) and the following nursing activities:

Assist with regular physical activities (e.g., ambulation, transfers, turning, and personal care), as needed.
Assist client to identify deficits in activity level.
Assist to focus on what client can do rather than on deficits.
Assist client to identify meaningful activities.
Assist to choose activities consistent with physical, psychological, and social capabilities.
Assist to identify and obtain resources required for the desired activity.
Refer to community centers or activity programs.
Assist to obtain transportation to activities, as appropriate.

- *Provide continuity of care* from nurse to nurse, from one nursing shift to the next, or from one unit/care setting to another.
- *Enhance communication* as the written plan becomes a permanent part of the client record and supplies consistent information for each person who reads it.
- *Assist with determination of agency or unit staffing needs* as well as setting of priorities for the work schedule and individual client assignments.
- *Document the nursing process* by providing reminders of what needs to be charted and when evaluations should be done.
- *Serve as a teaching tool* by sharing nurses' expertise and fostering professional growth as nurses learn what interventions are successful.
- *Coordinate provision of care among disciplines,* maximizing effort and use of resources to enhance quality of care and client outcomes.

The term *healthcare* is not synonymous with medicine or nursing; it includes many professional disciplines, each of which has its own definite characteristics and independent, but overlapping, functions. The fields of nursing and medicine are closely related. The relationship includes the exchange of data, the sharing of ideas, and the development of a plan of care that reflects all data pertinent to the individual client/family/significant others. The same type of relationship extends to all healthcare disciplines in which the provider has contact with the client.

The implication of this relationship is seen in what is contained in the plan of care; it is more than simply a description of the actions initiated by medical orders (collaborative actions). It also includes a combination of nursing orders (independent actions) and describes in writing the coordination of care given by all health-related disciplines. The nurse becomes the person responsible for ensuring that all the different activities are coordinated. This is essential to the delivery of holistic, cost-effective healthcare that promotes optimal client recovery in a timely manner.

Exercises in planning care are assigned to students to enhance their mastery of the nursing process and application of related knowledge from other scientific disciplines. The need to identify and prepare for every possible client need in a given situation results in the creation of a case study, instead of the more abbreviated and

JCAHO: Joint Commission on Accreditation of Healthcare Organizations; surveying body that certifies clinical and organizational performance of an institution according to established guidelines.

succinct plan of care that is usually found in the nursing unit Kardex or computer database in most hospitals or in the case plans maintained in community-based and/or home health agencies. However, the length of time and amount of detail required to complete these case studies often cause nursing students to develop a negative attitude toward planning care. It is important to keep this activity in perspective because nurses need to plan care for their clients, sometimes on a daily basis for the inpatient and for weeks, months, or even years in advance for community-based and/or home health clients. Mastery of the skills of planning care will allow you to complete this activity in a timely fashion as you gain experience.

The plan of care is primarily a communication tool that directs the client's care. Requirements of outside agencies (for example, **JCAHO**, CMS [Medicare and Medicaid] and private insurance companies) stipulate that the nurse is responsible for the planning of client care and that the plan is to be documented in the client's record. The plan of care is a permanent part of the client's record for these reasons and because it contains the outline for the care provided.

Discharge Planning

As you plan for the client's current needs, you must also consider future needs, especially eventual discharge from the healthcare facility. Discharge planning begins when the client enters the healthcare setting. It is crucial to take into account the anticipated discharge destination (e.g., home, rehabilitation center, assisted living, or skilled nursing facility). You are responsible for planning continuity of care between nursing personnel, between services within the care setting, and between the care setting and the community. You may also be responsible for initiating/cooperating in referrals to other community services and providing needed direction for client/family members who are learning to facilitate recovery and promote wellness.

Documenting the Plan of Care

CLINICAL PATHWAYS: a type of abbreviated plan of care; they provide outcome-based guidelines for goal achievement within a designated length of stay (see Appendix E).

CONCEPT/MIND MAPPING: a care planning technique that uses a graphic representation to illustrate the interconnections among all components of client care.

The plan of care may be recorded on a single page or on multiple pages, which may include one page for each diagnostic statement for a particular client. The page(s) may be kept in a folder (Kardex) at the nursing station, in the client's chart, or at the bedside to communicate and provide direction on a daily basis.

The format for documenting the plan of care is determined by agency policy. Student plans of care (case studies) are developed individually and are very detailed. Practicing professionals might use a computer with a plan of care database, standardized care plan forms, or **CLINICAL PATHWAYS** (e.g., critical pathway, care map, etc.). The plan of care must reflect the basic nursing standards of care; personal client data, nonroutine care, and qualifiers such as time or amount are added, as appropriate.

FOR EXAMPLE:

Measure intake and output [insert frequency]
Increase oral fluids [insert amount and frequency]
Medicate with [insert name of medication, dose, and frequency] for [insert reason]
Weigh with bedscale [insert time, frequency]

Some computerized systems for plans of care generate an updated plan at the beginning of each shift. The care provided during the new shift is recorded directly in the on-line plan of care throughout that shift. This method serves two purposes: (1) it documents the planning and implementation steps of the nursing process, and (2) it continuously updates the plan of care and the client's record. Other formats require the nurse to document updates to the plan of care through a notation on the Kardex or in the progress or nursing notes.

The plan of care enables visualization of the nursing process. As such, it is preserved as part of the client's permanent record. Therefore, all entries need to be dated and initialed or signed. Key words should be used instead of complete sentences, and only agency-approved abbreviations/symbols should be included (see end pages).

FOR EXAMPLE:

- 8/15 Routine urinary catheter care q (every) shift. RE
- 9/2 NPO (nothing by mouth) after 6 a.m., 9/3. PR
- 3/7 Maintain subarachnoid bolt per protocol. MT

Regardless of the format used, the plan of care contains identifying client data (including medical diagnosis), client diagnostic statements, goals/outcomes, and interventions; it also provides space for the healthcare provider to record the status of the outcomes (i.e., achieved, revised, or deleted) as shown in Figure 4–3. After reviewing the figure, complete Practice Activity 4–4.

Client: Donald Age: 46 DOB: 2/4/62 Gender: M   Admission 11/12/08 3:40 Dx: Acute Alcoholism/Depression

Date	Client Diagnostic Statement	Goal	Intervention	Outcomes	Status
11/12	Coping, ineffective, related to situational crisis of unemployment, personal vulnerability evidenced by reported inability to cope, use of alcohol, insomnia, and diminished problem-solving.	short term: Managing own situation effectively long term: Expresses sense of self-worth. Maintains sobriety.	1. Assess level of anxiety and Donald's perception of situation 2. Note verbal/nonverbal behaviors of anxiety 3. Look in q 2 hr and PRN 4. Encourage verbalization, expression of feelings of denial, depression/anger 5. Discuss normalcy of these feelings 6. Identify current coping mechanisms 7. Note effectiveness/ need for change 8. Discuss/refer to resources: social worker, alcohol counselor, support group, AA	Verbalizes awarenes of sources of anxiety (1000 11/14) Demonstrates congruency between feelings/behavior (1000 11/15) Demonstrates initial problem-solving skills (1000 11/15) Identifies options and resources available for assistance (1000 11/16) R. Smith, RN	Achieved 11/14 1030 R.S. Achieved 11/15 1000 P.D. Achieved 11/15 1000 P.D.

FIGURE 4–3. Sample documentation of a plan of care.

Instructions: Record the plan of care information from Box 4–4 on pages 88–89 using the following documentation format.

Date	Cleint Diagnostic Statement	Goal	Interventions	Outcomes	Status

Validating the Plan of Care

Before the plan of care is implemented, it should be reviewed to ensure that:

- It is based on accepted nursing practice, reflecting knowledge of scientific principles, nursing standards of care, and agency policies.
- It provides for the safety of the client by ensuring that the care provided will do no harm.
- The client diagnostic statements are supported by the client data.
- The goals and outcomes are measurable/observable and can be achieved.
- The interventions can benefit the client/family/significant others in a predictable way in achieving the identified outcomes and that they are arranged in a logical sequence.
- It demonstrates individualized client care by reflecting the concerns of the client and significant others as well as their physical, psychosocial, and cultural needs and capabilities.

Professional Concerns Related to the Plan of Care

Professional concerns associated with the identification of client needs in the construction of the plan of care include the following:

- What is the nurse's responsibility, once a nursing diagnosis is made, if the client is discharged from care before all short-term outcomes are met or problems are resolved?
- Who is responsible for follow-through in providing and evaluating care once the client has been discharged?
- Who is responsible for monitoring client progress toward long-term outcomes?
- Should this information be shared with the client's admitting/primary healthcare provider or office nurse?
- Is the nurse who has made a nursing diagnosis responsible for follow-through to its resolution?

On a national level, these questions are unresolved, and client outcomes may remain unmet. Ethically, it is up to the nursing community and the healthcare industry to formulate policies that promote optimal client recovery and health maintenance. It is important to remember that the plan of care is not developed in a vacuum but rather with input from the client and possibly the significant other/family. Therefore these individuals should be included in determining how to deal with unresolved needs. (Further discussion regarding termination of care is provided in Chapter 6.)

Putting It All Together

Practice Activity 4–5 presents the back page of the interactive plan-of-care worksheet described and used in Chapter 3. The information included on the worksheet and in the TIME OUT sections should give you another view of the steps of the nursing process described in this chapter. Return to Practice Activity 3–1 in Chapter 3 and see what portion of the information you can include based on the subjective and objective data of your client Robert, diagnosed with Activity

PRACTICE ACTIVITY 4–5
Interactive Care Plan Worksheet

Instructions: Record the plan of care information from Box 4–4 using the following documentation format.

PLANNING

Desired Outcome and Client Criteria: The Client will:

TIME OUT! The desired outcome must meet criteria to be accurate. The outcome must be specific, realistic, and measurable, and include a time frame for completion. Does the action verb describe the client's behavior to be evaluated? Can the outcome be used in the evaluation step of the nursing process to measure the client's response to the nursing interventions listed below?

Interventions	Rationale for Selected Intervention and References

EVALUATION

TIME OUT! Do your interventions assist the client in achieving outcomes? Do your interventions address further monitoring of the client's response to your interventions and to the achievement of the desired outcome? Are qualifiers: **when, how, amount, time,** and **frequency** used? Is the focus of the action's verb on the nurse's actions and not on the client? Do your rationales provide sufficient reason and directions?

What was your client's response to the interventions?

Was the desired outcome achieved? ☐ Yes ☐ No   If no, what revisions to either the desired outcome or interventions would you make?

DOCUMENTATION

Documentation Focus: Now that you have completed the evaluation, the next step is to document your care and the client's response. Use the areas below to enter your progress note information.

Reassessment Data:

Interventions Implemented:

Client's Response:

INSTRUCTOR'S COMMENTS:

Intolerance. What desired outcome would you identify for Robert? The TIME OUT sections will give you evaluation criteria to ensure that Robert's outcome statement is written correctly.

A Complementary Approach—Concept or Mind Mapping

Some educators (Mueller, Johnston & Bligh, 2002) have been concerned that their students spend so much time and energy focusing on filling the columns of traditional clinical care plans that a holistic view of the client never develops. These educators have addressed this concern by adding a new technique or learning tool, called "mind mapping," to the planning step. In this process, as the student analyzes the client's assessment data and identifies appropriate nursing diagnoses, a visual picture is formed, with the client at the center. The nurse no longer focuses on a single client need but considers how each need interacts with other identified needs. The left brain is useful in linear problem–based thinking; the visualization process promotes right-brain thinking and assists the student in recognizing relationships or interconnections between the data sets (signs and symptoms), the client's needs (nursing diagnoses), desired outcomes, and nursing actions, thus creating a "whole" picture of the client. The focus is always on the client rather than on a disease process. The client data, outcomes, nursing diagnoses, and interventions, along with evaluation data and collaborative treatments, are of equal importance and not subsumed under one another.

Mind or concept mapping facilitates the use of different learning styles. It also encourages students to maintain a holistic view of the client, with the client encouraged to participate in the care-planning process by sharing his or her own expectations, and students validate their findings. This supports the client's independence and enhances adherence to the plan, thus maximizing desired outcomes. Proponents believe that by combining concept mapping with care planning, students develop enhanced thinking skills; that is, critical, whole-brain thinking and client-centered thinking, which is so necessary for effective client care (Fig. 4–4). Regardless of the technique used (traditional clinical care plans or concept maps), an understanding of the nursing process remains essential if competent client care is to be provided.

Summary

Healthcare providers have a responsibility to plan care with the client and family, whether the desired outcome is an optimal state of wellness or a dignified death. Planning care by setting goals, determining outcomes, and choosing appropriate interventions is essential to the delivery of quality nursing care. These nursing activities make up the planning step of the nursing process, and they are documented in the plan of care for a particular client. As a part of the client's permanent record, the plan of care not only provides a means for the nurse who is actively caring for the client to be aware of the needs (nursing diagnoses), goals, and actions to be taken; it also substantiates the plan of care for third-party payers as well as for the accreditation process and legal review.

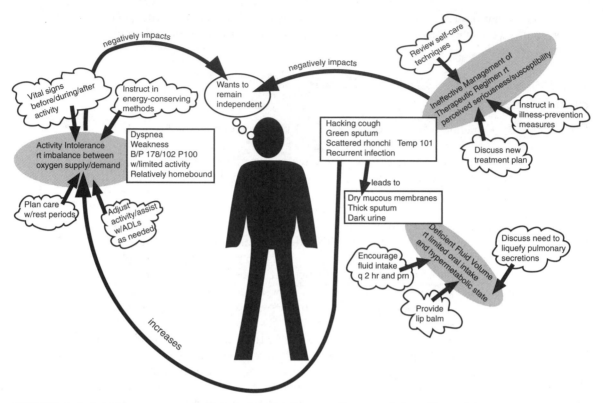

FIGURE 4–4. Initial concept map for Robert. Primary diagnosis: Recurrent bilateral lower lobe pneumonia.

This chapter introduced you to how the work of the Iowa Outcomes and Interventions Projects as well as the Omaha System can be used to assist you in providing a research-based approach to designing a plan of care. Both systems provide the structure, terms, and definitions to assist you in planning client care in any healthcare environment. In Chapter 6, The Evaluation Step: Determining Whether Desired Outcomes Have Been Met, you will see how helpful the standardized languages and accompanying rating and measurement scale are in evaluating the effectiveness of your plan of care.

Now, return to the third and fourth standards of the ANA Standard of Practice, and review the measurement criteria necessary to achieve and ensure compliance with each standard. The knowledge and skill required to meet the criteria listed in Box 4–7 have been described in this chapter.

The next chapter provides information on the fourth step of the nursing process, **implementation.** You will see how the plan of care can be implemented. You will learn what mechanisms help to prioritize the nursing interventions that were selected during the **planning** step. Finally, you will practice effective communication methods to help ensure the required continuity of care described in the client plan of care.

BOX 4–7

Measurement Criteria for ANA Standards 3 and 4

ANA Standard 3: Outcomes identification: The registered nurse identifies expected outcomes individualized to the client.

1. Involves the patient, family, and other healthcare providers in formulating expected outcomes when possible and appropriate.
2. Derives culturally appropriate expected outcomes from the diagnoses.
3. Considers associated risks, benefits, costs, current scientific evidence, and clinical expertise when formulating expected outcomes.
4. Defines expected outcomes in terms of the patient, patient values, ethical considerations, environment, or situation with such considerations as associated risks, benefits and costs, and current scientific evidence.
5. Includes a time estimate for attainment of expected outcomes.
6. Develops expected outcomes that provide direction for continuity of care.
7. Modifies expected outcomes based on changes in the status of the patient or evaluation of the situation.
8. Documents expected outcomes as measurable goals.

ANA Standard 4: Planning: The registered nurse develops a plan that prescribes strategies and alternatives to attain expected outcomes.

1. Develops an individualized plan considering patient characteristics or the situation (e.g., age and culturally appropriate, environmentally sensitive).
2. Develops the plan in conjunction with the patient, family, and others, as appropriate.
3. Includes strategies within the plan that address each of the identified diagnoses or issues, which may include strategies for promotion and restoration of health and prevention of illness, injury, and disease.
4. Provides for continuity within the plan.
5. Incorporates an implementation pathway or timeline within the plan.
6. Establishes the plan priorities with the patient, family, and others, as appropriate.
7. Utilizes the plan to provide direction to other members of the healthcare team.
8. Defines the plan to reflect current statutes, rules and regulations, and standards.
9. Integrates current trends and research affecting care in the planning process.
10. Considers the economic impact of the plan.
11. Uses standardized language or recognized terminology to document the plan.

1. List three reasons why the plan of care is important:

    a. _____

    b. _____

    c. _____

2. Briefly explain why setting priorities is necessary:

    _____

3. What is the difference between a goal and an outcome?

    _____

4. Identify five important components of client outcomes:

    a. _____

    b. _____

    c. _____

    d. _____

    e. _____

5. List four types of information that nursing interventions must contain:

    a. _____

    b. _____

    c. _____

    d. _____

6. Explain the difference between a measurable and a nonmeasurable verb, and give an example of each:

    _____

7. When does discharge planning begin?

    _____

8. How is the plan of care documented?

    _____

9. In the following vignette, identify two additional needs (human responses of concern) facing Michelle; then set a goal with one outcome and two interventions for each need.

    _____

VIGNETTE: Michelle, the 14-year-old female with compound fractures of the right lower leg and a mild concussion, has problems in addition to acute pain, as was previously discussed. Her wound was contaminated by dirt, and she had significant blood loss before paramedics arrived. Although the wound was flushed with sterile saline and antibiotic solution before being packed and dressed, a cast was not applied because of tissue swelling and concerns about the wound and bone. Instead, an external fixation device (a metal frame with pins extending through the skin and bone) is currently being used for immobilization of the tibia and fibula. The device is too heavy and awkward for Michelle to move without causing increased pain, and she is to remain on bedrest for 24 hours. In addition, IV antibiotics are to be administered every 4 hours.

1. Need:
   Goal:
   Outcome:
   Interventions:
   1.
   2.
2. Need:
   Goal:
   Outcome:
   Interventions:
   1.
   2.

BIBLIOGRAPHY

Bulechek, G. M., & McCloskey, J. C. (1989). Nursing interventions: Treatments for potential diagnoses. In R. M. Carrol-Johnson (Ed.). *Proceedings of Eighth Conference, North American Nursing Diagnosis Association.* Philadelphia: J. B. Lippincott.

Kalish, R. (1983). *The Psychology of Human Behavior,* ed 5. Monterey, CA: Brooks/Cole.

Martin K. S. (2005). *The Omaha System: A Key to Practice, Documentation, and Information Management,* ed 2. St. Louis: Elsevier.

Maslow, A. H. (1970). *Motivation and Personality,* ed 2. New York: Harper & Row.

McCloskey, J. C., & Bulechek, G. M. (1994). Standardizing the language of nursing treatments: An overview of the issues. *Nursing Outlook, 42*(10):56–63.

McCloskey Dochterman, J., & Bulechek, G. M. (Eds.). (2004). *Nursing Interventions Classification (NIC),* ed 4. St. Louis: Mosby.

Moorhead, S., Johnson, M., & Maas, M. (Eds.). (2004). *Iowa Outcomes Project: Nursing Outcomes Classification (NOC),* ed 3. St. Louis: Mosby.

Mueller, A, Johnston, M. & Bligh, D. (2002). Joining mind mapping and care planning to enhance student critical thinking and achieve holistic nursing care. *Nursing Diagnosis 13*(1):24–27.

SUGGESTED READINGS

Nursing Outcomes

Booten, D., & Naylor, M. D. (1995). Nurse's effect on changing patient outcomes. *Image: Journal of Nursing Scholarship, 27*:95–99.

Cox, R. A. (1998). Implementing nursing sensitive outcomes into care planning at a long-term facility. *Journal of Nursing Care Quality,* *12*(5):41–51.

Denehey, J. (1998). Integrating nursing outcomes classification into education. *Journal of Nursing Care Quality,* *12*(5):73–83.

Hajewski, C., Maupin, J. M., Rapp, D. A., & Pappas, J. (1998). Implementation and evaluation of Nursing Outcomes Classification in a patient education plan. *Journal of Nursing Care Quality,* *12*(5):30–40.

Head, B., et al. (1997). Outcomes for home and community nursing in integrated delivery systems. *Caring,* *16*(1):50–56.

Johnson, M., & Maas, M. (1998). The Nursing Outcomes Classification. *Journal of Nursing Care Quality,* *12*(5):9–20.

Lang, N. M., & Marek, K. D. (1990). The classification of patient outcomes. *Journal of Professional Nursing,* *6*(3):158–163.

Maas, M., et al. (1996). Classifying nursing-sensitive outcomes. *Image: Journal of Nursing Scholarship,* *28*:295–301.

Moorhead, S., Clarke, M., Willitis, M., & Tomsha, K. A. (1998). Nursing Outcomes Classification implementation projects across care continuum. *Journal of Nursing Care Quality,* *12*(5):51–63.

Pierce, S. L. (1997). Nurse-sensitive health care outcomes in acute care settings: An integrative analysis of the literature. *Journal of Nursing Care Quality,* *11*(4):60–72.

Prophet, C. M., & Delaney, C. W. (1998). Nursing Outcomes Classification: Implications for nursing information systems and the computer-based patient record. *Journal of Nursing Care Quality,* *12*(5):21–29.

Timm, J. A., & Behrenbech, J. G. (1998). Implementing the Nursing Outcomes Classification in clinical information system in a tertiary care setting. *Journal of Nursing Care Quality,* *12*(5):65–72.

Authors' Note: For an extensive listing of NOC-related publications, see Appendix H in Moorhead, S., Johnson, M., & Maas, M. (Eds.). (2004). *Iowa Outcomes Project: Nursing Outcomes Classification (NOC),* ed 3. St. Louis: Mosby.

Nursing Interventions

Daley, J., et al. (1995). Use of standardized nursing diagnoses and interventions in long-term care. *Journal of Gerontological Nursing,* *21*(8):29–36.

McCloskey, J. C., & Bulechek, G. M. (1993). The NIC taxonomy structure: Iowa Intervention Project. *Image: Journal of Nursing Scholarship,* *25*:178–192. St. Louis: Mosby.

Wakefield, B., et al. (1995). Nursing Interventions Classification: A standardized language for nursing care. *Journal of Health Care Quality,* *17*:26–33.

Authors' Note: For an extensive listing of NIC-related publications, see Appendix E in McCloskey Dochterman, J., & Bulechek, G. M. (Eds.). (2004). *Iowa Interventions Project: Nursing Interventions Classification (NIC),* ed 4. St. Louis: Mosby.

Nursing Language

Delaney, C., et al. (1992). Standardized nursing language for health care information systems. *Journal of Medical Systems,* *16*:145–159.

McCloskey, J. C., & Bulechek, G. M. (1994). Standardizing the language of nursing treatments: An overview of the issues. *Nursing Outlook,* *42*(10):56–63.

Werley, H., & Lang, N. (Eds.). (1988). *Identification of Nursing Minimum Data Set.* New York: Springer.

Chapter 5

The Implementation Step: Putting the Plan of Care Into Action

Identifying Caregiving Priorities

Ethical and Legal Concerns

Delivering Nursing Care

Ongoing Data Collection

Documentation

Verbal Communication With the Healthcare Team

Summary

■ **ANA STANDARD 5:** Implementation: The registered nurse implements the identified plan.

At this point in the nursing process, you are ready to perform the interventions and activities recorded in the client's plan of care. In order to **IMPLEMENT** this plan in a timely and cost-effective manner, first identify the priorities for providing client care. Then, as care is provided, monitor and document the client's response to each of the interventions and communicate this information to other healthcare providers as appropriate. Then, using the data, evaluate and revise the plan of care in the following step of the nursing process (see Chapter 6).

IMPLEMENTATION: fourth step of nursing process, in which the plan of care is put into action; performing identified interventions/ activities.

Identifying Caregiving Priorities

Regardless of how well a plan of care has been constructed, it cannot predict everything that will occur with a particular client on a daily basis. Your individual knowledge, expertise, and recognition of agency routines allow you the flexibility

Client	7	8	9	10	11	12	1	2	3	Comments
Rbt		Vital signs Chair	Med	Bed bath	IV	V.S. Chair	Med	I & O		

FIGURE 5–1. Sample worksheet for the 7 a.m. to 3 p.m. shift. While listening to the change-of-shift report, you review the plan of care and begin to plan how you will implement specific interventions. You notice that Robert is to eat meals sitting up in a chair; therefore, he should be helped out of bed before the meal trays arrive on the unit. You identify times for medications, times for expected change of the IV bottle, and the routine times for calculating the intake and output for the shift. In addition, you are aware that Robert's family usually visits at lunchtime, so you schedule hygiene needs appropriately while allowing Robert rest periods between activities.

necessary to adapt to the changing needs of the client. Paying close attention to the change-of-shift report, you will get the first clues where to begin. On a worksheet, such as the one in Figure 5–1, or a form supplied by the agency, you record specific information, interventions, and activities that are sequential or time-related.

Review the plan of care for outcomes that are to be evaluated during the shift and for routine procedures/treatments and medication administration. Now complete Practice Activity 5–1.

PRACTICE ACTIVITY 5–1
Setting Your Work Schedule for Implementing the Plan of Care

VIGNETTE: Michelle incurred a compound fracture of the right lower leg 2 days ago. In reviewing the plan of care, you note the following:
- Assist with bed bath
- Calculate input and output every 8 hours (2 p.m.)
- Change dressing twice a day and prn (9 a.m.)
- Assess vital signs every 4 hours (8 a.m., 12 noon)
- Monitor circulation/nerve function R lower leg every 4 hours (8 a.m., 12 noon) and prn
- IV medications (8 a.m., 2 p.m.)
- Up in chair with meals (7:30 a.m., 12 noon)
- Walk in halls 3 times a day after instructed in crutch walking

1. Organize the above interventions and activities on the worksheet below:

   Worksheet

Pt.	7	8	9	10	11	12	1	2	3	Comments

2. During nursing rounds, just after the change-of-shift report on 6/13, you find that Michelle is crying, and she reports sudden throbbing pain in her right lower leg. How will this affect your work plan? _____
   _____

After completion of the shift report, a baseline assessment of each client can provide clues about general physical status, equipment/supply needs, and safety concerns (e.g., patency of invasive lines [catheters/tubes] and intravenous [IV] flow rate). At this time, you may recognize a change in the significance or severity of a client need that could affect the plan of care.

FOR EXAMPLE: Robert, who is being treated for pneumonia, appears dyspneic at 7:30 a.m. You now need to do a more thorough focused assessment to determine his immediate needs. This could include obtaining pulse oximetry/arterial blood gases (ABGs) and restarting supplemental oxygen. In addition, you may decide against getting Robert up in a chair to eat his breakfast. Thus, interventions previously identified are not appropriate at this time, and new or alternate interventions are needed.

This is also the time to review the plan of care with the client/significant other to schedule activities and verify the client's responsibilities.

FOR EXAMPLE: Donald, admitted 48 hours ago for depression and alcohol withdrawal, displays coarse tremors of his hands and an unsteady gait and requires assistance with self-care. It is 7:30 a.m., and breakfast trays have arrived. He is required to attend the community meeting at 8:15 a.m. before proceeding to individually prescribed activities. He is ambivalent about his morning care but, in reviewing the scheduled activities, he decides that he will postpone his shower until his 10:30 a.m. break.

Ethical and Legal Concerns

Legal and ethical concerns related to the interventions need to be considered. The wishes of the client and family/significant others regarding what is being done need to be discussed and respected.

FOR EXAMPLE: Robert has decided that if he should suffer respiratory failure, he is not to be placed on a mechanical ventilator. This does not negate the need for intervention when you notice that he is developing problems. You still need to act promptly to prevent or limit further deterioration. Therefore, in addition to providing oxygen and assessing breath sounds and airway patency, you could elevate the head of Robert's bed, encourage Robert to deep-breathe and cough regularly, and notify other healthcare providers (e.g., physician and respiratory therapist) as appropriate, as well as Robert's significant other/contact person according to agency policy.

Consider the legal and ethical concerns of Robert's decision, and work through Practice Activity 5–2 before continuing with the next section. It is beyond the scope of this text to discuss these critical issues in detail. To assist you in your studies, an extensive bibliography on advance directives, ethics, and legal issues is included in the Suggested Readings. Also see Appendix A, Code for Nurses.

Delivering Nursing Care

Interventions may be composed of many activities, ranging from simple tasks to complex procedures. These activities may require direct "hands-on" care (such as complete bed bath), or they may merely require that the healthcare provider assist a client by setting up a basin of water and washing his back. Other frequent activities

PRACTICE ACTIVITY 5-2
Legal and Ethical Concerns of Care

As noted, Robert had completed a form directing healthcare providers to withhold advanced life-support measures, including the use of a mechanical ventilator.

1. Have you and your family members completed advance directives stating specific healthcare desires?

   If not, why?

   _____

2. As a nurse, how do you feel about adhering to advance directives as stipulated by an elderly client?

   _____

   For a premature infant as stipulated by the parents?

   _____

3. Review the Code of Ethics for Nurses (see Appendix A), and choose two principles you believe may address your responsibility to clients/guardians in regard to their decisions limiting care.

   _____

   _____

include instructing a client and/or significant other regarding the management of care and then supervising these efforts. The client and/or significant other may need to be counseled regarding psychosocial concerns, treatment regimens, or alternative ways to manage healthcare needs. Throughout these activities, you also monitor the client and such resources as diagnostic studies and/or progress reports from other healthcare providers for changes in health status/development of complications. Before implementing the interventions listed in the plan of care, you need to be sure that you:

- **Understand the reason for doing the intervention, its expected effect, and any associated potential hazards.** Without this knowledge, the nurse cannot be sure that the intervention will be beneficial. In addition, it will be difficult to determine if the desired effect is being achieved or if adaptations are required to provide for specific client needs/safety concerns.

   FOR EXAMPLE: You realize that a pulse oximetry/ABG study will provide information about Robert's current oxygenation status/needs and that he requires supplemental oxygen. That means you will implement these interventions in a slightly different sequence; that is, the diagnostic study (pulse oximetry/ABG) should be obtained before the supplemental oxygen is begun so that test results are not affected by the additional oxygen.

- **Provide an environment conducive to carrying out the planned interventions.** What is happening in the environment (e.g., noise, temperature, activities) is known to affect the client's physical and psychological self.

FOR EXAMPLE: Exposing Robert for a bed bath when the room is cold can cause him physical discomfort and affect his psychological response. *Or* Michelle has difficulty focusing on your instructions for administering medications when her roommate's TV is loud and visitors are talking loudly.

- **Consider which interventions can be combined to allow you to accomplish activities within your time constraints.** In some cases, shortcuts may be chosen or activities combined, which is acceptable as long as consideration is given to the successful accomplishment of the outcome.

FOR EXAMPLE: While administering Serax to Donald at 8 a.m., you can review the drug's actions, side effects, and adverse reactions. *Or* while assisting Sally with her sitz bath, you may choose to discuss her concerns about caring for herself and the new babies once she has been discharged.

As noted in Box 5–1, one simple intervention, such as providing a bedpan for a client, actually encompasses multiple nursing activities that, when listed individually, may appear to take considerable time and energy to perform. However, by prioritizing interventions and sequencing related activities, you can accomplish these tasks quickly.

Ongoing Data Collection

Once you have formulated the plan of care and put it into action, monitor the client to collect additional data. As you talk to the client, note changes in tone of voice and expression; when you reposition the client or provide a back rub, be aware of such abnormalities as a reddened area on the coccyx. All these data need to be noted and their meaning validated. This information will be used in decision making regarding the need for new goals, outcomes, and interventions and in reprioritizing the plan of care during the evaluation process.

DOCUMENTATION

It is legally required that professionals in all healthcare settings document nursing observations, the care provided, and the client's response. This record serves as a communication tool and a resource to aid in determining the effectiveness of care and to assist in setting priorities for ongoing care. In order to simplify record keeping and to promote timely and accurate charting, many agencies use flow sheets to document routine activities, monitoring, and ongoing client care (Fig. 5–2). Flow sheets reduce the need for writing detailed progress notes. Instead, only variations from the recorded baseline and any exceptions requiring additional explanation are written in the progress note. Further discussion about documentation and the use of progress notes is presented in Chapter 7.

VERBAL COMMUNICATION WITH THE HEALTHCARE TEAM

In addition to the written record, client information is shared verbally with other healthcare providers. Whether reporting to another nurse, reviewing with a physician, or discussing with professionals providing other resources (e.g., social worker, dietitian, or physical therapist), the manner in which information is conveyed, as well as the content itself, can affect the way in which this information is heard. This, in turn,

BOX 5–1

Simple Isn't Simple

Even "simple" nursing tasks require coordination and critical thinking—A seemingly simple task such as helping a client to perform the activity of elimination, whether by providing a bedpan or assistance to the commode, requires a complex series of nursing actions, judgments, and professional knowledge in order to provide optimal client care. The nurse:

Assesses:

Client's level of consciousness, ability to perform steps of activity

Mood and self-image in relation to dependence with this bodily function

Range of motion, strength, and any pain with movement

Respiratory pattern and rate, breath sounds, and ease of breathing before/during activity

Skin color, temperature, suppleness, presence of dermal irritation

Comfort level with passage of urine/stool

Performs actions including:

Promotion of self-esteem by acceptance of client in dependent position

Demonstrating proper technique, including disposal of waste material

Obtaining and processing necessary specimens for laboratory studies using correct procedure

Modeling good handwashing technique throughout activity

Providing skin/perineal care

Discussing disease process and affects on the client/elimination process

Identifying possible comfort measures for client

Reviewing ways to maintain or achieve normal functioning

Instructing client in symptoms to watch for and appropriate response/actions

Notes:

Urine color, amount, odor, and by-products (e.g., mucus, blood, sediment)

Stool color, amount, consistency, odor, and by-products (e.g., mucus, undigested food, blood)

Determines:

Does urine/stool assessment reveal effects of medications (e.g., for urine—Lasix, Pyridium, aminoglycosides; for stool—antibiotics, barium sulfate, narcotics), fluid/food intake (including rate/type of enteral feeding), disease process (e.g., for urine—diabetes, dehydration, renal failure; for stool—cholelithiasis, irritable bowel syndrome, peptic ulcer), or presence of infection; or decreased activity

What additional actions are indicated—does the physician/healthcare provider need to be notified, are changes required in current plan of care

Evaluates:

Client's understanding of teaching provided

Adapted from "The Truth about Bedpans" by Karen Tolin, RN, Joplin, Mo., printed by *RN* Magazine.

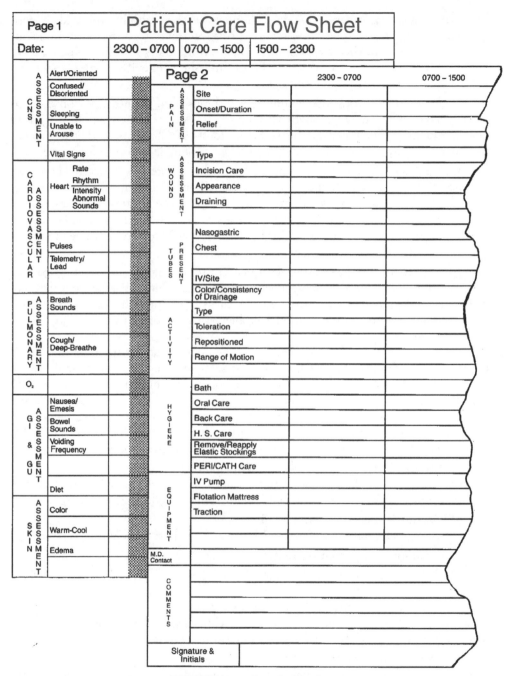

Patient Care Flow Sheet

Page 1

Date:	2300 – 0700	0700 – 1500	1500 – 2300

CNS ASSESSMENT	Alert/Oriented		
	Confused/Disoriented		
	Sleeping		
	Unable to Arouse		
	Vital Signs		
CARDIOVASCULAR ASSESSMENT	Heart: Rate		
	Rhythm		
	Intensity		
	Abnormal Sounds		
	Pulses		
	Telemetry/Lead		
PULMONARY ASSESSMENT	Breath Sounds		
	Cough/Deep-Breathe		
	O₂		
GI & GU ASSESSMENT	Nausea/Emesis		
	Bowel Sounds		
	Voiding Frequency		
	Diet		
SKIN ASSESSMENT	Color		
	Warm-Cool		
	Edema		

Page 2

		2300 – 0700	0700 – 1500
PAIN ASSESSMENT	Site		
	Onset/Duration		
	Relief		
WOUND ASSESSMENT	Type		
	Incision Care		
	Appearance		
	Draining		
TUBES PRESENT	Nasogastric		
	Chest		
	IV/Site		
	Color/Consistency of Drainage		
ACTIVITY	Type		
	Toleration		
	Repositioned		
	Range of Motion		
HYGIENE	Bath		
	Oral Care		
	Back Care		
	H. S. Care		
	Remove/Reapply Elastic Stockings		
	PERI/CATH Care		
EQUIPMENT	IV Pump		
	Flotation Mattress		
	Traction		
M.D. Contact			
COMMENTS			
Signature & Initials			

FIGURE 5–2. Sample flow sheet.

can have an impact on the quality of the healthcare provided. For this reason, it is important to avoid judgmental language and to be conscious of tone of voice and body language. Presenting information in an objective and accurate manner reduces the likelihood of being misunderstood or of influencing the client's care negatively.

FOR EXAMPLE: When Sally talked to the nurse, she tearfully expressed concern about going home. The nurse reported this information to the oncoming shift personnel and to the physician by saying: "I think Sally is trying to manipulate us. She says she's not ready to go home, and she thinks if she 'acts weak,' she won't have to leave the hospital."

After listening to this judgmental report, the oncoming nurse's response might be defensive, and that nurse might be inclined to "show" Sally that she is indeed ready to go home. The nurse may also subconsciously stop listening and be less receptive to what Sally is saying. Contrast the previous example with the following.

FOR EXAMPLE: The nurse reports: "Sally has expressed concern about her ability to manage at home. She was weak when we got her up this morning, requiring assistance with walking. Then she spent the afternoon talking on the telephone, at one point ignoring the cries of Baby B until I responded to the room. We need information about her situation at home and her need for assistance with newborn care of twins."

In this report, the nurse expresses a need in terms that challenge colleagues to find a solution. This need is approached with an open mind as additional data are gathered and appropriate resources are identified. This provides opportunities for creating solutions instead of additional problems, thus promoting a positive client/ nurse experience.

The primary format for communicating the client's current situation and needs in the acute care setting is the nursing change-of-shift report. This type of report may be done either in person or via tape recorder. Because time for this activity is usually limited, it is necessary for staff members to be brief and organized while still providing pertinent data. After basic client data (e.g., room number, name, age, diagnosis, and physician) are supplied, reporting may be done "by exception." This means that only occurrences that are out of the ordinary are reported. You report:

- **Abnormalities/changes in assessment findings**

"Robert became short of breath during a.m. rounds and required supplemental oxygen at 2 L/min by nasal cannula." "Michelle's right lower leg edema is resolving."

- **Diagnostic procedures and results**

"Robert's oxygen saturation is 92% on 2 L of oxygen; chest x-ray report is pending."

- **Variations from usual routine**

"Robert was not out of bed this a.m. but was up for lunch and tolerated sitting up in a chair for 45 minutes without difficulty."

- **Activities not completed on your shift**

"The crutches are in Michelle's room; a physical therapist will return at 4 p.m. to instruct her in their use; then we can begin getting her out of bed."

- **Status of invasive treatments**

"Sally's IV of lactated Ringer's with 2 amps of pitocin is infusing in the left forearm at 60 mL/hr with 300 mL remaining."

- **Additions or changes to the plan of care** (this includes evaluation of outcomes and the status of client needs)

"Robert's Airway Clearance need has recurred, requiring aggressive pulmonary toilet every 2 hours and use of incentive spirometer."

Change-of-shift reports may include nursing rounds, with each client being visited by the offgoing and oncoming nurse together. Nursing rounds are beneficial in verifying the status of invasive treatments, the appearance of wounds/dressings, and the current condition of the client (e.g., extent of jaundice, level of coolness of an extremity, etc.). It is imperative for nurses to maintain the confidentiality of client information, and usually it is preferable to review the change-of-shift information before leaving the report room and going to the client's bedside.

Client confidentiality is an ethical/moral concern that must be respected by each professional at all times. These concerns are extended to conversations at the nursing station, on the telephone, or wherever client information is discussed. This includes refraining from discussions with those not directly involved in the client's care (e.g., staff on other units, your own family, friends and acquaintances of the client).

Before concluding this chapter, complete Practice Activity 5–3.

Summary

In putting the plan of care into action and providing effective client care, you review resources to determine priorities, consulting with and considering the desires of the client during this implementation step of the nursing process. You identify who is responsible for the actions to be taken and set realistic time frames for carrying out actions. Changes in the client's needs must be monitored continually because client care takes place in a dynamic environment. The relevance of new data collected in each interaction with the client is determined according to what is already known. This newly gathered information is documented and shared with other healthcare providers as appropriate. Throughout these activities, flexibility is important to allow for changed circumstances, interruptions, and so forth.

Return to the fifth standard of the ANA Standards of Practice at the beginning of this chapter, and review the measurement criteria necessary to achieve and ensure compliance with the standard. The knowledge and skill required to meet the criteria listed in Box 5–2 were described in this chapter on the **implementation** step of the nursing process.

Chapter 6 will enable you to see how continuous evaluation of nursing actions helps you determine whether specific interventions are leading to achievement of the desired outcomes. In addition, evaluation of client plans of care serves as a mechanism for review of the care provided on a unit or within an agency. This review process addresses professional issues of overall quality of care and provides a means by which outside agencies can evaluate the institution.

PRACTICE ACTIVITY 5–3
Communicating Nursing Information to Other Caregivers

1. Two methods of communicating your observations about client care and activities to other nurses are by:

   a. _____

   b. _____

Continued

Communicating Nursing Information to Other Caregivers *(Continued)*

2. Discuss the benefits of nursing rounds.

_____

_____

3. Underline the information listed below that you would include in your change-of-shift report:
Sally ate well
Age 20
Dr. Jefferson
Second day postpartum
Weak and unsteady while up in hall
Episiotomy reddened, slight edema, no drainage
Scheduled for discharge tomorrow
Received oral pain medication at 11 a.m. with reported relief
Does not want to go home
Sister in to visit at lunchtime
Coordination for home-care services in progress with the discharge planner
Spent afternoon talking on phone
Has not named Baby B
 At times has ignored infant cues

4. The wife of a prominent local politician is admitted for treatment of alcoholism. You could discuss her admission and course of therapy with which of the following people?
Attending/primary physician
Nursing supervisor
The pediatric nurse (who is her best friend)
Your husband
The client's son
A newspaper reporter
Other nurses on your unit

BOX 5-2

Measurement Criteria for ANA Standard 5

ANA Standard 5: Implementation: The registered nurse implements the identified plan.

1. Implements the plan in a safe and timely manor.

2. Documents implementation and any modifications, including changes or omissions, of the identified plan.

3. Utilizes evidence-based interventions and treatments specific to the diagnosis or problem.

4. Utilizes community resources and systems to implement the plan.

5. Collaborates with nursing colleagues and others to implement the plan.

1. Identify three activities involved in implementing the plan of care:

   a. _____

   b. _____

   c. _____

2. Discuss the importance of understanding the expected effect and potential hazards of the interventions you will implement:

   _____

   _____

   _____

3. Explain the purpose for ongoing data collection throughout the **implementation** step of the nursing process:

   _____

   _____

4. List two reasons why documentation of care provided is important:

   a. _____

   b. _____

5. Name three activities you might use to carry out interventions for planned client care:

   a. _____

   b. _____

   c. _____

6. What is the advantage of reporting "by exception"?

   _____

7. When and where is client confidentiality important?

   _____

8. Flexibility in providing client care is important because:

   _____

VIGNETTE: Robert signed advance directives asking that no extraordinary means (e.g., intubation and mechanical ventilation) be used to prolong his life. When his condition deteriorated, his daughter was notified as required. While visiting with her father, she is surprised to learn of his decision. She is very upset, and a confrontation develops. Robert tells her, "it is none of your business," and refuses to enter into further conversation.

What can you do now?

_____

_____

_____

SUGGESTED READINGS

Cowen, C. S., & Moorhead, S. (Eds.). (2006). *Current Issues in Nursing*, ed 7. St. Louis: Mosby.

Doenges, M. E., Moorhouse, M. F., & Murr, A. C. (2008). *Nurse's Pocket Guide: Nursing Diagnoses with Interventions*, ed 11. Philadelphia: F. A. Davis.

Advance Directives, Ethics, and Legal Aspects

Aiken, T. D. (2004). *Legal, Ethical, and Political Issues in Nursing*, ed 2. Philadelphia: F. A. Davis.

American Nurses Association. (1998). *Legal Aspects of Standards and Guidelines for Clinical Nursing Practice*. Washington, DC: Author.

Arras, J. D. (1995). (Ed.). *Bringing the Hospital Home: Ethical and Social Implications of High-Tech Home Car.* Baltimore: Johns Hopkins University.

Bandman, E. L., & Bandman, B. (2001). *Nursing Ethics Through the Life Span*, ed 4. Upper Saddle River, NJ: Prentice Hall.

Beckmann, J. P. (1996). *Nursing Negligence: Analyzing Malpractice in the Hospital Setting*. Thousand Oaks, CA: Sage Publications.

Benner, P. A., Tanner, C. A., & Chesla, C. A. (1998). *Expertise in Nursing Practice: Caring, Clinical Judgment, and Ethics*. New York: Springer.

Berger, A. S. (1995). *When Life Ends: Legal Overviews, Medicolegal Forms, and Hospital Policies*. Westport, CT: Praeger.

Bishop, A. H., & Scudder, J. R. (1996). *Nursing Ethics: Therapeutic Caring*. Boston: Jones & Bartlett.

Brent, N. J. (2000). *Nurses and the Law: A Guide to Principles and Applications*, ed 2. Philadelphia: W. B. Saunders.

Burkhardt, M. A., & Nathaniel, A. K. (2007). *Ethics and Issues in Contemporary Nursing*, ed 3. Albany, N.Y: Cengage Delmar.

Cantor, N. L. (1993). *Advance Directives and the Pursuit of Death With Dignity*. Bloomington: Indiana University Press.

Catalano, J. T. (1995). *Ethical and Legal Aspects of Nursing*, ed 2. Springhouse, PA: Springhouse.

Concern for Dying. (1991). *Advance Directive Protocols and the Patient Self-Determination Act*. New York: Author.

Davis, A. J., Arosker, M. A., & Liaschinko, J. (1997). *Ethical Dilemmas and Nursing Practice*, ed 4. Stamford, CT: Prentice Hall.

Dougas, D. J., & McCullough, L. B. (1991). The values history: The evaluation of the patient's values and advanced directives. *Journal of Family Practice, 32*:145–153.

Doukas, D. J., & Reichel, W. (1993). *Planning for Uncertainty: A Guide to Living Wills and Other Advance Directives for Health Care*. Baltimore: Johns Hopkins University.

English, D. D. (1994). *Bioethics: A Clinical Guide for Medical Students*. New York: W. W. Norton.

Fiesta, J. (1997). *Legal Implications in Long-Term Care*. Albany, N.Y: Delmar.

Guido, G. W. (2005). *Legal and Ethical Issues in Nursing*, ed 4. Upper Saddle River, N.J.: Prentice Hall.

Hall, J. K. (1996). *Nursing Ethics and Law*. Philadelphia: W. B. Saunders.

Husted, G. L., & Husted, J. H. (2001). *Ethical Decision Making in Nursing and Healthcare*, ed 3. New York: Springer.

Kapp, M. B. (1994). (Ed.). *Patient Self-Determination in Long-Term Care: Implementing the PSDA in Medical Decisions*. New York: Springer.

Kikuchi, H., & Simmons, D. R. (1996). (Eds.). *Truth in Nursing Inquiry*. Thousand Oaks, CA: Sage Publications.

King, N. M. P. (1996). *Making Sense of Advance Directives*. Washington, D.C.: Georgetown University Press.

Lashley, F. R. (Ed.). (1997). *The Genetics Revolution: Implications for Nursing*. Washington, D.C.: American Academy of Nursing.

Martin, S., & Vitello, J. M. (1992). Making a critical decision before it becomes critical. *Heart Lung, 21*:15A–18A.

Monarch, M. (2002). *Nursing and The Law: Issues and Trends*. Washington, D.C.: American Nurses Association.

Reigle, J. (1992). Preserving patient self-determination through advance directives. *Heart Lung, 21*:196–198.

Salipante, D. M. (1998). Cultural diversity: Refusal of blood by a critically ill patient: A healthcare challenge. *Critical Care Nurse, 18*(2):68–76.

Scanlon, C., & Fibison, W. (1995). *Managing Genetic Information: Implications of Nursing Practice*. Washington, DC: American Nurses Publishing.

Silverman, H. J., Fry, S. T., & Armistead, N. (1994). Nurses' perspective on implementation of the Patient Self-Determination Act. *Journal of Clinical Ethics, 5*:30–37.

Silverman, H. J., Vinicky, J. K., & Gasner, M. R. (1992). Advance directives: Implications for critical care. *Critical Care Medicine, 20*:1027–1031.

Singleton, K. A., Dever, R., & Donner, T. A. (1992). Durable power of attorney: Nursing implications. *Dimensions of Critical Care Nursing, 11*:41–46.

Snider, G. L. (1995). Withholding and withdrawing life-sustaining therapy: All systems are not yet "go." *American Journal of Critical Care Medicine, 151*:279–281.

Springhouse. (2004). *Nurse's Legal Handbook*, ed 5. Philadelphia: Lippincott Williams & Wilkins.

Sullivan, G. H. & Mattera, M. D. (1997). *RN's Legally Speaking: How to Protect Your Patients and Your License*. Montvale, NJ: Medical Economics.

Summers, S. K., & Krohm, C. (2001). *Advance Health Care Directives: A Handbook for Professionals*. American Bar Association.

Trandel-Korenchuk, D. M., & Trandel-Korenchuk, K. M. (1997). *Nursing and the Law*, ed 5. Gaithersburg, MD: Aspen.

Veins, D. C. (1989). A history of nursing's code of ethics. *Nursing Outlook, 37*(1):43–49.

White, G. B. (1992). *Ethical Dilemmas in Contemporary Nursing Practice*. Washington, DC: American Nurses Publishing.

White, P. D. (1997). The role of the critical care nurse in counseling families about advance directives. *Critical Care Nursing Clinics of North America, 9*:53–61.

Zucker, M. B., & Zucker, H. D. (1997). (Eds.). *Medical Futility and the Evaluation of Life-Sustaining Interventions*. Cambridge, NY: Cambridge University Press.

Change-of-Shift Report

Barbera, M. L. (1994). Giving report: How to sidestep common pitfalls. *Nursing, 24*(9):41.

Benson, E., Rippin-Sisler, C., Jabusch, K., & Keast, K. (2007). Improving nursing shift-to-shift report. *Journal of Nursing Care Quality, 22*(1):80–84.

Bosek, M. S. D., & Fugate, K. (1994). Intershift report: A quality improvement project. *MEDSURG Nursing, 3*(2):128–132.

Coleman, S., & Henneman, E. A. (1991). Comprehensive patient care and documentation through unit-based nursing rounds. *Clinical Nurse Specialist, 5*(2):117–120.

Copp, L. A. (1998). Change of shift report. *Journal of Professional Nursing, 14*(2):63–64.

Cox, S. S. (1994). Taping report tips to record by. *Nursing, 24*(3):64.

Fraser, L. E., O'Brien, K., Tobar, I., & Waller, D. M. (1991). Patient care plans for intershift report. *Journal of Pediatric Nursing: Nursing Care of Children and Families, 6*(5):310–316.

Guido, G. W. (1988). Legal commentary: Shift reports. *Dimensions of Critical Care Nursing, 7*:380.

Hays, M. M. (2002). An exploratory study of supportive communication during shift report. *Southern Online Journal of Nursing Research, 3*(3). Accessed Sept 2007 at http://www.snrs.org/publications/SOJNR_articles/iss03vol03.pdf

Howell, M. (1994). Confidentiality during staff reports at the bedside. *Nursing Times, 90*(34):44–45.

Liukkonen, A. (1993). The content of nurses' oral shift reports in homes for elderly people. *Journal of Advanced Nursing, 18*(7):1095–1100.

McMahon, R. (1990). What are we saying? *Nursing Times, 86*(30):38–40.

Monahan, M. L., et al. (1998). Change of shift report: A time for communication with patients. *Nursing Management, 19*(2):80.

Mosher, C., & Bontomasi, R. (1996). How to improve your shift report. *American Journal of Nursing, 96*(8):32–43.

Patterson, P. K., Blehm, R., Foster, J., Fuglee, K., & Moore, J. (1995). Nurse information needs for efficient care continuity across patient units. *Journal of Nursing Administration, 25*(10):28–36.

Reiley, P. J., & Stengrevics, S. S. (1989). Change-of-shift report: Put it in writing! *Nursing Management, 20*(9):54–56.

Taylor, C. (1993). Intershift report: Oral communication using a quality assurance approach. *Journal of Clinical Nursing, 2*(5):266–267.

Wolf, Z. R. Learning the professional jargon of nursing during change of shift report. *Holistic Nursing Practice, 4*(1):78–83.

Chapter 6

The Evaluation Step: Determining Whether Desired Outcomes Have Been Met

Reassessment

Modification of the Plan of Care

Termination of Services

Enhancing Delivery of Quality Care

Summary

■ **ANA STANDARD 6:** Evaluation: The registered nurse evaluates progress toward attainment of outcomes.

The final step of the nursing process is evaluating the client's response to the care delivered, to make sure the desired outcomes developed in the **planning** step and documented in the plan of care have been achieved. **EVALUATION**, which is an ongoing process, is necessary for determining how well the plan of care is working. As the client's condition changes, information is added to the client database, requiring revision and updating of the plan of care; this is an essential component of the **evaluation** step.

Although the process of evaluation may seem similar to the activity of assessment, there are important differences. Instead of identifying the client's general status and needs, the evaluation focuses on the appropriateness of the care provided and the client's progress or lack of progress toward the desired outcomes. Evaluation is

EVALUATION: final step of the nursing process. A continuous process essential to ensuring the quality and appropriateness of the care provided; it is done by reviewing client responses to determine effectiveness of the plan of care in meeting client needs.

an interactive, continuous process. As each nursing action is performed, the client's response is noted and evaluated in relation to the identified outcomes. Then, based on the client's response, appropriate revisions of nursing interventions and/or client outcomes may be necessary.

Although it is frequently considered simplistically as a pass-or-fail judgment, evaluation should actually be a constructive opportunity to provide positive feedback to the client and caregivers for their efforts and to encourage them to continue to strive for a higher level of functioning or wellness. It is an opportunity for problem solving and personal growth. The evaluation step has three components: reassessment, modification of the plan of care, and termination of services. The first two components form a continuous loop of recurring assessment and reaction, which eventually leads to the third component. "Termination of services" may sound rather abrupt, but this final part of the evaluation step is in reality the next step for the client in looking toward the future and moving on. Termination, in part, includes completion of discharge planning; it addresses those client nursing diagnoses or client needs that were not fully attained during the time frame when nursing care was provided. Further description of this part of the evaluation step is presented later in this chapter.

Reassessment

Reassessment is a constant "measuring and monitoring" of the client's status that evaluates the client's response to nursing interventions and progress toward attaining the desired outcome. This process is ongoing; it does not occur only when an outcome is to be reviewed or a determination made of the client's readiness for discharge. Data collected as the plan of care was implemented in step 4 of the nursing process are now reassessed. Evaluation of the data determines:

- **The appropriateness of the nursing actions**

FOR EXAMPLE: Robert's dyspnea has resolved with the provision of oxygen and attention to pulmonary toilet (i.e., periodic deep-breathing exercises, effective cough, position changes, use of the incentive spirometer). Or Donald's tremors have lessened since he received his a.m. dose of Serax.

- **The need to revise the interventions**

FOR EXAMPLE: Robert was kept in bed for breakfast but should be able to be out of bed for lunch. Or while you were assisting Michelle to walk the length of the hall, you noted that she is unsteady on her crutches and will initially require the assistance of two individuals to provide for client and employee safety.

- **The development of new client needs**

FOR EXAMPLE: Sally is scheduled for discharge tomorrow. Her current weakness and lack of attention to her infant's cues raise concerns about her coping abilities and the potential for parenting/attachment problems as well as issues of self-care.

- **The need for referral to other resources**

FOR EXAMPLE: Sally's physician is notified of your observations, and possible solutions are discussed. A family meeting may be requested to clarify roles/responsibilities and availability of assistance. The home health nurse is to be contacted to arrange self-care and homemaker assistance and to supervise Sally's situation after discharge. Referrals to community support groups (such as Mothers of Twins) may be made to provide additional assistance and problem-solving options.

- **The need to rearrange priorities to meet the changing demands of care**

FOR EXAMPLE: You had planned to get Robert up in the chair for breakfast, but the focused assessment revealed a change in his respiratory status, requiring new interventions and revision of the plan. *Or* external factors may occur, such as the emergency department calling to say that it has a new client requiring admission. You need to review and reschedule the activities planned for Robert in order to accommodate these additional and unplanned responsibilities.

While evaluating the client's response to care, you note progress toward the specified outcomes. In addition, because each outcome has an identified time frame, achievement of the outcomes is reviewed periodically. You must now determine whether the outcomes have been met completely, partially, or not at all, and whether the plan of care needs to be revised. Outcome(s) may be evaluated by:

- **Direct observation**

FOR EXAMPLE: Did the client ambulate the length of the hall without developing dyspnea? Did the client demonstrate proper technique for the administration of insulin? Is the client free of skin breakdown?

- **Client interview**

FOR EXAMPLE: Does the client report decreased level of pain after administration of oral pain medication? Can the client list available community resources? Is the client able to verbalize the signs/symptoms that require medical evaluation or follow-up?

- **Review of records** (e.g., progress notes, flow sheets, medication record)

FOR EXAMPLE: Has the client's temperature remained within normal range? Are the intake and output balanced? Has the client gained weight? Has a laxative been required for constipation?

An important aspect of this process is the involvement of the client. How does the client believe he or she is doing? Inclusion of the client's point of view can reveal important insights that may provide additional data for evaluating and revising the plan of care.

As mentioned in Chapter 4, the Omaha System's Problem Rating Scale for Outcomes provides three levels of evaluation. Box 6–1 lists the three system concepts of knowledge, behavior, and status. A similar five-point system is used by Nursing Outcomes Classification (NOC) to evaluate its outcome indicators (NOC uses 11 different scales). For example:

BOX 6–1

Omaha Problem-Rating Scale for Outcomes

Concept	1	2	3	4	5
Knowledge	No knowledge	Minimal knowledge	Basic knowledge	Adequate knowledge	Superior knowledge
Behavior	Not appropriate	Rarely appropriate	Inconsistently appropriate	Usually appropriate	Consistently appropriate
Status	Extreme signs/ symptoms	Severe signs/ symptoms	Moderate signs/ symptoms	Minimal signs/ symptoms	No signs/ symptoms

Martin, K. S., & Scheet, N. J. (1992). *The Omaha System: A Pocket Guide for Community Health Nursing*. Philadelphia: W. B. Saunders.

Scale A: 1 = severely compromised to 5 = not compromised, for outcomes such as Ambulation, Memory, Spiritual health.

Scale I: 1 = none to 5 = extensive, for outcomes such as Abuse recovery: Physical, Knowledge: Infant Care, Neglect Cessation

Scale M: 1 = never domonstrated to 5 = consistently demonstrated, for outcomes such as Aggression Self-control, Hope, Suicide Self-restraint. See Box 6–2.

If the outcomes were achieved completely, ask yourself the following questions: "Do any interventions need to be continued, or which interventions can be terminated?" "How easily were the outcomes achieved?" "Can the time frame be shortened?" In determining why a desired outcome was not met completely, the following questions may help provide clarification:

BOX 6–2

NOC Rating Scale for Outcome Knowledge: Diet

Indicator	1—None	2—Limited	3—Moderate	4—Substantial	5—Extensive
Description of diet			X		
Description of diet goals				X	
Description of foods to be avoided		X			

- Were the outcomes realistic and appropriate?
- Was the client involved in setting the outcomes?
- Does the client believe the outcomes were important?
- Does the client know why the outcomes have not been met?
- Have all the interventions that were identified been carried out and in the time frame specified? If not, why not? Were they too vague or misinterpreted?
- What variables may have affected achievement of the outcomes?
- Were new needs/adverse client responses detected early enough to allow appropriate changes to be made in the plan of care?

In addition, review the orders and progress notes of all healthcare providers, and identify factors that helped or hindered achievement of outcomes. Document your findings on the plan of care and/or progress notes, as appropriate, and share them with the client.

Modification of the Plan of Care

When you have completely evaluated the outcomes and the plan of care, you may find that the client's condition has changed in a direction that was not anticipated, regardless of your nursing interventions and the client's desire to achieve the stated outcomes. At this point, a change in treatment approach is indicated, and the plan of care must be modified to reflect these changes.

As basic physiological needs, such as air, water, and food; and safety/security-level needs, such as coping, protection, management of anxiety, are met, nursing care can progress to such higher-level concerns as self-esteem. Alternatively, higher-level needs may be delayed while those associated with newly emerging basic needs are addressed. At any time, the nurse may identify or activate additional client diagnostic statements, goals, and/or desired outcomes and corresponding interventions. An earlier chapter discussed the difficulty of dealing with more than three to five client problems at one time. The actual number varies from client to client and the complexity of the nursing diagnoses present/level of care required, but the point is that there may simply be too many client needs to be addressed in the initial plan of care. Priority setting is required when this situation exists, with progression to higher-level needs as the client's condition permits.

When the desired outcomes are evaluated and found to be unmet, the reasons need to be identified and documented and the outcomes then revised or new ones written. When revising client outcomes, keep in mind that they may need simply to be restated or their time frames lengthened so the client can successfully achieve them.

FOR EXAMPLE: When Donald was first admitted for acute alcoholism and depression, initial concerns focused on issues of client safety/potential for injury, changes in sensory interpretation, anxiety, and general nutrition. When Donald completed his initial withdrawal from alcohol and his physical condition stabilized, nursing attention shifted to focus on previously identified problems concerning individual coping and role performance.

As the plan of care is modified, remember to address the changing needs of the client/significant others and the changes in the client's health status, environment, and therapeutic regimen. To assist in this process, a client care conference may be scheduled, or a consultation with a colleague or other resource people with special knowledge may be necessary to gain additional insight and to problem-solve solutions.

Practice Activity 6–1 provides an opportunity for you to review and evaluate the plan of care for Michelle. Read the narrative accompanying Michelle's plan of care, and follow the directions for evaluating whether Michelle has attained the stated outcomes. Write your evaluations in the STATUS column of the plan of care. Once you have completed Practice Activity 6–1, go on to Practice Activity 6–2, and add your modifications to Michelle's plan of care in the space provided.

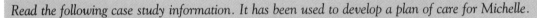

PRACTICE ACTIVITY 6-1
Evaluating Client Outcomes

Read the following case study information. It has been used to develop a plan of care for Michelle.

When Michelle was admitted to the hospital the evening of 6/11, a physiological (Maslow's) or survival (Kalish) need of pain avoidance was identified (i.e., acute Pain). A higher-level need of safety or stimulation was noted (i.e., impaired physical Mobility), as was a safety need of protection (i.e., risk for Infection).

The following morning (6/12) during the 8 a.m. assessment, Michelle indicated that she was successful in obtaining relief of pain with the morphine sulfate PCA and occasional bolus injections. Michelle also found that deep-breathing exercises and focusing her attention on the scenic picture at the foot of her bed helped minimize the severity of recurrent muscle spasms in her right leg. In addition, frequent weight shifts using the overhead trapeze and range-of-motion exercises reduced general aches and joint stiffness, and meditation enhanced general relaxation.

The nurse noticed that most of Michelle's breakfast was untouched. Michelle reported she was not very hungry but did want fruit juice and other fluids. After the morning bed bath, the dressings were changed, and the right leg wound was evaluated. Skin edges were pink, and serous drainage was odorless. Pin sites were also cleaned, and no signs of inflammation were noted. At lunch, Michelle's intake was poor. She indicated that she was having difficulty opening her mouth and chewing, and she had an aching sensation located in her right temple and ear.

During the afternoon assessment at 4:30 p.m., Michelle's nurse verified that Michelle understood and was using infection control techniques of proper handwashing and avoidance of contact with wound and pin sites.

When Michelle was set up on the side of the bed before her dinner, she reported dizziness and sharp pain in her right leg, and she became pale and diaphoretic. She was returned to the supine position, and a focused assessment was performed, revealing a blood pressure of 92/60. Within 20 minutes, Michelle's color had improved, the dizziness was gone, blood pressure had improved to 110/72, and the pain was relieved with an additional bolus of medication.

In reviewing the excerpts from Michelle's plan of care, complete the status column denoting whether the outcomes have been met (m), partially met (pm), or not met (nm) appropriately for the time frames indicated.

PLAN OF CARE: MICHELLE

Client: Michelle   Age: 14—3/2/94   Gender: F   Admission: 6/11/08   5:30 p.m.   Dx: Compound Fx R tibia/fibula, closed head injury/mild concussion

Date	Client Diagnostic Statement	Goal	Interventions	Outcomes	Status
	Acute Pain: related to movement of bone fragments, soft tissue injury/edema, and use of external fixator, as evidenced by verbal reports, guarding, muscle tension, narrowed focus, and tachycardia	Pain-free or controlled by discharge	1. Maintain limb rest R leg × 24 hr to 5 p.m. 6/12 2. Elevate lower leg with folded blanket 3. Apply ice to area as tolerated × 48 hr to 5 p.m. 6/13 4. Place cradle over foot of bed 5. Document reports and characteristics of pain 6. Morphine sulfate PCA IV w/bolus, advance to Vicodin 5 mg PO q4h prn 7. Demonstrate/encourage use of progressive relaxation techniques, deep-breathing exercises, visualization 8. Provide alternate comfort measures, position change, back rub 9. Encourage use of diversional activities— TV, music, texting friends	Verbalizes relief of pain within 5 min (IV) or 45 min (PO) of administration of medication Identifies methods that provide relief by 9 a.m., 6/12 Uses relaxation skills to reduce level of pain by 9 a.m., 6/12	

Based on your evaluation, how would you alter Michelle's plan of care from Practice Activity 6–1?

_____

_____

_____

PLAN OF CARE: MICHELLE

Client: Michelle   Age: 14—3/2/94   Gender: F   Admission: 6/11/08 5:30 p.m.   Dx: Compound Fx R tibia/fibula, closed head injury/mild concussion

Date	Client Diagnostic Statement	Goal	Interventions	Outcomes	Status
	Risk for Infection: risk factors of broken skin, traumatized tissues, decreased hemoglobin levels, invasive procedures, environmental exposure	Free of infection	1. Monitor temp, VS q4h 2. Aseptic dressing change bid 9 a.m., 9 p.m., and prn. 3. Pin care per protocol bid 9 a.m., 9 p.m. 4. Routine IV site care daily 5. Document condition of wound, IV, and pin sites q4h 6. Review ways client can reduce risk of infection 7. Administer cefoxitin 2 g IV piggyback q8h (8 a.m., 4 p.m., 12 a.m.).	Identifies and practices interventions to reduce risk of infection by 5 p.m., 6/12 Identifies signs/symptoms requiring medical evaluation by 9 a.m., 6/13 Displays initial wound healing free of purulent drainage/signs of infection by discharge	
	Impaired physical Mobility: related to loss of integrity of bone structures, imposed restrictions of movement (external fixator), pain, and reluctance to initiate movement as evidenced by limited range of motion, difficulty turning, slowed movement	Ambulates safely with assistive device	1. Monitor circulation/nerve function R leg q1h × 24 hr to 5 p.m., 6/12, then q4h and prn. 2. Support R leg fixator during movement. 3. Support feet with footboard. 4. Encourage use of side rails/overhead trapeze for position change. 5. Demonstrate/assist with ROM exercises to unaffected limbs q2h. 6. Assist out of bed, nonweight-bearing R leg 6 p.m., 6/12. 7. Instruct in/monitor use of crutches 6/13. 5 p.m., 6/12.	Participates in activities to maintain muscle strength by 9 a.m., 6/12 Increases level of activity beginning 6 p.m., 6/12 and ongoing Demonstrates techniques/behaviors that enable resumption of activities by 6 p.m., 6/13 Maintains position of function R leg, free of foot drop—ongoing	

Termination of Services

When the desired outcomes have been achieved and the broader goals met, termination of care is planned. The focus at this point is on how the client will manage on his or her own. Although termination of care ideally occurs when all goals/outcomes are met, it is possible that some will not be met before discharge. The goals/outcomes that have not been met need to be reviewed, and the reasons why they were not met should be documented. Some nursing diagnoses, such as Anxiety or imbalanced Nutrition, may require months or years to be completely resolved. Because the hospitalization or home care episode is only one point along the client's health continuum, it is realistic that not all outcomes will be achieved or all nursing diagnoses resolved.

The discharge plans that began at the time of admission and were updated periodically are finalized and put into action. It must be verified that the client or significant other has received written and verbal instructions regarding treatments, medications, and activities to be followed at home. Signs and symptoms indicating the need for continued contact with the healthcare providers are reviewed. When necessary, referrals/phone numbers and other information about resources (including appropriate Web sites) are given to the client/significant other. It must also be determined whether contact has been made with appropriate providers (e.g., social worker, home health nurse, or equipment suppliers) for follow-up care, as indicated.

Concerns regarding unmet needs, the importance of follow-up monitoring, and progress toward long-term goals after discharge were discussed in Chapter 4. Depending on how your facility or agency has decided to deal with these issues, you may choose to document your findings and client instructions in a discharge summary, which also identifies additional suggestions for the client and family to resolve unmet needs and achieve long-range outcomes/goals. A copy of this nursing discharge summary may be given to the client. Box 6–3 shows how client teaching information can be organized and conveyed to the client/significant other.

BOX 6–3

Example of Client Teaching Information for Client Going Home on Antidysrhythmic Medication

---

Dear Client:

This drug has been prescribed for you. This is what you should know about your drug to get the most from your therapy:

1. Antidysrhythmics are taken to regulate your heart rhythm.
2. Antidysrhythmics may have to be taken for the rest of your life.
3. Quinidine, procainamide hydrochloride (Pronestyl), propranolol (Inderal), and phenytoin (Dilantin) are taken with meals.
4. Do not take your antidysrhythmics concurrently with [fill in appropriate drugs].

Continued

Example of Client Teaching Information for Client Going Home on Antidysrhythmic Medication (Continued)

5. Always check with your doctor or pharmacist before taking other drugs because interactions may occur. Drugs known to cause interactions include over-the-counter products for nasal congestion, allergy, pain, or obesity. Drugs of abuse, such as marijuana, may raise blood pressure and stimulate heart activity and thus increase abnormal heart rhythm.

6. If you forget to take your antidysrhythmic, take it as soon as you remember. **Do not,** however, try to catch up by taking two doses at the same time.

7. Do not stop taking your drug unless directed by your doctor.

8. If you have any side effects from your drug, call your doctor. Side effects from taking antidysrhythmics include low blood pressure, lightheadedness, gastrointestinal distress, changes in rate or rhythm of the heart, and often blurred vision. Keep a written log of the effects that are noted and the time of day, such as in the morning upon awaking, with meals, or with activity.

9. Weigh yourself weekly. A gain of 1–2 lb a week may be a sign of increased water retention. Call your doctor if this occurs.

10. Check your feet and ankles for swelling. If this occurs, call your doctor.

11. Limit your coffee, tea, or cola drinks because caffeine may cause an increase in abnormal heart rhythm.

12. Store these drugs in a tight, light-resistant bottle to prevent breakdown of drug.

Kuhn, M. A. (1998). *Pharmacotherapeutics: A Nursing Process Approach,* ed 4. Philadelphia: F. A. Davis.

Even though the client has been discharged, it is important for the client and family to know what has been accomplished and how they can continue to enhance the client's future health status. In addition, the discharge summary may be shared with the home care nurse or the nurse practitioner/primary physician for inclusion in the office record to promote continuity of care with continued work toward goals and monitoring of progress/changing needs.

Enhancing Delivery of Quality Care

Evaluation is an important step for determining the success of the plan of care because it involves a review of all the steps of the nursing process. Although client care is evaluated on an individual basis, unit and/or general agency-based nursing audit committees focus attention on selected groups of clients, such as those receiving chemotherapy or those with longer than normal stay. Comparing overall outcomes and noting the effectiveness of specific interventions are the clinical components of evaluation that can become the bases of research for validating the nursing process. This external evaluation process is the key for refining standards of care and determining the protocols, policies, and procedures necessary for the provision of quality nursing care in a particular agency.

Summary

During the **evaluation** step of the nursing process, the nurse monitors and reports on the current status of the identified client needs according to the outcomes that were developed in the planning step. The evaluation process includes the client, significant others, and whoever else is involved in the care of the client. This process is a positive one in which the client's responses to the nursing interventions are evaluated to determine whether the desired outcomes were achieved. When the findings are analyzed and it is determined that the outcomes have been met, termination of services is begun, and discharge planning is completed. However, if the outcomes have not been met (totally or in part), reassessment is required to determine why this is the case. Consideration must be given to factors such as new information, unexpected complications, or the choice of the wrong nursing diagnosis. At this point, the nursing process should be reinitiated and the plan of care modified to include the newly identified nursing diagnoses, outcomes, and/or interventions. This modification, in turn, will be re-evaluated at an appropriate time.

The evaluation process can also be more broadly applied at an institutional level to measure the overall quality of care. It is used increasingly to set standards and to supply client information about many facets of the care provided by healthcare agencies. The evaluation step needs to be viewed positively as an opportunity for growth, both for individuals and for the profession. It is essential for the effective delivery of client care and so is a process to be valued rather than avoided and/or glossed over quickly.

Now, return to the sixth standard of the ANA Standards of Practice, and review the measurement criteria necessary to achieve and ensure compliance. The knowledge and skill required to meet the criteria listed in Box 6–4 were described in this

---

BOX 6–4

Measurement Criteria for ANA Standard 6

ANA Standard 6 Evaluation: The registered nurse evaluates progress toward attainment of outcomes.
Measurement Criteria
1. Conducts a systematic, ongoing, and criteron-based evaluation of the outcomes in relation to the structures and processes prescribed by the plan and the indicated timeline.
2. Includes the patient and others involved in the care or situation in the evaluation process.

Continued

Measurement Criteria for ANA Standard 6 *(Continued)*

3. Evaluates the effectiveness of the planned strategies in relation to patient responses and the attainment of the expected outcomes.
4. Documents the results of the evaluation.
5. Uses ongoing assessment data to revise the diagnoses, outcomes, the plan, and the implementation, as needed.
6. Disseminates the results to the patient and others involved in the care or situation, as appropriate, in accordance with state and federal laws and regulations.

---

chapter. The measurement criteria for this standard, combined with the previous standards, provide a valuable tool for evaluating your understanding and application of the nursing process.

Accurate documentation of the findings of the evaluation step is essential for ensuring the continuity of care described in the plan of care. This topic is discussed in Chapter 7.

1. What is the difference between assessment and evaluation?

   _____

2. What is the primary purpose of the evaluation process?

   _____

3. The evaluation process provides what three opportunities for the client and nurse?

   a. _____

   b. _____

   c. _____

4. List the three methods in which client outcomes may be evaluated, and give an example for each:

   Method of Evaluation   **Example**

   a. _____   _____

   b. _____   _____

   c. _____   _____

5. Because it is advisable to deal with only three to five nursing diagnoses at a time, how are needs prioritized?

   _____

6. When is consideration of discharge planning begun?

   _____

VIGNETTE: Today is Donald's fifth in-patient day. At the start of the shift, you have completed a focused assessment to evaluate progress/changes in status of the identified client needs. Donald's initial nausea has resolved, and his intake yesterday was approximately 3000 calories. During rounds, you notice he has eaten all the food on his breakfast tray. He fills out the next day's menu, neglecting to include any vegetables and selecting only one fruit.

Later, during group, Donald talks about his options for employment and says he knows an employment agency and a business where he can check about possible jobs. He also mentions a friend who he believes might be willing to help him. He says he is realizing that he is really doing well, even though the loss of his job was a devastating event for him so soon after his divorce. He acknowledges that his feelings of anxiety led to an increase in his drinking. He further says he still has feelings of sadness and occasionally feels a sense of despair but believes he will feel better as he begins to get his life back together again. He seems tentative about accepting his need to be involved in AA, saying he does not know "where they meet or anyone who attends the meetings."

a. **Evaluation:** Based on the previous information, evaluate Donald's progress regarding his problems of imbalanced Nutrition: less than body requirements, ineffective Coping, and ineffective Role Performance, as outlined in the plan of care.

_____

_____

_____

b. **Modification:** How would you change Donald's plan of care?

_____

_____

c. **Termination:** How might new concerns regarding the client affect your discharge plans?

_____

_____

BIBLIOGRAPHY

Kuhn, M. A. (1998). *Pharmacotherapeutics: A Nursing Process Approach,* ed 4. Philadelphia: F. A. Davis.

Martin, K. S., & Scheet, N. J. (1992). *The Omaha System: A Pocket Guide for Community Health Nursing.* Philadelphia: W. B. Saunders.

SUGGESTED READINGS

Ackley, B. J., & Ladwig, G. B. (2003). *Nursing Diagnosis Handbook: A Guide to Planning Care.* St. Louis: Mosby.

Carpenito-Moyet, L. J. (2003). *Nursing Care Plans and Documentation,* ed 4. Philadelphia: Lippincott Williams & Wilkins.

Craft-Rosenberg, M. J., & Denehy, J. A. (Eds.). (2000). *Nursing Interventions for Infants, Children, and Families.* Philadelphia: W. B. Saunders.

Doenges, M. E., Moorhouse, M. F., & Murr, A. C. (2006). *Nursing Care Plans: Guidelines for Planning and Documenting Client Care,* ed 7. Philadelphia: F. A. Davis.

Doenges, M. E., Moorhouse, M. F., & Murr, A. C. (2008). *Nurse's Pocket Guide: Nursing Diagnoses with Interventions,* ed 11. Philadelphia: F. A. Davis.

Holloway, N. M. (2003). *Medical-Surgical Care Planning,* ed 4. Philadelphia: Lippincott Williams & Wilkins.

Joint Commission on Accreditation of Healthcare Organizations. (1997). *Nursing Practice and Nursing Outcomes Measurement.* Oakbrook Terrace, IL: Author.

Leuner, J. D., Manton, A. K., Kelliher, D. B., Sullivan, S. P., et al. (1990). *Mastering the Nursing Process: A Case Study Approach.* Philadelphia: F. A. Davis.

Maas, M., Buckwalter, K. C., & Hardy, M. (1991). *Nursing Diagnosis and Interventions for the Elderly.* Menlo Park, CA: Addison-Wesley.

Newfield, S., et al. (2007). *Cox's Clinical Applications of Nursing Diagnosis: Adult, Child, Women's, Psychiatric, and Home Health Considerations,* ed 5. Philadelphia: F. A. Davis.

Chapter 7

Documenting the Nursing Process

■ **JCAHO STANDARD:** Patient-Specific Data/Information

■ **IM.7.1.** A medical record is initiated and maintained for every individual assessed or treated. The medical record incorporates information from subsequent contacts between the patient and the organization.

■ **IM.7.2.** The medical record contains sufficient information to identify the patient, support the diagnosis, justify the treatment, document the course and results accurately, and facilitate continuity of care among healthcare providers.

Role of Documentation

Documentation is not only a requirement for accreditation; it is also a legal requirement in any healthcare setting. From a nursing focus, documentation provides a record of the use of the nursing process for the delivery of individualized client care. The initial **assessment** is recorded in the client history or database.

The **identification** of client needs and the **planning** of client care are recorded in the plan of care. The **implementation** of the plan is recorded in the progress notes and/or flow sheets. Finally, the **evaluation** of care may be documented in the progress notes and/or plan of care. The goals of the documentation system are to:

- Facilitate the delivery of quality client care
- Ensure documentation of progress with regard to client-focused outcomes
- Facilitate interdisciplinary consistency and the communication of treatment goals and progress

Progress Notes

The plan of care serves as a framework or outline for the charting of administered care. As noted, this information may be recorded on flow sheets and/or progress notes. Progress notes are an integral component of the overall medical record and should include all significant events that occur during the client's hospitalization/treatment program. The notes should be written in a clear and objective fashion and in a manner that reflects progress toward desired measurable outcomes with the use of planned staff interventions. Progress notes have seven major functions, and any given note may be written to address one function more than another:

1. Staff communication
2. Evaluation
3. Relationship monitoring
4. Reimbursement
5. Legal documentation
6. Accreditation
7. Training and supervision

STAFF COMMUNICATION

Staff members arriving for the next and subsequent shifts need to know what has occurred during the current shift so they can make appropriate judgments regarding client management. Colleague-to-colleague communication is the most obvious function of the progress note, yet it is only a piece of the communication picture. Nursing staff members are in the unique position of being in contact with the client for extended periods and in a variety of situations. As a nurse, your observations of your client's behavior and response to therapy provide invaluable information to the physician or other providers who may see the client for only a few minutes each day. Whether the client's current desired outcomes and interventions are discontinued or revised or new ones developed, depends on the information gathered.

EVALUATION

Periodic review of the client's progress and the effectiveness of the treatment plan is performed by the nurse and/or the treatment team. An evaluation of the client's progress may be documented on the plan of care and/or in the progress notes.

For the purposes of review (e.g., nursing audit committees and state, federal, and private agencies such as the board of health, Medicare, Joint Committee on the Accreditation of Healthcare Organizations [JCAHO]), the medical record should be written to facilitate an assessment of the care given the client. Progress notes need to be written to reflect the client's progress toward measurable outcomes and the interventions used. Someone not associated with the healthcare facility should be able to read the notes, determine if the plan of care is being implemented, and assess whether progress is being made toward the measurable outcomes. The medical record should serve as a method of tracking the client's response to treatment and, consequently, as a means for evaluating the quality of care provided.

RELATIONSHIP MONITORING

The therapeutic relationship between staff and client is an important aspect of treatment in any setting. The **NURSE/CLIENT RELATIONSHIP** is the tool used by the nurse to help the client make the most of his or her own abilities. In the psychiatric setting, many of the client's pathologies are manifested in these relationships, and indications of progress are first identified through the client's ability to relate more positively and openly with staff as well as with peers and family. Therefore, monitoring the client's relationships is essential, and notes detailing observations of these relationships (how the client interacts in group situations, in competitive settings, in one-on-one interactions, etc.) have important clinical implications in any setting.

Finally, regardless of the setting, the client's relationship with significant other(s) can have an impact on general well-being, progress toward recovery, independence in self-care, and (ultimately) a successful transition to the home setting. Thus, observation and monitoring of these interactions are important components of nursing care.

NURSE/CLIENT RELATIONSHIP: a therapeutic relationship built on a series of interactions, developing over time and meeting the needs of the client.

REIMBURSEMENT

Third-party payers are insistent that the "why, when, where, how, what, and who" of services be clearly documented. An absence of such documentation may result in termination of funding for individual clients and, therefore, termination of treatment. The medical record is a primary site for maintaining information about the client's treatment and associated revenues; it provides proof of services. Therefore, progress notes must document any significant observations about what is happening to the client during illness, treatment, and recovery. Data about medications, details about equipment used, and any other pertinent information must be recorded.

LEGAL DOCUMENTATION

Nurses have a legal and moral duty to do no harm to clients. Harm can result from a nurse's action or inaction. Careful attention to all the steps of the nursing process reduces the possibility that harm will result from errors of omission (failing to take appropriate action as a result of missing an actual nursing diagnosis) or errors of commission (taking inappropriate action because of misdiagnosis or overdiagnosis).

In our litigious society, with its pervasive threat of malpractice lawsuits, all aspects of the medical record (including the information contained in daily progress notes) may be important for legal documentation. Both the implementation of interventions and progress toward the measurable outcomes should be documented in the progress notes of the client's medical or health record. Progress notes and flow sheets need to document that appropriate actions have been carried out and precautions have been taken, as required, to implement the treatment plan. These notations must be specific about date and time and must be signed by the person who makes the entry. In addition, the time an entry is written needs to be noted, along with the time the activity actually occurred (when charting is delayed). Errors in the document must be crossed out with one line so that it is still legible; they must be identified by the author as "error" and then initialed. White-outs or cross-outs that make the information unreadable are not acceptable because they could be construed that the individual or facility is trying to alter the facts. When charting by computer, remember that additions or changes made to the record can be tracked as to actual date/time of the entry and the author.

ACCREDITATION

One of the essential requirements for healthcare facilities (as determined by JCAHO and/or other accreditation and licensing agencies) is maintenance of a medical/health record. JCAHO standards state that the medical record must be documented accurately and in a timely manner. Therefore, it is important that notes be completed on schedule and in a manner that facilitates retrieval of data. In addition, JCAHO standards specify that, "Nursing care data related to patient assessments, nursing diagnoses and/or patient needs, nursing interventions, and patient outcomes are permanently integrated into the medical record."

TRAINING AND SUPERVISION

An often underestimated aspect of note writing is the value of notes for training and supervision purposes. An experienced nurse's description of how a complicated situation was handled, a supervisor's analysis of the problems presented by a new admission, and a description of patterns noted in a particular client's response to care are all examples of notes that provide models for the remainder of the staff. Supervisors also gain insight into an employee's abilities by reading her or his progress notes and may be able to isolate areas in which additional supervision or training/education would be beneficial.

Complete Practice Activity 7–1 before proceeding to the next section.

Techniques for Descriptive Note Writing

Potential readers for notes written into the health record might include coworkers, clinical nurse specialists, nurse practitioners, physicians, therapists, psychiatrists,

PRACTICE ACTIVITY 7–1
Elements of Progress Notes

Give a brief explanation of how progress notes provide for the following elements of the nurse/client relationship.

1. Staff communication: _____

    _____

    _____

2. Evaluation: _____

    _____

    _____

3. Relationship monitoring: _____

    _____

    _____

4. Reimbursement: _____

    _____

    _____

5. Legal documentation: _____

    _____

    _____

6. Accreditation: _____

    _____

    _____

7. Training/Supervision: _____

    _____

    _____

psychologists, social workers, nurse reviewers, lawyers, judges, utilization reviewers, insurance personnel, surveyors, agency representatives, parents or guardians, and the client. Because of the number of possible readers, the need for clarity and accuracy in the progress notes is a priority.

From the notes, the reader should be able to form a clear picture of what occurred with the client. The best way to ensure the clarity of progress notes is through the use of descriptive (or observational) statements. The following guideline for writing observation-based notes compares and contrasts judgmental and descriptive language.

JUDGMENTAL LANGUAGE

We are all aware of the possibilities for miscommunication that exist in ordinary conversation. The dangers of miscommunication may be even greater when information is written, and the opportunities for clarification that are available in face-to-face communication are absent in the written word. We are accustomed to speaking and writing in a judgmental (and therefore ambiguous) manner without being aware of it. Judgmental statements include phrases that:

- Make reference to undefined periods of time
- Refer to undefined quantities
- Refer to unsupported qualities
- Fail to specify any objective basis for the judgment made

For examples, consider the following statements:

- "She asks for pain medication *too often*."
- "He is *uncooperative* today."
- "She did a *good job* on her incentive spirometer today."
- "He is a *manipulative* client."
- "The new client is really *difficult*."
- "He has a *poor* outlook."
- "She had a *bad attitude* about doing her physical therapy this morning."

The italicized words in each of the previous statements represent judgments (or conclusions), not facts. Without any elaboration or basis for comparison, each of the statements is a statement of opinion, open to varying interpretations. Contrast these with the statements in Box 7–1.

Undefined Periods of Time

Statements that refer to undefined periods of time may contain words or phrases such as the following:

often/almost always/most of the time
rarely/frequently/now and then
seldom/occasionally/every so often

Use of these and similar phrases without clarification leave statements unclear and judgmental. How often, for example, is "every so often"? Is it every 5 minutes, once an hour, or three times per shift? This is not to say that the staff member must time each and every interaction or occurrence. Rather, be aware of the potential for confusion in these words. Ask yourself: Do I need to be more specific about the time of the event mentioned in this note? If you are documenting for potential legal purposes (an injury, for example), specificity is essential; however, for routine communication purposes, this may not be the case. For example, if you note, "The client

---

BOX 7-1

Comparison of Judgmental and Behavioral Notes

The important thing to know about judgmental statements is that they can be translated into more precise terms. For example:

Judgmental: The client did pretty well today.

Behavioral: The client followed directions for drawing up and administering his insulin without any mistakes.

Judgmental: The meeting with the physical therapist did not go very well.

Behavioral: The client stated she "could not do the exercises that were to be started today."

Judgmental: The client had a bad attitude all day.

Behavioral: The client argued with staff five times during the shift.

Judgmental: The client became aggressive.

Behavioral: The client clenched his fists and yelled at the nurse, "I'd like to hit you." He then hit the wall twice with his right fist.

Judgmental: The client would not follow directions.

Behavioral: The client drank a glass of water 30 minutes before his scheduled surgery in spite of reminders to remain NPO.

Judgmental: The client ate poorly.

Behavioral: The client ate one third of her lunch (all of the broccoli and corn; no meat, potatoes, or bread) and drank 50 mL of apple juice.

As you can see from the previous examples, it often takes a bit more thought to write a note that is objectively descriptive. However, the benefits in clarity of communication make the effort essential for the many purposes of progress notes.

---

was quiet for most of the shift today," it is not necessary to record the exact number of minutes during which he or she was quiet or not quiet for reasonably accurate communication to occur.

Undefined Quantities

Statements that refer to undefined quantities may use such words or phrases as the following:

> some/enough/a great deal/too much
> a lot/many/very little/large amount

Each of these terms is open to interpretation. "A lot" of complaints to one person, for example, might mean 5; to another it might mean 20. "A moderate amount of bloody drainage" could be 200 mL or 50 mL of fluid. It is generally advisable to avoid undefined quantities.

Unsupported Qualities

All descriptive adjectives applied to clients have the potential to fall under this category because they may involve making subjective judgments beforehand. Of most concern, however, are words that could be called "semitechnical" in nature such as:

> passive/irritating/incompetent
> nervous/manipulative/overprotective
> demanding/alcoholic/disturbed

Because these kinds of words have connotations in the health field beyond the scope of their ordinary definitions, more common adjectives may pose less of a problem and may have less potential for misunderstanding. However, observed behaviors may call for conclusions that are influenced by your own biases and cultural background. It is best to verify the connotations of the following terms with others, and particularly with the client, before you use them:

> friendly/unhappy/enthusiastic/proud
> attentive/excited/bored/observant
> aloof/apathetic/cheerful/happy

Finally, slang words, which are used informally and mostly by small subcultural groups, are unclear and should not be included in a professionally written note in any case. For example:

> hyped-up/spaced-out/bummed/crazy
> loose/pushy/cool/tanked-up

Objective Basis for Judgments

Some statements clearly express a judgment on the part of the observer and are offered without any objective basis. Such statements may cause the reader to ask "How do you know that this client . . . ":

- is improving?
- has a good attitude?
- enjoys reading?
- dislikes his roommate?

Recording your observations and providing an objective basis for your judgment reduces the possibility of miscommunication or misinterpretation, and the reader will not have to look elsewhere for clarification. Consider the following statements. Although the italicized words represent a judgment or conclusion, objective facts or behavioral observations are provided to support or substantiate the judgment.

- Michelle is *improving;* she walked the length of the hall using her crutches unassisted.
- Robert has a *good attitude*, expressing optimism that he will be able to prevent a recurrence of pneumonia.
- Sally *enjoys reading*, spending 1 to 2 hours a day in this activity.
- Donald *expresses anger* about his roommate's smoking, loud conversations with visitors, and commandeering of the TV. (**Note:** Making the inference that Donald hates his roommate because of his expression of anger results in an unclear or unsupported judgment.)

DESCRIPTIVE LANGUAGE

As noted previously, descriptive language includes observations only and avoids statements that are evaluative or judgmental, unless observational evidence can be presented to support the judgment. Remember that being able to actually observe the client doing something is the criterion of a well-written outcome. The situation is similar for observation-based progress notes; properly written objective statements refer to specific observable or measurable events. Descriptive statements:

- **Contain measurable periods of time**

FOR EXAMPLE:

10 times in 1 hour/every half hour/15 minutes
48 hours/four times a day/once

- **Contain measurable quantities**

FOR EXAMPLE:

20% of the diet/all the group members
six out of eight/completely saturated
none/5 mL

- **Provide a basis or rationale for qualities named in the note**

FOR EXAMPLE:

Sally's lochia flow is moderate to heavy, saturating one peripad in approximately
 1 hour on two separate occasions.
Donald's intake at lunch was poor, consisting of 1/2 cup of soup, 2 bites of sandwich, and 1/2 glass of milk.

You may have gotten the impression in the preceding section that you can never use adjectives in your notes. This is far from the case. In fact, you should give your impressions of the client.

Statements in which you note that the client "seemed" or "appeared" to be exhibiting a certain physical/emotional state are inferential statements. These include a subset of descriptive statements in which you infer the client's state based on your observations of the client's behavior and interactions, your knowledge of the client's patterns, and the connections you make between behavior/affect and what has been happening during the illness. Such statements are often of great value.

However, do not allow your subjective impressions to stand alone, particularly if your observation involves some of the more "semitechnical" qualities noted earlier. Provide some reasons why you believe the client is "improving," "demanding," "manipulative," and so on.

FOR EXAMPLE:

Robert was upset by his daughter's objections to his advance directive choices,
 cutting off the discussion and instructing her to "mind her own business."
Donald is passive, responding to the nurse's questions regarding scheduling of
 his care by replying: "whatever you want to do."
Sally appears distressed, expressing concern about how she will manage two
 newborns when she already has two children at home, needs to return to
 work, and has no energy to do anything.

Michelle's mother is oversolicitous, refusing to leave her daughter's bedside and performing care activities that Michelle is capable of doing herself.

When comparisons or judgments are made, a descriptive statement should state the source or basis of judgment.

FOR EXAMPLE:

According to the client's laboratory report,...
Psychological testing showed that....
The roommate stated that....
Judging by the fact that....

Also note that whenever the source of a judgment is specified, the statement becomes a behavioral report. Because such a report can be observed, this type of statement is an observation and is therefore descriptive. Consider the differences between the following two statements:

The client is stronger today.
The physical therapist reports, "Michelle is stronger today."

The first statement is clearly judgmental because of the undefined phrase "stronger today." The second, however, is an observable event. Obviously (although the physical therapist may be wrong), it is an objective fact that the physical therapist said that the client is stronger today. It may help to think of such statements as quotations. What the physical therapist said does not influence the ability to observe the therapist saying it and then objectively reporting that observation. However, physical therapy notes should reflect measurable descriptions of the client situation.

Finally, you can chart observations in a nonjudgmental manner: "Michelle displayed increased endurance, walked the length of the hall without assistance, appeared more confident with crutch use." In Box 7–1, additional examples further illustrate how judgmental statements may be interpreted and restated more objectively. To further assist you in your understanding of how to document descriptive progress notes, complete Practice Activity 7–2.

CONTENT OF NOTE/ENTRY

The term *progress note* indicates that the client's progress is to be documented, along with the implementation of the treatment plan. Contents should be as specific and accurate as possible.

For communication purposes, it is important to record in the progress notes any information that is of importance to oncoming shifts as well as observations you have made that may be significant for other healthcare providers. Box 7–2 profiles the information that should be included. You are charting for future reference. You know what is happening today. However, the reader tomorrow, next week, or next year must rely on your written words to share your understanding of the client's situation at a given moment.

For example, when applying restraints, which constitutes a major event with both therapeutic and legal ramifications, you need to document the exact time the procedure was initiated, whether any injuries resulted, and so forth. It is also

PRACTICE ACTIVITY 7–2
Writing Nonjudgmental Statements

Circle either J or O/B for each of the following statements to identify either judgmental (J) or observational/behavioral (O/B) documented statements. If the statement is judgmental, rewrite to reflect observational/behavioral language.

1. Mrs. Jewel has a poor body image since undergoing a mastectomy. **J O/B**

_____

2. Mr. Dunn needs to be evaluated regarding his competence to manage his household affairs because of his left-sided weakness following his stroke. **J O/B**

_____

3. Miss Janus does a good job of breast self-examination. **J O/B**

_____

4. Mary Bird does not eat enough for her current level of activity. **J O/B**

_____

5. Mr. Lambert stops taking his medication; then, when he has a seizure, he presents at the doctor's office for treatment. **J O/B**

_____

6. It has been a long time since Mr. Babbitt had his medication evaluated. **J O/B**

_____

necessary to document what led up to the situation, how staff and other participants reacted, what less restrictive measures were tried, and any significant observations regarding the incident. An example of how to document a therapeutic event is presented in Box 7–3.

Other tools that promote accurate communication include the use of correct grammar and spelling, legible handwriting, and nonerasable ink. To promote clarity, avoid repeating data when possible. Because this is "the client's record," it is not necessary to use the term "the client"; however, periodically using the client's name can help the reader to identify the proper chart and prevent problems of charting on the wrong record, especially when you chart on several clients' records at a time. Use abbreviations with caution, or avoid them in most instances. Although some institutions provide a list of approved abbreviations that identifies the correct meaning (such as those noted on the end pages of this textbook), abbreviations can be misleading or easily misinterpreted, resulting in misunderstandings and errors with serious consequences. For example, a client reading his record might not realize that SOB means "short of breath."

BOX 7–2

Content of Successful Progress Notes

Examples of the kind of information important to record in the progress notes include:

- **Unsettled or unclear problems or "issues"** that need to be considered, including attempts to contact other healthcare providers
- **Noteworthy incidents or interviews** involving the client that would benefit from a more detailed recording
- **Other pertinent data**, such as notes on phone calls, home visits, and family interactions
- **Additional critical incident data**, such as seemingly significant or revealing statements made by the client, an insight you have into a client's patterns of behavior, client injuries, the use of any special treatment procedure, or other major events such as episodes of pain, respiratory distress, panic attacks, medication reactions, suicidal comments
- **Administered care activities or observations**, if not recorded elsewhere on flow sheets (physician visits, completion of ordered tests, nonroutine medications, etc.)

BOX 7–3

Documenting a Therapeutic Event

Twenty-four hours after Donald was admitted to the unit with a diagnosis of acute alcoholism, he became disoriented to time, place, and person; was extremely agitated; and was "picking in the air," saying he was trying to "catch the bugs." He was given medication and placed in restraints in a seclusion room with the door open. This was charted as follows:

4:00 p.m.: Suddenly became agitated. Medicated with Valium, reoriented to place/events in quiet tones as staff paced with him and reinforced that he would be kept safe. Agitation escalated, unable to remain in one place for longer than 60 seconds, expressed fear of "things" he was seeing. Agreed to use of restraints to help keep him safe until he could regain control and/or medication becomes effective.

4:15 p.m.: Procedure explained as Donald put in seclusion room C and placed in 4-point wrist/ankle restraints without incident or injury. He was informed that door would remain open and a staff member would check on him every 10 minutes or more frequently as needed. Vital signs: B/P 150/90; P, 120; respirations, 32.

4:20 p.m.: Dr. Carter notified of current events.

4:30 p.m.: Level of agitation reassessed. Donald reports feeling less anxious but still "jumpy." Remains restless. Restraints continued.

Finally, be brief. Entries need to be concise, short, succinct sentences or phrases that provide enough information to communicate your observations, thoughts, and plans. The entries must be consistent in style and format to avoid confusion and to comply with agency policies. Avoid repetition. Do not rewrite what is already recorded on flow sheets; use the progress note to expand on the flow sheet as appropriate and to note the client's response. For example: when documenting your repeat assessment of a wound, you may chart "no change" (if that is the case) if your baseline or previous observations are recorded.

FORMAT OF NOTE/ENTRY

Several charting formats have been used for documentation. These include block notes, with a single entry covering an entire shift (e.g., 7 a.m.–3 p.m.); narrative timed notes (e.g., 8:30 a.m., Ate entire breakfast); the problem-oriented medical record system (**POMR** or **PORS**) using the **SOAP/SOAPIER** approach (Box 7–4) and PIE/ADPIE based on the steps of the nursing process as defined by each facility or agency, to name a few. The **POMR** format can provide thorough documentation, but it was designed by physicians for episodic care and requires that entries be tied to a client problem identified from a problem list.

A system format created by nurses for documentation of frequent/repetitive care is **FOCUS** CHARTING™. It was designed to encourage looking at the client from a positive rather than a negative (or problem-oriented) perspective by using precise documentation to record the nursing process. Recording assessment, intervention, and evaluation information in a **DAR** (data, action, and response) format (Box 7–5) facilitates tracking and following what is happening to the client at any given moment. Charting focuses on client and nursing concerns. The focal point is client status and the associated nursing care. The "focus" is always stated to reflect the client's concern/need rather than a nursing task or medical diagnosis. Box 7–6 highlights some of the distinguishing features of a Focus.

POMR or **PORS**: problem-oriented medical record—a method of recording data about the health status of a client by focusing on the client's problems.

SOAP/SOAPIER: format for documentation— subjective, objective, analysis, plan/ implementation, evaluation, revision.

DAR: format for documentation—data, action, response.

BOX 7–4

Components of the SOAP/SOAPIER Charting Format

The SOAP format is generally used for the initial assessment of the client. Once the plan of care is implemented and the evaluation process begun, the SOAPIER format becomes more appropriate.

Subjective: Statements from client/others

Objective: Measurable or observable data

Analysis: Interpretations/conclusions based on the subjective and/or objective data

Plan: What is to be done about the identified problem(s)

Implementation: How plan is carried out

Evaluation: Client's response to the interventions

Revision: How the plan of care will be changed

BOX 7–5

Components of the FOCUS CHARTING™ Format

Focus: Nursing diagnosis, client need/concern, sign/symptom, event
Data: Subjective/objective information describing and/or supporting the focus
Action: Immediate/future nursing actions based on assessment and consistent with/complementary to the goals and nursing action recorded in the client plan of care
Response: Describes the effects of interventions and whether the goal/outcome was met

BOX 7–6

What Is a Focus?

The nurse often speaks of "a focus" for assessment, diagnosis, and planning of care.

- A client need/concern or nursing diagnosis

For example:

Airway	Nutrition	Fluid excess

Deficient Knowledge regarding wound care
The "stem" or diagnostic label is taken from the plan of care. You do not need to use time and space to repeat the entire diagnostic statement.

- Signs/symptoms of potential importance

For example:

Fever	Confusion
Hypotension	Nausea
Dysrhythmia	Edema

These require monitoring or limited intervention, but if the signs and symptoms persist, a client need will be identified and added to the plan of care.

FOR EXAMPLE: Continued nausea can affect fluid volume; sustained dysrhythmias and hypotension may develop into a cardiac output concern.

- Significant event or change in status

For example:

Admission/transfer	Seizure activity
Fall out of bed	Respiratory arrest

- A single incident may evolve into a client need for inclusion in the plan of care.

For example: A fall raises concerns about risk for Injury, or, possibly, disturbed Thought Processes, if client is disoriented; or a respiratory arrest may be related to ineffective Airway Clearance or ineffective Breathing Pattern.

- Specific standards of care/hospital policy

For example:

Admission/discharge	Preoperative visit
Summary	Discharge planning
Routine shift assessment	

Whatever documentation system you use, an organized format is a method of identifying, working through, and solving the client's needs. **SOAP, DAR,** and **ADPIE** help organize your thinking and provide structure, which can promote creative problem solving. Structured communication facilitates consistency between various services and healthcare providers. Compare the charting examples for SOAP and DAR in Tables 7–1 and 7–2 for a client with type 2 diabetes (non–insulin-dependent diabetes mellitus) who has an ulceration of the left foot.

ADPIE/PIE: documentation format—assessment, diagnosis (problem), plan (goals), implementation (intervention), evaluation/problem, intervention, evaluation.

TABLE 7–1. **Sample SOAP/IER Charting Format for Richard**

Date	Time	Number/Problem*	SOAP Format†
6/29/08	1900	1 (Skin Integrity)	**S:** "That hurts" (when tissue surrounding wound is palpated).
			O: Scant amount serous drainage on dressing. Wound borders pink. No odor present.
			A: Wound shows early signs of healing, free of infection.
			P: Continue skin care per plan.

In order to document more of the nursing process, some institutions have added the following: Implementation, Evaluation, and Review (if plan were to be altered).

			I: NS irrigation as ordered. Applied wet sterile dressing with paper tape.
			E: Wound clean, no drainage present.
			Signed: *E. Moore, RN*
6/29/08	2100	2 (acute Pain)	**S:** "Dull, throbbing pain (in left foot), no radiation to other areas."
			O: Muscles tense. Moving about bed, appears uncomfortable.

Continued

TABLE 7–1. Sample SOAP/IER Charting Format for Richard *(Continued)*			
Date	**Time**	**Number/Problem***	**SOAP Format†**
			A: Persistent pain.
			P: Per plan of care.
			I: Foot cradle placed on bed.
			Darvocet-N 100 mg given PO.
			Signed: *M. Siskin, RN*
		2200	**E:** Reports pain relieved. Appears relaxed.
			Signed: *M. Siskin, RN*
6/30/08	1100	3 (deficient Knowledge, diabetic teaching)	**S:** "My wife and I have some questions and concerns we wish to discuss."
			O: Copy of list of questions attached to teaching plan.
			A: R.S. and wife need review of information and practice for insulin administration.
			P: Attended group teaching session with wife and read "Understanding Your Diabetes." To meet with dietitian.
			I: Richard demonstrated insulin administration techniques for wife to observe. Procedure handout sheet for future reference provided to couple. Scheduled meeting for them with dietitian at 1300 today to discuss remaining questions.
			E: More confident in demonstration; performed activity without hesitation, correctly and without hand tremors. Richard explained steps of procedure and reasons for actions to wife. Couple identified resources to contact if questions/problems arise.
			Signed: *B. Briner, RN*

*As noted on plan of care.
† S = Subjective: Statements from client/others.
 O = Objective: Measurable or observable data.
 A = Analysis: Interpretations/conclusions based on the subjective and/or objective data.
 P = Plan: What is to be done about the identified problem(s).
 I = Implementation: How plan is carried out.
 E = Evaluation: Client's response to the interventions.
 R = Revision: How the plan of care will be changed.

TABLE 7–2. **Sample of DAR for Richard**			
Date	**Time**	**Focus**	**DAR Format***
6/29/08	1900	Skin integrity L foot	**D:** Scant amount serous drainage on dressing, wound borders pink, no odor present, denies discomfort except with direct palpation of surrounding tissue. **A:** NS irrigation as ordered. Sterile wet dressing applied with paper tape. **R:** Wound clean—no drainage present. Signed: *E. Moore, RN*
6/29/08	2100	Pain L foot	**D:** Reports dull/throbbing ache L foot—no radiation. Muscles tense, restless in bed. **A:** Foot cradle placed on bed. Darvocet-N 100 mg given PO. Signed: *M. Siskin, RN*
6/29/08	2200	Pain L foot	**R:** Reports pain relieved. Appears relaxed. Signed: *M. Siskin, RN*
6/30/08	1100	Learning Need, diabetic teaching	**D:** Attended group teaching session with wife. Both have read "Understanding Your Diabetes." **A:** Reviewed list of questions/concerns from Richard and wife (copy attached to teaching plan). Richard demonstrated insulin administration technique for wife to observe. Procedure handout sheet for future reference provided to couple. Scheduled meeting with dietitian for 1300 today to discuss remaining questions. **R:** Richard more confident in demonstration, performed activity without hesitation, correctly and without hand tremors. He explained steps of procedure and reasons for actions to wife.

Continued

Date	Time	Focus	DAR Format*

TABLE 7–2. **Sample of DAR for Richard** *(Continued)*

Date	Time	Focus	DAR Format*
			Couple identified resources to contact if questions/problems arise. Signed: *B. Briner, RN*

The following is an example of documentation of a client need/concern that currently does not require identification as a client problem (nursing diagnosis) or inclusion in the plan of care and therefore is not easily documented in the SOAP format:

Date	Time	Focus	DAR Format*
6/28/08	2120	Gastric distress	**D:** Awakened from light sleep by "indigestion/burning sensation." Places hand over epigastric area. Skin warm/dry, color pink, vital signs unchanged. **A:** Given Mylanta 30 mL PO. Head of bed elevated approximately 15°. **R:** Reports pain relieved. Appears relaxed, resting quietly. Signed: *E Moore, RN*

*D = Data: subjective/objective information describing and/or supporting the focus.
A = Action: immediate or future nursing actions that address the focus; any changes required for the plan of care.
R = Response: description of client responses to care provided and whether goals/outcomes are met.
Lampe, S. S. (1997). *Focus Charting™*. Minneapolis: Creative Nursing Management.

A copy of the back page of the interactive plan-of-care worksheet is included in Figure 7–1. It is an example of one method of documenting by focusing on certain aspects of the nursing process. The **documentation** section of the interactive plan-of-care worksheet is divided into three possible areas for which documentation is appropriate and may be required in certain agencies.

The first section is reassessment data. In this area, you will review the client's initial assessment data to note any changes. Also, data derived from **monitoring-**focused nursing interventions ("monitor vital signs every shift" or "monitor serum potassium level every 8 hours") are documented in this section.

The second documentation area directs attention to the nursing interventions implemented to assist clients in attaining their stated desired outcomes. Examples are "Assisted client with ambulation bid" and "Instructed in proper use of a walker."

The third section is the client's response to your interventions: How well did the client tolerate assisted ambulation? Did the client use the walker in the correct manner as demonstrated?

	Desired Outcome and Client Criteria:	The Client will:	
P L A N N I N G	**TIME OUT!**	The desired outcome must meet criteria to be accurate. The outcome must be specific, realistic, measurable, and include a time frame for completion. Does the action verb describe the client's behavior to be evaluated? Can the outcome be used in the evaluation step of the nursing process to measure the client's response to the nursing interventions listed below?	
	Interventions		**Rationale for Selected Intervention and References**
E V A L U A T I O N	**TIME OUT!**	Do your interventions assist in achieving the desired outcome? Do your interventions address further monitoring of the client's response to your interventions and to the achievement of the desired outcome? Are qualifiers: when, how, amount, time, and frequency used? Is the focus of the action's verb on the nurse's actions and not on the client? Do your rationales provide sufficient reason and directions?	
	What was your client's response to the interventions?		
	Was the desired outcome achieved? □ Yes □ No	If no, what revisions to either the desired outcome or interventions would you make?	
D O C U M E N T A T I O N	**Documentation Focus:** Now that you have completed the evaluation, the next step is to document your care and the client's response. Use the areas below to enter your progress note information.		
	Reassessment Data:		
	Interventions Implemented:		
	Client's Response:		

INSTRUCTOR'S COMMENTS:

FIGURE 7–1. Reverse side of the interaction plan worksheet previously introduced, providing documentation of the nursing process.

Summary

Documentation of client care information communicates and reflects the individualized care you provide. Documentation promotes continuity of client care among the varied healthcare providers and serves as a basis for evaluation of the care provided. Finally, the documentation process continually reinforces your accountability and responsibility to implement and evaluate the nursing process. As your documentation skills improve, you will save time by consistently using a documentation system that focuses on specific issues. Accurate documentation can also help the clinician in meeting legal and accreditation requirements.

The last chapter in this text includes a client case study to help you bring all the steps of the nursing process together. The case study provides information about a new client, Mr. R. Simmons. His completed client database and the physician's admitting orders are provided to assist you in identifying possible nursing diagnoses, developing appropriate desired outcomes for Mr. Simmons, and selecting nursing interventions that will assist him in attaining the desired outcomes.

The final chapter also presents an evaluation checklist that was developed to include the important aspects of all the American Nurses Association's Standards of Practice detailed throughout this text. This comprehensive evaluation checklist serves as a helpful tool for your self-evaluation and ensures that your assigned written care-planning tasks are accomplished correctly.

1. You are writing a paper regarding documentation. Identify three goals of the documentation process that you will include:

   a. _____

   b _____

   c. _____

2. Steps of the nursing process are documented on which form?

Steps	Form
Assessment	a. Plan of care
Diagnosis/Need Identification	b. Progress notes
Planning	c. Client database
Implementation	d. Flow sheets
Evaluation	

3. List five functions of progress notes:

   a. _____

   b. _____

   c. _____

   d. _____

   e. _____

4. Complete the following statements describing the JCAHO's standards for documentation.

   a. A medical record is _____ and _____ for every individual assessed or treated. The medical record incorporates information from subsequent contacts between the _____ and the _____.

   b. The medical record contains _____ to _____ the client, support the _____, justify the _____, document the course and results accurately, and facilitate _____ of care among healthcare providers.

5. When the healthcare provider is documenting for reimbursement, five factors need to be included. These are:

   _____

6. Two ways in which the plan of care can be used for supervision are:

   _____

7. The best way to ensure clarity of the progress notes is:

_____

8. Rewrite the following judgmental statements to make them nonjudgmental:

a. He is uncooperative today.

_____

b. He is a manipulative client.

_____

c. She had a bad attitude about taking her medication this morning.

_____

d. The new client is really difficult.

_____

9. List three types of judgmental statements:

a. _____

b. _____

c. _____

10. Name three types of data that are important to record in the progress notes:

a. _____

b. _____

c. _____

11. List five additional factors that can enhance accurate communication:

a. _____

b. _____

c. _____

d. _____

e. _____

12. What actions can be taken to correct an error in charting?

_____

13. Name three charting formats:

a. _____

b. _____

c. _____

Read the following vignette, and record the client data using the SOAP and DAR formats as well as the format used in your facility/agency, if different.

VIGNETTE: Sally was discharged home with the twins on the evening of her third postpartal day. On the morning of day 5, she is visited by the public health nurse who specializes in maternal/newborn care.

Sally is dressed in a robe and slippers, her hair is uncombed, her color is pale, and she has dark circles under her eyes. She is sitting in a recliner, bottle-feeding Baby A (Laura). Her mother is sitting on the couch, feeding Baby B (unnamed). The living area is noted to be clean and neat with comfortable ambient temperature. The two older children are reported to be at preschool from 9:00 a.m. to 2:30 p.m. daily.

The postpartal assessment form is completed, with physical findings within normal limits. Sally reports that her bowels are working "slowly" (small, firm bowel movements this a.m.) with fluid intake of approximately 2 L/day and moderate appetite—"just too tired to really eat or do anything else." Sally's mother indicates that she is providing household assistance—cooking, cleaning, and child care. Sally and her mother agree that fatigue is a major concern for Sally. Both Sally and her mother are up twice during the night to feed the twins. Sally takes short naps during the day. Sally is observed to display usual attachment behaviors toward Laura; however, her interaction with unnamed Baby B is of short duration, appears to lack warmth, and is restricted to care-taking activities.

You provide Sally with a teaching sheet that describes postpartal fatigue and discusses dietary needs/supplements, energy conservation techniques, and the importance of balanced activity/exercise and rest. You suggest that Sally's husband might get up for one feeding during the night to allow her a longer period of uninterrupted sleep and to provide him with additional opportunity for interaction with his daughters.

Next, you ask Sally how she feels about being the mother of twins. Sally becomes tearful and states, "I just don't know what I'm going to do when Mom goes home." You ask if she would like to have a visit from a member of the Mothers of Multiples group. You also suggest that she hold a family meeting to problem-solve her concerns. You then discuss your observation that Sally appears more comfortable with Laura than with her twin, asking Sally to describe her perceptions of and feelings for Baby B. After reflecting on the question, Sally says she has felt so overwhelmed that she has not truly accepted the reality of having twins. She is visibly upset, berating herself for being a "poor mother." You tell her that it is not unusual to be overwhelmed by the reality of a multiple birth, even when it is planned in advance of delivery.

You ask Sally to think about what she needs to help her resolve this situation. Sally states that she needs to spend more time getting to know Baby B, allowing other family members to care for and interact with Laura. Following a discussion about the individual characteristics of her other children, Sally says Baby B is unique in her level of alertness and her "acceptance" of anyone who cares for her. "She deserves a name reflecting family ties and thanksgiving for the special gift of twins." You encourage Sally to read the literature about twins provided before her discharge and to apply techniques she has previously found successful in dealing with stressful situations. You schedule a follow-up visit for 1 week later and leave a contact number in case Sally should have any questions or need assistance before your next visit. When you depart, Sally appears focused on ways to improve her current situation—smiling, displaying a lighter mood, and giving a firm handshake.

15.
POMR/SOAP FORMAT: Problem:
S:
O:
A:
P:
I:
E:
R:
DAR FORMAT: Focus:
D:
A:
R:
FORMAT USED IN YOUR INSTITUTION/AGENCY, if different:

BIBLIOGRAPHY

Lampe, S. S. (1997). *Focus Charting*™. Minneapolis: Creative Nursing Management.

SUGGESTED READINGS

Author. (2006). *Mosby's Surefire Documentation: How, What, and When Nurses Need to Document*, ed 2. St. Louis: Mosby.

Burke, L. J. (1995). *Charting by Exception Applications: Making It Work in Clinical Settings*. Albany: Delmar.

Burke, L. J. (1998). *Charting Made Incredibly Easy*. Springhouse, PA: Springhouse.

Eggland, E. T., & Eggland, N. H. (1994). *Nursing Documentation: Charting, Recording, and Reporting*. Philadelphia: Lippincott Williams & Wilkins.

Fischbach, F. T. (1991). *Documenting Care: Communication, the Nursing Process and Documentation Standards*. Philadelphia: F. A. Davis.

Iyer, P. W., & Camp, N. H. (1999). *Nursing Documentation: A Nursing Process Approach*, ed 3. St. Louis: Mosby.

Kerr, S. D. (1992). A comparison of four nursing documentation systems. *Journal of Nursing Staff Development*, 8(1):26–31.

Marrelli, T. M. (2000). *Nursing Documentation Handbook*, ed 3. St. Louis: Mosby.

Meiner, S. (1999). *Nursing Documentation: Legal Focus Across Practice Settings*. Thousand Oaks, CA: Sage Publications.

Springhouse. (2006). *Chart Smart*, ed 2. Philadelphia: Lippincott Williams & Wilkins.

Springhouse. (2007). *Complete Guide to Documentation*, ed 2. Philadelphia: Lippincott Williams & Wilkins.

Yocum, F. (1993). *Documentation Skills for Quality Patient Care*. Tipp City, OH: Awareness Productions.

Chapter 8

Interactive Care Planning: From Assessment to Client Response

Instructions for Case Study

Case Study Care-Planning Worksheet

Care-Planning Evaluation Checklist

Practicing Critical Thinking

Conclusion

Putting Together What You Have Learned About the Nursing Process

This final chapter provides you with the opportunity to evaluate and apply the steps of the nursing process presented in the previous chapters. A case study based on simulated assessment data gathered on your client, Mr. Simmons, and the inclusion of physician admission orders add to the realism of this nursing process exercise. The objective and subjective data are organized within the Doenges and Moorhouse 13 Diagnostic Divisions assessment tool, which was described in Chapter 2. (The complete assessment tool is available in Appendix B.)

Instructions for Case Study

First, read over the admitting physician's orders, and reflect on how your implementation of these orders will assist you in structuring Mr. Simmons' plan of care. After reviewing the physician's orders, review the extensive client database gathered on Mr. Simmons. As you study the database, start to record or highlight those subjective and objective cues that suggest a client need (or problem) and that may be similar to the defining characteristics of possible nursing diagnoses for Mr. Simmons.

One purpose of this exercise is for you to identify two accurate nursing diagnoses. The accuracy of your nursing diagnoses depends on the availability of the subjective and objective data gathered during the admission history and physical examination and the subsequent matching of these data with the defining characteristics of the nursing diagnoses described by NANDA-I. The NANDA-I nursing diagnoses, their related risk factors, and their defining characteristics are in Appendix I.

To further assist you in comparing Mr. Simmons' assessment data with the defining characteristics of possible nursing diagnoses, Table 8–1 presents the 13 diagnostic divisions, with selected associated NANDA-I nursing diagnoses. By reviewing this information, you will be able to better visualize the relationship between the varied nursing diagnoses and the focused assessments of the different diagnostic divisions.

For example, when the client's assessment data gathered in the **elimination** diagnostic division are analyzed, if abnormal subjective and/or objective data are present, your next step would be to direct your attention to Table 8–1. Review the 15 NANDA-I nursing diagnoses associated with the **elimination** diagnostic division. Once you have identified a possible nursing diagnosis from the **elimination** division, your next task is to review the defining characteristics of that nursing diagnosis (see Appendix I) and determine if there is an accurate match with your data. Box 8–1 provides an abbreviated checklist to assist you as you begin diagnosing and constructing plans of care.

TABLE 8–1. Nursing Diagnoses Organized According to Diagnostic Divisions

After data have been collected and areas of concern/need have been identified, consult the Diagnostic Divisions framework to review the list of nursing diagnoses that fall within the individual categories. This will assist you with the choice of the specific diagnostic labels to describe the data accurately from the client database. Then, with the addition of etiology (when known) and signs and symptoms, the client diagnostic statement emerges.

Diagnostic Division

ACTIVITY/REST: Ability to engage in necessary/desired activities of life (work and leisure) and to obtain adequate sleep/rest

Diagnoses

Activity Intolerance	Mobility, impaired bed
Activity Intolerance, risk for	Mobility, impaired wheelchair
Disuse Syndrome, risk for	Sleep, readiness for enhanced
Diversional Activity, deficient	Sleep Deprivation
Fatigue	Transfer Ability, impaired
Insomnia	Walking, impaired
Lifestyle, sedentary	

CIRCULATION—Ability to transport oxygen and nutrients necessary to meet cellular needs

Diagnoses
Autonomic Dysreflexia
Autonomic Dysreflexia, risk for
Cardiac Output, decreased
Intracranial Adaptive Capacity, decreased
Tissue Perfusion, ineffective (specify type: renal, cerebral, cardiopulmonary, gastrointestinal, peripheral)

EGO INTEGRITY—Ability to develop and use skills and behaviors to integrate and manage life experiences

Diagnoses

Anxiety [specify level]
Anxiety, death
Behavior, risk-prone health
Body Image, disturbed
Conflict, decisional (specify)
Coping, defensive
Coping, ineffective
Coping, readiness for enhanced
Decision Making, readiness for enhanced
Denial, ineffective
Dignity, risk for compromised human
Distress, moral
Energy Field, disturbed
Fear
Grieving
Grieving, complicated
Grieving, risk for complicated
Hope, readiness for enhanced
Hopelessness
Identity, disturbed personal
Post-Trauma Syndrome
Post-Trauma Syndrome, risk for

Power, readiness for enhanced
Powerlessness
Powerlessness, risk for
Rape-Trauma Syndrome
Rape-Trauma Syndrome: compound reaction
Rape-Trauma Syndrome: silent reaction
Religiosity, impaired
Religiosity, ready for enhanced
Religiosity, risk for impaired
Relocation Stress Syndrome
Relocation Stress Syndrome, risk for
Self-Concept, readiness for enhanced
Self-Esteem, chronic low
Self-Esteem, situational low
Self-Esteem, risk for situational low
Sorrow, chronic
Spiritual Distress
Spiritual Distress, risk for
Spiritual Well-being, readiness for enhanced

ELIMINATION—Ability to excrete waste products

Diagnoses

Bowel Incontinence
Constipation
Constipation, perceived
Constipation, risk for
Diarrhea
Urinary Elimination, impaired
Urinary Elimination, readiness for enhanced

Urinary Incontinence, functional
Urinary Incontinence, overflow
Urinary Incontinence, reflex
Urinary Incontinence, stress
Urinary Incontinence, total
Urinary Incontinence, urge
Urinary Incontinence, risk for urge
Urinary Retention [acute/chronic]

FOOD/FLUID—Ability to maintain intake of and utilize nutrients and liquids to meet physiological needs

Diagnoses

Breastfeeding, effective
Breastfeeding, ineffective
Breastfeeding, interrupted
Dentition, impaired
Failure to Thrive, adult
Fluid Balance, readiness for enhanced
[Fluid Volume, deficient hyper/hypotonic]
Fluid Volume, deficient [isotonic]
Fluid Volume, excess
Fluid Volume, risk for deficient
Fluid Volume, risk for imbalanced
Glucose, risk for unstable blood

Infant Feeding Pattern, ineffective
Liver Function, risk for impaired
Nausea
Nutrition: less than body requirements, imbalanced
Nutrition: more than body requirements, imbalanced
Nutrition: more than body requirements, risk for imbalanced
Nutrition, readiness for enhanced
Oral Mucous Membrane, impaired
Swallowing, impaired

HYGIENE—Ability to perform basic activities of daily living

Continued

TABLE 8–1. **Nursing Diagnoses Organized According to Diagnostic Divisions** *(Continued)*

Diagnoses
Self-Care, readiness for enhanced
Self-Care Deficit: bathing/hygiene
Self-Care Deficit: dressing/grooming
Self-Care Deficit: feeding
Self-Care Deficit: toileting

NEUROSENSORY—Ability to perceive, integrate, and respond to internal and external cues
Diagnoses

Confusion, acute
Confusion, chronic
Confusion, risk for acute
Infant Behavior, disorganized
Infant Behavior, risk for disorganized
Infant Behavior, readiness for enhanced
  organized
Memory, impaired
Neglect, unilateral

Peripheral Neurovascular Dysfunction,
  risk for
Sensory Perception, disturbed (specify:
  visual, auditory, kinesthetic, gustatory,
  tactile, olfactory)
Stress Overload
Thought Processes, disturbed

PAIN/DISCOMFORT—Ability to control internal/external environment to maintain comfort
Diagnoses
Comfort, readiness for enhanced
Pain, acute
Pain, chronic

RESPIRATION—Ability to provide and use oxygen to meet physiological needs
Diagnoses
Airway Clearance, ineffective
Aspiration, risk for
Breathing Pattern, ineffective
Gas Exchange, impaired
Ventilation, impaired spontaneous
Ventilatory Weaning Response, dysfunctional

SAFETY—Ability to provide safe, growth-promoting environment

Allergy Response, latex
Allergy Response, risk for latex
Body Temperature, risk for imbalanced
Contamination
Contamination, risk for
Death Syndrome, risk for sudden infant
Environmental Interpretation Syndrome,
  impaired
Falls, risk for
Health Maintenance, ineffective
Home Maintenance, impaired
Hyperthermia
Hypothermia
Immunization Status, readiness for
  enhanced
Infection, risk for
Injury, risk for

Injury, risk for perioperative positioning
Mobility, impaired physical
Poisoning, risk for
Protection, ineffective
Self-Mutilation
Self-Mutilation, risk for
Skin Integrity, impaired
Skin Integrity, risk for impaired
Suffocation, risk for
Suicide, risk for
Surgical Recovery, delayed
Thermoregulation, ineffective
Tissue Integrity, impaired
Trauma, risk for
Violence, [actual/]risk for other-directed
Violence, [actual/]risk for self-directed
Wandering [specify sporadic or continual]

SEXUALITY—[Component of Ego Integrity and Social Interaction]—**Diagnoses**
Ability to meet requirements/characteristics of male/female role
Sexual Dysfunction
Sexuality Pattern, ineffective

SOCIAL INTERACTION—Ability to establish and maintain relationships

Diagnoses

Attachment, risk for impaired parent/child
Caregiver Role Strain
Caregiver Role Strain, risk for
Communication, impaired verbal
Communication, readiness for enhanced
Conflict, parental role
Coping, compromised family
Coping, disabled family
Coping, ineffective community
Coping, readiness for enhanced
  community

Coping, readiness for enhanced family
Family Processes: alcoholism,
  dysfunctional
Family Processes, interrupted
Family Processes, readiness for enhanced
Loneliness, risk for
Parenting, impaired
Parenting, risk for impaired
Role Performance, ineffective
Social Interaction, impaired
Social Isolation

TEACHING/LEARNING—Ability to incorporate and use information to achieve healthy lifestyle/optimal wellness

Diagnoses

Development, risk for delayed
Growth, risk for disproportionate
Growth and Development, delayed
Health-Seeking Behaviors (specify)
Knowledge, deficient [Learning Need]
  (specify)
Knowledge (specify), readiness for
  enhanced
Noncompliance [Adherence, ineffective]
  (specify)

Therapeutic Regimen Management,
  effective
Therapeutic Regimen Management,
  ineffective
Therapeutic Regimen Management:
  ineffective community
Therapeutic Regimen Management:
  ineffective family
Therapeutic Regimen Management,
  readiness for enhanced

BOX 8-1

Diagnostic Decision Making

1. Read the physician's admitting orders.
2. Review all of the data included in the 13 Diagnostic Divisions. Pay particular attention to Mr. Simmons' subjective data, which describe his perception of his illness and his responses to the various healthcare problems described.
3. Review the discharge considerations section at the end of the assessment tool. Can this information assist you in identifying his nursing diagnoses accurately?
4. Record or highlight any abnormal responses or observations identified while reviewing Mr. Simmons' assessment data.
5. Review the assessment tool's individual Diagnostic Divisions where you recorded or highlighted abnormal data.

Continued

BOX 8–1

Diagnostic Decision Making (*Continued*)

6. In those divisions where abnormal data were highlighted, review the nursing diagnoses associated with the Diagnostic Division (see Table 8–1).
7. Select a possible nursing diagnosis from the Diagnostic Division.
8. Review the defining characteristics of your selected possible nursing diagnosis (see Appendix I).
9. Compare the recorded or highlighted data with the selected nursing diagnosis' defining characteristics. Is there sufficient match? (Refer to Appendix C, Lunney's Scale.) "Yes": Move to step 10. "No": Return to the assessment tool, and ensure you have reviewed all the appropriate data. If your review is sufficient, then return to step 6 because another possible nursing diagnosis may be appropriate for consideration.
10. Once you have decided on an accurate nursing diagnosis, complete the client diagnostic statement by adding the related factor(s) specific to Mr. Simmons' situation (refer again to Appendix I).
11. Now develop a client outcome statement for Mr. Simmons' identified nursing diagnosis. Two options are available for this step.
    a. Look at the nursing diagnosis, and define how Mr. Simmons could resolve this identified response to his healthcare problem. For example, if his nursing diagnosis is Anxiety, an appropriate path in the development of an outcome statement would include "a reduction or elimination of his identified anxiety."
    b. A second strategy in outcome statement development is to review the *related factor(s)*, and develop an outcome reflecting either elimination or reduction of the related factor(s). For example, if the Anxiety is determined to be related to a change in health status, then his outcome statement could reflect a correction in health status or return to premorbid state, or in this case, more appropriately, an increase in Mr. Simmons' control of his condition.
12. Once you have developed the outcome statements for Mr. Simmons, select appropriate nursing interventions to assist him in achieving the desired outcome. Several methods can be employed to assist you in selecting nursing interventions.

    For example: Your assigned medical-surgical or fundamentals texts are excellent resources for nursing interventions and their rationales. Other resources include care planning guides (such as Doenges, Moorhouse, and Murr's *Nursing Care Plans*, ed 7, 2006) or nursing diagnosis handbooks (such as Doenges, Moorhouse, and Murr's *Nurse's Pocket Guide*, ed 11, 2008) that provide outcome statements and nursing interventions for each NANDA-I nursing diagnosis.
13. Repeat steps 6–12 for your second nursing diagnosis.

Case Study Care-Planning Worksheet

Use the case study care-planning worksheets to enter your two client diagnostic statements (NANDA-I nursing diagnosis label, the related factors [etiologies], and evidence of signs/symptoms you used in making the diagnosis) for Mr. Simmons. Then, use the worksheets to list two outcome statements for each of the diagnostic statements you identify for Mr. Simmons. Next, select at least three nursing interventions that will assist Mr. Simmons in achieving the two measurable outcome statements you have listed, and record them in the space provided on the worksheets.

The two-page Interactive Care Plan Worksheet can also assist you during this care-planning and evaluation exercise. Review the Time Out sections; information provided here will further assist you in accurately complying with the criteria required for developing accurate diagnostic statements, constructing client outcome statements, and selecting appropriate nursing interventions.

Care-Planning Evaluation Checklist

The evaluation checklist is included in this chapter to provide a workable guide for constructing Mr. Simmons' plan of care as well as for future use in care-planning assignments. The evaluation checklist was designed to include the criteria presented in the TIME OUT sections of the Interactive Care Plan Worksheets, the requirements of the ANA's Standards of Practice presented in the previous chapters, and the standards for JCAHO Management of Information. An additional copy of the checklist is included so that you will be able to take it with you to your assigned nursing unit and use it to help construct plans of care and evaluate your implementation of the steps of the nursing process. See Figure 8–1.

CRITERIA:	Yes	No	Instructor's Comments
1. Client assessment data include areas of biophysical, psychosocial, environmental, self-care, and/or discharge planning.			
2. Appropriate assessment techniques used (interviewing, questioning).			
3. Assessment data are documented in appropriate manner (nursing history form, progress note, flow sheet).			
4. Client diagnostic statement is accurately derived from assessment data.			
5. Client diagnostic statement is verified against NANDA-I defining characteristics and related factors.			
6. Client diagnostic statement is verified with client, significant other(s), and/or other healthcare providers.			
7. Client's desired outcome is derived from the identified diagnostic statement.			

Continued

FIGURE 8–1.   Evaluation checklist for Interactive Care Plan Worksheets. (Adapted in part from ANA Standards of Practice and the Joint Commission Standards for Management of Information.)

CRITERIA:	Yes	No	Instructor's Comments
8. Outcome is specific to the identified diagnostic statement.			
9. Outcome is realistic in relation to the client's current and potential resources and capabilities.			
10. Outcome is attainable in relation to the client's current and potential resources and capabilities.			
11. Outcome includes a realistic timeframe for attainment.			
12. Outcome is mutually formulated with client and/or significant other(s).			
13. Plan of care includes nursing interventions based on the identified client diagnostic statement and the desired outcome.			
14. Selected nursing interventions assist the client in attaining the desired outcome.			
15. Interventions include monitoring the client's response to the implemented nursing interventions.			
16. Interventions include monitoring the client's response toward the attainment of the outcome.			
17. Interventions include the qualifiers of who, what, how, amount, time, and frequency.			
18. The action verb describing the nursing intervention focuses on the nurse's behavior, not the client's.			
19. Interventions are implemented in a safe manner.			
20. Rationale included for a selected nursing intervention thoroughly explains the reason for selection and the desired effect of implementation.			
21. Reassessment is used to revise client diagnostic statements, desired outcomes, and/or nursing interventions.			
22. Evaluation includes the client's response to implemented nursing interventions.			
23. Evaluation includes the client's progress toward desired outcome attainment.			
24. Documentation of client care includes reassessment data.			
25. Documentation of client care includes reference to nursing interventions implemented.			
26. Documentation of client care includes reference to the client's response to nursing interventions.			

FIGURE 8–1. *Continued*

Use the evaluation checklist after you have documented your first attempts at identifying Mr. Simmons' two nursing diagnoses, his two measurable outcome statements, and the appropriate nursing interventions for each outcome statement.

Review the checklist's criteria against your completed case study care plan worksheet for feedback on how well your plan of care for Mr. Simmons is being accomplished.

Practicing Critical Thinking

Once you have worked through the exercise and completed your plan of care for Mr. Simmons, construct a mind map that demonstrates any linkages you have identified.

Conclusion

The nursing process steps described in this text are an integral part of the day-to-day science and practice of nursing. Regardless of the nursing practice setting you choose, the steps of the nursing process are universal in their application.

It is our hope that this interactive approach has been helpful in stimulating critical thinking and providing instruction on how to use the steps of the nursing process. The several interactive approaches were all designed to assist you in developing the necessary cognitive, affective, and psychomotor learning skills required to successfully apply the decision-making steps in the nursing process. We extend our best wishes to you as you begin your nursing career.

Putting Together What You Have Learned About the Nursing Process

Review the following vignette and nursing history. Then, create a plan of care for your client, Mr. Simmons. Identify two client needs, and write the client diagnostic statement and two outcomes. Choose three interventions for each client diagnostic statement.

VIGNETTE: Mr. R. Simmons, who has had type 2 diabetes for 10 years, presented to his physician with a nonhealing ulcer on his left foot of 3 weeks' duration. Screening studies done in the physician's office revealed blood glucose (BG) of 356 per fingerstick and urine Chemstix of 2%. Because of distance from a medical provider and lack of local community services, Mr. Simmons is admitted to the hospital.

Admitting Physician's Orders
Culture/sensitivity and Gram stain of foot ulcer
Random blood glucose on admission and fingerstick BG qid
CBC, electrolytes, serum lipid profile, glycosylated Hb in a.m.
Chest x-ray and ECG in a.m.
Diabeta 10 mg PO bid
Glucophage 500 mg PO daily to start—will increase gradually
Humulin N 10 U q a.m. and hs. Begin insulin instruction for post-discharge self-care if necessary
Dicloxacillin 500 mg PO q6h; start after culture obtained
Darvocet-N 100 mg PO q4h prn for pain
Diet—2400 calories/3 meals with 2 snacks

Arrange consultation with dietitian
Up in chair ad lib with feet elevated
Foot cradle for bed
Irrigate lesion L foot with NS tid, then cover with wet-to-dry sterile dressing
Vital signs qid

Client Assessment Database

Name: R. Simmons **Informant:** Client
Reliability (Scale 1–4): 3
Age: 70   **DOB:** 5/3/37   **Race:** Caucasian   **Gender:** M
Adm. date: 6/28/08 **Time:** 7 p.m.   **From:** Home

ACTIVITY/REST

Reports (Subjective)

Occupation: Farmer
Usual activities/hobbies: Reading, playing cards. "Don't have time to do much. Anyway, I'm
  too tired most of the time to do anything after the chores."
Limitations imposed by illness: "I have to watch what I order if I eat out."
Sleep: Hours: 6–8 hr/night
Naps: No
Aids: No
Insomnia: "Not unless I drink coffee after supper." Usually feels rested when awakens at
  4:30 a.m. but has been feeling fatigued last several weeks. Up 1 or 2 times at night to void.

Exhibits (Objective)

Observed response to activity: Limps, favors L foot when walking
Mental status: Alert/active
Neuro/muscular assessment: Muscle mass/tone: Bilaterally equal/firm
Posture: Erect
ROM: Full, all extremities
Strength: Equal three extremities/favors L leg & foot currently

CIRCULATION

Reports (Subjective)

History of slow healing: Lesion L foot, 3 weeks' duration
Extremities: Numbness/tingling: "My feet feel cold and tingling like sharp pins poking the
  bottom of my feet when I walk the quarter mile to the mailbox."
Cough/character of sputum: Occ./white
Change in frequency/amount of urine: Yes/voiding more lately

Exhibits (Objective)

Peripheral pulses: Radials 3+; popliteal, dorsalis, postibial/pedal, all 1+
B/P: R: Lying: 146/90/**Sit:** 140/86/**Stand:** 138/90
    L: Lying: 142/88/**Sit:** 138/88/**Stand:** 138/84
Pulse: Apical: 86/**Radial:** 86/**Quality:** Strong/**Rhythm:** Regular
Chest auscultations: Few wheezes clear with cough, no murmurs/rubs
Jugular vein distention: -0-
Extremities:
  Temperature: Feet cool bilat./legs warm

Color: Skin: Legs pale
Capillary refill: Slow both feet (approx 4 sec)
Homans' sign: -0-
Varicosities: Few enlarged superficial veins both calves
Nails: Toenails thickened, yellow, brittle
Distribution and quality of hair: Coarse hair to midcalf, none on ankles/toes
Color:
　General: Ruddy face/arms
　Mucous membranes/lips: Pink
　Nailbeds: Blanch well
　Conjunctiva and sclera: White

EGO INTEGRITY
Reports (Subjective)
Stress factors: "Normal farmer's problems: weather, pests, bankers, etc."
Ways of handling stress: "I get busy with the chores and talk things over with my livestock, they listen pretty good."
Financial concerns: Has Medicare but no supplemental or disability insurance; needs to hire someone to do chores while in hospital.
Relationship status: Married
Cultural factors: Rural/agrarian, eastern European descent, "American, no ethnic ties."
Religion: Protestant/practicing
Lifestyle: Middle class/self-sufficient farmer
Recent changes: No
Feelings: "I'm in control of most things, except the weather and this diabetes now." Concerned about possible therapy change "from pills to shots."
Exhibits (Objective)
Emotional status: Generally calm; appears frustrated at times
Observed physiological response(s): Occasionally sighs deeply/frowns, shrugs shoulders/throws up hands, shoulders tense, fidgeting with coin

ELIMINATION
Reports (Subjective)
Usual bowel pattern: Most every p.m.
Last BM: Last night
Character of stool: Firm/brown
Bleeding: -0-
Hemorrhoids: -0-
Constipation: Occ.
Laxative used: Hot prune juice on occ.
Urinary: No problems; has been voiding more frequently/gets up 1 or 2 times to void during night
Character of urine: Pale yellow
Exhibits (Objective)
Abd. tender: No/**Soft/firm:** Soft/**Palpable mass:** None
Bowel sounds: Active all four quads

FOOD/FLUID

Reports (Subjective)

Usual diet (type): 2400 ADA (occ. "cheats" with dessert; "My wife watches it pretty closely.")

No. of meals daily: 3/1 snack

Dietary pattern:

B: Fruit juice/toast/ham/decaf coffee

L: Meat/potatoes/veg/fruit/milk

D: Meat sandwich/soup/fruit/decaf coffee

Snack: Milk/crackers at hs.

Usual beverage: skim milk, 2 to 3 cups decaf coffee, and drinks "a lot of water—several qts"

Last meal/intake: Dinner: Hot roast beef sandwich, vegetable soup, pear with cheese, decaf coffee

Loss of appetite: "Never, but lately I don't feel as hungry as usual."

Nausea/vomiting: -0- **Food allergies:** None

Heartburn/food intolerance: Cabbage causes gas, coffee after supper causes heartburn

Mastication/swallowing probs: No/**Dentures:** Partial upper plate—fits well

Usual weight: around 175/**Recent changes:** Has lost about 6 lb this month

Diuretic therapy: No

Exhibits (Objective)

Wt: 170 lb/**Ht:** 5'10"/**Build:** Stocky/**Skin turgor:** Good/leathery

Appearance of tongue: Midline, pink/**Mucous membranes:** Pink, moist

Condition of teeth/gums: Good, no irritation/bleeding noted

Breath sounds: Few wheezes cleared with cough

Bowel sounds: Active all four quads

Urine Chemstix 2%/Fingerstick 356 (physician office) 450 random BG drawn on adm

HYGIENE

Reports (Subjective)

Activities of daily living: Independent in all areas

Preferred time of bath: p.m.

Exhibits (Objective)

General appearance: Clean, shaven, short cut hair, hands rough and dry, skin on feet dry, cracked, and scaly; no body odor

Scalp & eyebrows: Scaly white patches

NEUROSENSORY

Reports (Subjective)

Headache: "Occasionally behind my eyes when I worry too much."

Tingling/Numbness: Feet, 4 or 5 times/week (as noted)

Eyes: Vision loss; far-sighted, "seems a little blurry now"

Exam: 2 yr ago

Ears: Hearing loss/**R:** "Some"/**L:** No (has not been tested)

Nose: Epistaxis: -0-

Sense of smell: "No problem"

Exhibits (Objective)

Mental status: Alert; oriented to time, place, person, situation

Affect: Concerned

Memory: Remote/Recent: Clear and intact
Speech: Clear/coherent, appropriate
Pupil reaction: PERLA/small
Glasses: Reading
Hearing Aid: No
Handgrip/release: Strong/equal
PAIN/DISCOMFORT
Reports (Subjective)
Primary focus: Medial aspect, heel of L foot
Intensity (0–10): 4–5/**Quality:** Dull ache with occ. sharp stabbing sensation
Frequency/duration: "Seems like all the time."
Radiation: No
Precipitating factors: Shoes, walking
How relieved: ASA, not helping
Additional concerns: Sometimes has back pain following chores/heavy lifting, relieved by ASA/ liniment rubdown; knees ache at times, uses topical heat ointment
Exhibits (Objective)
Facial grimacing: When lesion border palpated
Guarding affected area: Pulls foot away
Narrowed focus: No
Emotional response: Tense, irritated
RESPIRATION
Reports (Subjective)
Dyspnea: -0-
Cough: occ. morning cough, white sputum
Emphysema: -0-/**Bronchitis:** -0-/**Asthma:** -0-/**Tuberculosis:** -0-
Smoker: Filters/**Pack/day:** 1/2/**No. of pack years:** 25+
Use of respiratory aids: -0-
Exhibits (Objective)
Respiratory rate: 22/**Depth:** Good/**Symmetry:** Equal, bilateral
Auscultation: Few wheezes, clear with cough
Cyanosis: -0-
Clubbing of fingers: -0-
Sputum characteristics: None to observe
Mentation/restlessness: Alert/oriented/relaxed
SAFETY
Reports (Subjective)
Allergies: -0-
Blood transfusions: -0-
Sexually transmitted disease: None
Risk behavior: Wears seat belt
Fractures/dislocations: L clavicle, 1967/age 40, fell getting off tractor
Arthritis/unstable joints: "I think I've got some in my knees."
Back problems: Occ. lower back pain
Vision impaired: Requires glasses for reading

Hearing impaired: Slightly (R), compensates by turning "good ear" toward speaker

Exhibits (Objective)

Temperature: 99.4°F (37.4°C) tympanic

Skin integrity: Impaired L foot

Scars: R inguinal, surgical

Rashes: -0-/**Bruises:** -0-/**Lacerations:** -0-/**Blisters:** -0-

Ulcerations: Medial aspect L heel, 2.5 cm diameter, approx. 3 mm deep, wound edges inflamed, draining sm. amt. cream-color/pink-tinged matter, slight musty odor noted

Strength (general): Equal all extremities

Muscle tone: firm

ROM: Good/**Gait:** Favors L foot/**Paresthesia/Paralysis:** Tingling, prickly sensation in feet after walking ¼ mile

Immunizations: Current flu/pneumonia 3 yr ago/tetanus 8 yr ago "maybe"

SEXUALITY: MALE

Reports (Subjective)

Sexually active: Yes

Use of condoms: No (monogamous)

Recent changes in frequency/interest: "I've been too tired lately."

Penile discharge: -0-

Prostate disorder: -0-

Vasectomy: -0-

Last proctoscopic exam: about 2 yr ago

Prostate exam: about 1 yr ago

Practice self-exam: Breast/testicles: No

Problems/concerns: "I don't have any problems, but you'd have to ask my wife if there are any complaints."

Exhibits (Objective)

Exam: Breast: no masses/**Testicles:** deferred/**Prostate:** deferred

SOCIAL INTERACTION

Reports (Subjective)

Marital status: Married 45 yr/**Living with:** Wife

Report of problems: None

Extended family: One daughter lives in town (30 miles away); one daughter married/grandson, living out of state

Other: Several couples; wife and he play cards/socialize 2–3 times/month

Role: Works farm alone; husband/father/grandfather

Report of concerns related to illness/condition: None until now

Coping behaviors: "My wife and I have always talked things out. You know the 11th commandment is 'Thou shalt not go to bed angry.'"

Exhibits (Objective)

Speech: Clear, intelligible

Verbal/nonverbal communication with family/SO(s): Speaks quietly with wife, looking her in the eye; relaxed posture

Family interaction patterns: Wife sitting at bedside, relaxed, both reading paper, making occasional comments to each other

TEACHING/LEARNING
Reports (Subjective)
Dominant language: English/**Second language:** no/**Literate:** Yes

Education level: 2 years of college

Health and illness beliefs/practices/customs: "I take care of the minor problems and see the doctor only when something's broken."

Advance directives: Yes—wife to bring in

Durable medical power of attorney: Wife

Familial risk factors/relationship:
  Diabetes: Maternal uncle/**Tuberculosis:** Brother died age 27
  Heart disease: Father died, age 78, heart attack
  Strokes: Mother died age 81/**High B/P:** Mother

Prescribed medications: Drug: Diabeta/**Dose:** 10 mg/**Schedule:** 8 a.m./6 p.m. Last dose 6 p.m. today/**Purpose:** Control diabetes

Does client take medications regularly? Yes

Home glucose monitoring: "Only using Tes Tape, stopped some months ago when I ran out of TesTape. It was always negative anyway."

Nonprescription (OTC) drugs: Occ. ASA

Herbals/supplements: None

Use of alcohol (amount/frequency): Socially, occ. beer

Tobacco: Smokes 1/2 pack/day **Smokeless:** No

Admitting diagnosis (physician): Hyperglycemia with nonhealing lesion L foot

Reason for hospitalization (client): "Sore on foot, and the doctor is concerned about my blood sugar, and says I'm supposed to learn this fingerstick test now."

History of current concern: "Three weeks ago I got a blister on my foot from breaking in my new boots. It got sore so I lanced it, but it isn't getting any better."

Client's expectations of this hospitalization: "Clear up this infection and control my diabetes."

Other relevant illness and/or previous hospitalizations/surgeries: 1969 R inguinal hernia repair

Evidence of failure to improve: Lesion L foot, 3 wk

Last physical exam: Complete about 1 yr ago, office follow-up 5 mo ago

DISCHARGE CONSIDERATIONS (AS OF 6/28)
Anticipated discharge: 7/1/08 (3 days)

Resources: Self; wife

Financial: "If this doesn't take too long to heal, we got some savings to cover things."

Community supports: Diabetic Support Group (has not participated)

Anticipated lifestyle changes: Become more involved in management of condition

Assistance needed: May require farm help for several days

Teaching: Learn new medication regimen and wound care; review diet, encourage smoking cessation

Referral: Supplies: Downtown pharmacy or AARP

Equipment: Glucometer—AARP

Follow-up: Primary care provider 1 wk after discharge to evaluate wound healing and potential need for additional changes in diabetic regimen

INTERACTIVE CARE PLAN WORKSHEET

Student Name:

NURSING DIAGNOSIS	Client's Medical Diagnosis:
DEFINITION:	
DEFINITION: CHARACTERISTICS:	
RELATED FACTORS:	
STUDENT INSTRUCTIONS:	In the space below, enter the subjective and objective data gathered during your client assessment.

ASSESSMENT

Subjective Data Entry	Objective Data Entry

TIME OUT!

Student Instructions: To be sure your client diagnostic statement written below is accurate you need to review the defining characteristics and related factors associated with the nursing diagnosis and see how your client data match. Do you have an accurate match or are additional data required, or does another nursing diagnosis need to be investigated?

DIAGNOSIS

CLIENT DIAGNOSTIC STATEMENT:	Nursing Diagnosis (specify) _____
	_____
	Related to _____
	_____
	_____

FIGURE 8–2a.

Desired Outcome The Client will:
and Client Criteria:

P L A N N I N G

TIME OUT!	The desired outcome must meet criteria to be accurate. The outcome must be specific, realistic, measurable, and include a time frame for completion. Does the action verb describe the client's behavior to be evaluated? Can the outcome be used in the evaluation step of the nursing process to measure the client's response to the nursing interventions listed below?
Interventions	**Rationale for Selected Intervention and References**

E V A L U A T I O N

TIME OUT!	Do your interventions assist in achieving the desired outcome? Do your interventions address further monitoring of the client's response to your interventions and to the achievement of the desired outcome? Are qualifiers: when, how, amount, time, and frequency used? Is the focus of the action's verb on the nurse's actions and not on the client? Do your rationales provide sufficient reason and directions?

What was your client's response to the interventions?

Was the desired outcome achieved? If no, what revisions to either the desired outcome or interventions would you make?
☐ Yes ☐ No

D O C U M E N T A T I O N

Documentation Focus: Now that you have completed the evaluation, the next step is to document your care and the client's response. Use the areas below to enter your progress note information.

Reassessment Data:

Interventions Implemented:

Client's Response:

INSTRUCTOR'S COMMENTS:

FIGURE 8–2b.

INTERACTIVE CARE PLAN WORKSHEET

Student Name:

Client's Medical Diagnosis:

NURSING DIAGNOSIS	
DEFINITION:	
DEFINITION: CHARACTERISTICS:	
RELATED FACTORS:	
STUDENT INSTRUCTIONS:	In the space below, enter the subjective and objective data gathered during your client assessment.

A S S E S S M E N T	Subjective Data Entry	Objective Data Entry

TIME OUT!	**Student Instructions:** To be sure your client diagnostic statement written below is accurate you need to review the defining characteristics and related factors associated with the nursing diagnosis and see how your client data match. Do you have an accurate match or are additional data required, or does another nursing diagnosis need to be investigated?

D I A G N O S I S	**CLIENT DIAGNOSTIC STATEMENT:**	**Nursing Diagnosis (specify)** _____ _____ **Related to** _____ _____

FIGURE 8–3a.

Desired Outcome and Client Criteria: The Client will:		
TIME OUT!	The desired outcome must meet criteria to be accurate. The outcome must be specific, realistic, measurable, and include a time frame for completion. Does the action verb describe the client's behavior to be evaluated? Can the outcome be used in the evaluation step of the nursing process to measure the client's response to the nursing interventions listed below?	
	Interventions	**Rationale for Selected Intervention and References**
TIME OUT!	Do your interventions assist in achieving the desired outcome? Do your interventions address further monitoring of the client's response to your interventions and to the achievement of the desired outcome? Are qualifiers: when, how, amount, time, and frequency used? Is the focus of the action's verb on the nurse's actions and not on the client? Do your rationales provide sufficient reason and directions?	
What was your client's response to the interventions?		
Was the desired outcome achieved? ☐ Yes ☐ No If no, what revisions to either the desired outcome or interventions would you make?		
Documentation Focus: Now that you have completed the evaluation, the next step is to document your care and the client's response. Use the areas below to enter your progress note information.		
Reassessment Data:		
Interventions Implemented:		
Client's Response:		

P L A N N I N G

E V A L U A T I O N

D O C U M E N T A T I O N

INSTRUCTOR'S COMMENTS:

FIGURE 8–3b.

INTERACTIVE CARE PLAN WORKSHEET   **Student Name:**

NURSING DIAGNOSIS   Client's Medical Diagnosis:

DEFINITION:

DEFINITION: CHARACTERISTICS:

RELATED FACTORS:

STUDENT INSTRUCTIONS: In the space below, enter the subjective and objective data gathered during your client assessment.

Subjective Data Entry

Objective Data Entry

A S S E S S M E N T

TIME OUT!

Student Instructions: To be sure your client diagnostic statement written below is accurate you need to review the defining characteristics and related factors associated with the nursing diagnosis and see how your client data match. Do you have an accurate match or are additional data required, or does another nursing diagnosis need to be investigated?

CLIENT DIAGNOSTIC STATEMENT:

Nursing Diagnosis (specify) _____

_____

Related to _____

_____

D I A G N O S I S

FIGURE 8–4a.

P L A N N I N G

Desired Outcome and Client Criteria: The Client will:

TIME OUT! The desired outcome must meet criteria to be accurate. The outcome must be specific, realistic, measurable, and include a time frame for completion. Does the action verb describe the client's behavior to be evaluated? Can the outcome be used in the evaluation step of the nursing process to measure the client's response to the nursing interventions listed below?

Interventions	Rationale for Selected Intervention and References

E V A L U A T I O N

TIME OUT! Do your interventions assist in achieving the desired outcome? Do your interventions address further monitoring of the client's response to your interventions and to the achievement of the desired outcome? Are qualifiers: when, how, amount, time, and frequency used? Is the focus of the action's verb on the nurse's actions and not on the client? Do your rationales provide sufficient reason and directions?

What was your client's response to the interventions?

Was the desired outcome achieved?   If no, what revisions to either the desired outcome or interventions would you make?
☐ Yes ☐ No

D O C U M E N T A T I O N

Documentation Focus: Now that you have completed the evaluation, the next step is to document your care and the client's response. Use the areas below to enter your progress note information.

Reassessment Data:

Interventions Implemented:

Client's Response:

INSTRUCTOR'S COMMENTS:

FIGURE 8–4b.

Appendix A

Code for Nurses

1. The nurse, in all professional relationships, practices with compassion and respect for the inherent dignity, worth, and uniqueness of every individual, unrestricted by considerations of social or economic status, personal attributes, or the nature of health problems.
2. The nurse's primary commitment is to the patient, whether an individual, family, group, or community.
3. The nurse promotes, advocates for, and strives to protect the health, safety, and rights of the patient.
4. The nurse is responsible and accountable for individual nursing practice and determines the appropriate delegation of tasks consistent with the nurse's obligation to provide optimum patient care.
5. The nurse owes the same duties to self as to others, including the responsibility to preserve integrity and safety, to maintain competence, and to continue personal and professional growth.
6. The nurse participates in establishing, maintaining, and improving health care environments and conditions of employment conducive to the provision of quality health care and consistent with the values of the profession through individual and collective action.
7. The nurse participates in the advancement of the profession through contributions to practice, education, administration, and knowledge development.
8. The nurse collaborates with other health professionals and the public in promoting community, national, and international efforts to meet health needs.
9. The profession of nursing, as represented by associations and their members, is responsible for articulating nursing values, for maintaining the integrity of the profession and its practice, and for shaping social policy.

Reprinted with permission from Code of Ethics for Nurses, 2001, American Nurses Association, Washington, DC.

General Assessment Tool

This is a suggested guideline/tool that may be used in most care settings for creating a client database. It provides a nursing focus (Doenges & Moorhouse's Diagnostic Divisions of Nursing Diagnoses) that will facilitate planning client care. Although the sections are alphabetized for ease of presentation, they can be prioritized or rearranged to meet individual needs.

ADULT MEDICAL/SURGICAL ASSESSMENT TOOL

General Information
Name:_____ Age:_____ DOB:_____
Gender:_____ Race: _____
Admission Date:_____ Time:_____ From:_____
Reason for this visit/admission (primary concern):_____
Source of Information:_____
Reliability (1–4 with 4 = very reliable):_____

Activity/Rest

SUBJECTIVE (REPORTS)
Occupation:_____
Able to participate in usual activities/hobbies:__
Leisure time/diversional activities:_____
Ambulatory:_____ Gait (describe):_____
Activity level (sedentary to very active):_____
Daily exercise (type):_____
Changes in muscle mass/tone/strength:_____
History of problems/limitations imposed by condition (e.g, immobility, weakness, breathlessness, fatigue):_____
Feelings (e.g., exhaustion, restlessness, boredom, dissatisfaction):_____
Developmental factors (e.g., delayed/age):_____
_____
Sleep: Hours:_____ Naps:_____ Aids:_____
  Insomnia:_____ Related to:_____
  Difficulty falling asleep:_____
  Difficulty staying asleep:_____
  Rested on awakening:_____

Excessive grogginess:____ Bedtime rituals:_____
Relaxation techniques:_____
Sleeps on more than one pillow:_____
Use of oxygen (type):_____
  When used:_____
Medications or herbals for/affecting sleep:_____

OBJECTIVE (EXHIBITS)

Observed response to activity: Heart rate:_____
  Rhythm (reg/irreg):_____
  Blood pressure:_____ Respiratory rate:____
  Pulse oximetry:_____
Mental status (e.g., cognitive impairment, with-
  drawn/lethargic):_____
Neuromuscular assessment: Muscle mass/tone:___
_____
Posture (e.g., normal, stooped, curved spine):___
_____ Tremors (location):_____
ROM:_____ Strength:_____
Deformity:_____
Mobility aids (list):_____

Circulation

SUBJECTIVE (REPORTS)

History of/treatment for: High blood pressure:___
  Brain injury:_____ Stroke:_____
  Heart condition/surgery:_____
  Rheumatic fever:_____ Palpitations:_____
  Syncope:_____ Claudication:_____
  Ankle/leg edema:_____ Blood clots:_____
  Bleeding tendencies:_____
  Dysreflexia episodes (describe):_____
  Slow healing (describe):_____
Extremities: Numbness (location):_____
Tingling (location):_____
Cough (describe)/hemoptysis:_____
Change in frequency/amount of urine:_____
_____
Medications/herbals:_____
_____

OBJECTIVE (EXHIBITS)

Color (e.g., pale, cyanotic, jaundiced, mottled,
  ruddy): Skin:_____
  Mucous membranes:_____ Lips:_____
  Nailbeds:____ Conjunctiva: ____ Sclera:____
Skin moisture: (e.g., dry, diaphoretic):_____

BP: (R & L): Lying:_____ Sitting:_____
  Standing:_____ Pulse pressure:_____
Auscultatory gap:_____
Pulses (Palpated 1–4 strength): Carotid:_____
  Temporal:_____ Jugular:____ Radial: _____
  Femoral:____ Popliteal:_____ Post-tibial:____
  Dorsalis pedis: _____
Cardiac (palpation): Thrill:_____
  Heaves:_____
  Heart sounds (auscultation): Rate:_____
  Rhythm:____ Quality:____ Friction rub:_____
  Murmur (describe location/sounds):_____
Vascular bruit (location):_____
Jugular vein distention:_____
Breath sounds (describe location & sounds):____
_____
Extremities: Temperature:_____ Color:_____
  Capillary refill (1–3 sec):_____
  Homan's sign (+ or –):_____
  Varicosities (location):_____
  Nail abnormalities:_____
  Edema (+1 to +4): _____
  Distibution/quality of hair:_____
  Trophic skin changes: _____

Ego Integrity

SUBJECTIVE (REPORTS)

Relationship status:_____
Expressed concerns (e.g., financial, relationships;
  recent or anticipated lifestyle or role changes):
_____
Stress factors:_____
Usual ways of handling stress:_____
Expression of feelings of: Anger:_____
  Anxiety:_____ Fear:_____
  Grief: _____ Helplessness:_____
  Hopelessness:_____ Powerlessness:_____
Cultural factors/ethnic ties:_____
Religious affiliation:_____ Active/practicing:___
Practices prayer/meditation:_____
Religious/Spiritual concerns:_____
Desires clergy visit:_____
Expression of sense of connectedness/harmony
  with self and others:_____
Medications/herbals:_____

OBJECTIVE (EXHIBITS)
Emotional status (check those that apply):
Calm:__ Anxious:___ Angry:___ Withdrawn:__
  Fearful:__ Irritable:__ Restive:__ Euphoric:__
Observed body language:_____
Observed physiological responses (e.g., crying, change in voice quality/volume):_____
Changes in energy field: Temperature:_____
  Color:_____ Distribution:_____
  Movement: _____ Sounds:_____

Elimination

SUBJECTIVE (REPORTS)
Usual bowel elimination pattern _____
  Character of stool (e.g., hard, soft, liquid): ___
  Stool color (e.g., brown, black, yellow, clay colored, tarry):_____
Last BM and character of stool:_____
History of bleeding:____ Hemorrhoids/fistula:___
  Constipation (acute/chronic):_____
  Diarrhea (acute/chronic):_____
  Bowel incontinence:_____
Laxative use:_____ How often:_____
  Enema/suppository:_____ How often:_____
Usual voiding pattern _____
  Urgency:_____ Frequency:_____
  Difficulty voiding: _____ Retention:_____
  Bladder spasms:_____ Pain/burning:_____
  Urinary incontinence (associated activity/time of day, etc.):_____
Character of urine:_____
History of kidney/bladder disease:_____
Diuretic use:_____
Other medications/herbals:_____

OBJECTIVE (EXHIBITS)
Abdomen (palpation): Soft/firm:_____
  Distention:_____
  Tenderness/pain (quadrant location):_____
  Palpable mass:_____ CVA tenderness:___
  Size/girth:_____
Abdomen (auscultation): Bowel sounds (Location/type):_____
Bladder palpable:____ Residual (per scan):_____

Overflow voiding:_____
Rectal sphincter tone (describe):_____
Hemorrhoids/fistulas:_____
Stool in rectum:_____
Impaction:_____
Occult blood: (+ or –):_____
Presence/use of catheter or continence devices:
  _____
Ostomy appliances (describe appliance and location):_____

Food/Fluid

SUBJECTIVE (REPORTS)
Usual diet (type):_____ Calorie/carbohydrate/protein/fat-g/day:_____
No. meals daily:_____ Snacks (no. daily, time consumed & type):_____
Last meal consumed/content:_____
Food preferences:_____
Food allergies/intolerances:_____
Cultural or religious food preparation concerns/prohibitions:_____
Usual appetite:_____ Change in appetite:_____
Usual weight:_____ Unexpected/undesired weight loss or gain:_____
Nausea/vomiting:_____ Related to?_____
Heartburn/indigestion:_____ Related to?_____
  Relieved by?_____
Chewing/swallowing problems:_____
Gag/swallow reflex (present):_____
Facial injury/surgery:_____ Stroke/other neurological deficit:_____
Teeth: Normal:_____ Dentures (full/partial):___
Loose/absent teeth:___ Sore mouth/gums:_____
Dental hygiene practices:_____
Professional dental care/frequency:_____
Diabetes/type:_____ Controlled with diet/pills/insulin:_____
Vitamin/food supplement use:_____
Medications/herbals:_____

OBJECTIVE (EXHIBITS)
Current weight:_____ Height:_____
Body build:_____ Body fat %:_____
Skin turgor (e.g, firm, supple, dehydrated):_____

Mucous membranes (moist/dry):_____
Edema (describe): Generalized:_____
    Dependent:_____ Feet/ankles:_____
    Periorbital:_____ Abdominal/ascites:_____
Jugular vein distention:_____
Breath sounds (auscultation)/location: Normal:
    _____ Faint/distant:_____ Crackles:_____
    Wheezes:_____
Condition of teeth/gums:_____ Appearance of
    tongue:_____ Mucous membranes:_____
Abdomen: Bowel sounds (quadrant location/
    type):_____ Hernia/masses:_____
Urine S/A or Chemstix:_____
Serum glucose (Glucometer):_____

Hygiene

SUBJECTIVE (REPORTS)
Ability to carry out activities of daily living:
Independent/dependent (level 1, no assistance
needed; to level 4, completely dependent):
Mobility:____ Needs assistance (describe):_____
    Assistance provided by:_____
    Equipment/prosthetic devices required:_____
Feeding:_____ Needs assistance (describe):_____
    Assistive devices:_____
    Hygiene:_____
    Needs assistance (describe):_____
    Preferred time of personal care/bath:_____
Dressing/grooming:_____
    Needs assistance (describe):_____
Toileting:_____ Needs assistance with
    (describe): _____

OBJECTIVE (EXHIBITS)
General appearance: Manner of dress:_____
Grooming/personal habits:_____
Condition of hair/scalp:_____ Body odor:_____
Presence of vermin (e.g., lice, scabies):_____

Neurosensory

SUBJECTIVE (REPORTS)
History of brain injury, trauma, stroke (residual
    effects):_____
Fainting spells/dizziness:_____
Headaches (location/type/frequency):_____

Tingling/numbness/weakness (location):_____
Seizures:_____ History/onset:_____
    Type (e.g., generalized, partial):_____
    Frequency:_____ Aura (describe):_____
    Postictal state:_____ How controlled:_____
Vision loss/changes:_____
Glasses/contacts: _____ Last exam:_____
Glaucoma: _____ Cataract:_____
Eye surgery (type/date): _____
Hearing loss:_____ Sudden or gradual:_____
Hearing aids:_____ Last exam:_____
Sense of smell (changes):_____
Epistaxis:_____
Sense of taste (changes):_____
Other:_____

OBJECTIVE (EXHIBITS)
Mental status (note duration of change):
    Oriented/disoriented: Time:_____ Place:____
    Person:_____ Situation:_____
    Check all that apply: Alert:_____ Drowsy:_____
    Lethargic:_____ Stuporous:_____ Comatose:____
    Cooperative:_____ Follows commands:_____
    Agitated/Restless:_____ Combative:_____
    Delusions (describe):_____
    Hallucinations (describe):_____
    Affect (describe):_____ Speech:_____
    Memory: Recent:_____ Remote:_____
Pupil shape:_____ Size/Reaction: R/L:_____
Accommodation:_____ Facial droop:_____
Swallowing: _____
Handgrasp/release, R/L:_____ Deep tendon
    reflexes (present/absent/location):_____
Coordination:_____ Balance:_____
Walking:_____ Tremors:_____
Posturing:_____ Paralysis (L/R):_____

Pain/Discomfort

SUBJECTIVE (REPORTS)
Primary focus: Location:_____
Intensity (use pain scale or pictures):_____
Quality (e.g., stabbing, aching, burning):_____
    Radiation:_____ Frequency:_____
    Duration:_____ Acceptable/manageable
    pain level:_____

Precipitating/aggravating factors:_____
How relieved (including nonpharmaceuticals/
therapies):_____
Associated symptoms (e.g., nausea, sleep problems,
photosensitivity):_____
Effect on daily activities:_____
    Relationships: _____ Job:_____
    Enjoyment of life:_____
Additional pain focus/describe:_____
Cultural expectations regarding pain perception
and expression:_____

OBJECTIVE (EXHIBITS)
Facial grimacing:_____
Guarding affected area:_____ Posturing:_____
Behaviors:_____ Narrowed focus:_____
Emotional response (e.g., crying, withdrawal,
anger):_____
Vitals sign changes (acute pain): BP:_____
    Pulse:_____ Respirations:_____

Respiration

SUBJECTIVE (REPORTS)
Dyspnea/related to:___ Precipitating factors:___
Relieving factors:_____ Airway clearance (e.g.,
spontaneous/device):_____
Cough/describe (e.g., hard, persistent, croupy): __
Produces sputum (describe color/character):____
Requires suctioning:_____
History of (year): Bronchitis:____ Asthma:____
    Emphysema:_____ Tuberculosis:_____
    Recurrent pneumonia:_____ Exposure to
noxious fumes/allergens, infectious agents/
diseases, poisons:_____
Smoker:____ packs/day:____ No. pack years:___
Cigar use:_____
Use of respiratory aids:_____
Oxygen (type & frequency):_____
Medications/herbals:_____

OBJECTIVE (EXHIBITS)
Respirations (spontaneous/assisted):___ Rate:___
    Depth:_____Chest excursion (e.g., equal/
symmetrical):_____ Use of accessory muscles:
_____ Nasal flaring:____ Fremitus:____ Breath
sounds (describe):_____ Egophony:_____

Skin/mucous membrane color (e.g., pale, cya-
notic):_____ Clubbing of fingers:_____
Sputum characteristics:_____
Mentation (e.g., calm, anxious, restless):_____
Pulse oximetry:_____

Safety

SUBJECTIVE REPORTS
Allergies/sensitivity (medications, foods, environ-
ment, latex):_____
    Type of reaction:_____
Blood transfusion/number:_____ Date:_____
    Reaction (describe):_____
Exposure to infectious diseases (e.g., measles,
influenza, pink eye):_____
Exposure to pollution, toxins, poisons/pesticides,
radiation (describe reactions):_____
Geographic areas lived in/recent travel:_____
Immunization history/date: Tetanus:_____
    MMR: _____ Polio:_____ Hepatitis:_____
    Pneumonia:_____Influenza:_____
    HPV:_____
Altered/suppressed immune system (list cause):
_____
History of sexually transmitted disease (date/
type):_____ Testing:_____
High-risk behaviors (specify):_____
Uses seat belt regularly:_____ Uses helmets/other
safety devices:_____
Workplace safety/health issues (describe):_____
Occupation:_____ Currently working:_____
Rate working conditions (e.g., safety, noise,
heating, water, ventilation, etc.):_____
History of accidental injuries:_____
Fractures/dislocations:_____
Arthritis/unstable joints:_____
Back problems:_____
Skin problems (e.g., rashes, lesions, moles, breast
lumps, enlarged nodes)/describe:_____
Delayed healing (describe):_____
Cognitive limitations (e.g., disorientation, con-
fusion):_____
Sensory limitations (e.g., impaired vision/hearing,
detecting heat/cold, taste, smell, touch):_____
_____

Prosthesis:_____
Ambulatory devices: _____
Violence (episodes or tendencies):_____

OBJECTIVE (EXHIBITS)
Body temperature/method (e.g., oral, rectal, tympanic):_____
Skin integrity (mark location on diagram):
    Scars:_____ Rashes:_____ Lacerations:_____
    Ulcerations:_____ Bruises:_____ Blisters:____
    Drainage:___ Burns (degree/% of surface):___
Musculoskeletal: General strength:_____
    Muscle tone:_____ Gait:_____ ROM:_____
    Paresthesia/paralysis:_____
Results of testing (e.g., cultures, immune function, TB, hepatitis):_____

Sexuality [Component of Social Interaction]

SUBJECTIVE REPORTS
Sexually active:_____ Monogamous/Committed relationship: ____ Use of condoms:___
Birth control method:_____
Sexual concerns/difficulties:_____
Pain/discomfort:_____
Recent change in frequency/interest:_____

OBJECTIVE (EXHIBITS)
Comfort level with subject matter:_____

FEMALE: SUBJECTIVE (REPORTS)
Menstruation: Age at menarche:_____
Length of cycle:_____ Duration:_____
Number of pads/tampons used/day:_____
Last menstrual period:_____
Bleeding between periods:____ Menopausal:___
Last period:____ Hysterectomy (type/date):____
Problems with: Hot flashes:_____
Vaginal lubrication:_____ Vaginal discharge:___
Related surgeries (type and date):_____
Infertility concerns:_____ Type of therapy:_____
Pregnant now:_____ Para:_____ Gravida:_____
Due date:_____
Practices breast self-examination:_____
Last mammogram:___Last Pap smear/results:___
Hormonal therapy:_____ Supplemental calcium:
    _____ Other medications/herbals:_____

OBJECTIVE (EXHIBITS)
Breast examination:_____
Genitalia:_____ Warts/lesions:_____
Vaginal bleeding/discharge:_____
STD test results:_____

MALE: SUBJECTIVE (REPORTS)
Penis: Circumcised:____ Lesions/discharge:____
Vasectomy:_____
Prostate disorder:_____
Practice self-exam: Breast:_____ Testicles:____
Last proctoscopic/prostate examination:_____
Last PSA:_____
Medications/herbals:_____

OBJECTIVE (EXHIBITS)
Genitalia: Penis:_____ Warts/lesions: _____
Bleeding/discharge:____ Testicles (e.g., descended,
    lumps):_____ Prostate:_____
Breast examination:_____
STD test results:_____ PSA:_____

Social Interactions

SUBJECTIVE REPORTS
Relationship status: Single:____ Married:_____
Living with partner:_____ Divorced:_____
    Widowed:_____
Years in relationship:_____
Perception of relationship:_____
Concerns/stresses:_____
Role within family structure:_____
Number/age of children:_____
Individuals living in home:_____
Caregiver (to whom & how long):_____
Extended family/availability:_____
Other support person(s):_____
Perception of relationship with family members:
_____
Ethnic/cultural affiliation:_____
Strength of ethnic identity:_____
Lives in ethnic community:_____
Feelings of (describe): Mistrust:_____
    Rejection:_____ Unhappiness:_____
    Loneliness/isolation:_____

Problems related to illness/condition:_____

Difficulties with communication (e.g., speech, another language, brain injury):_____

Use of communication aids (list):_____

Requires interpreter:_____

Genogram: (complete on separate form)

OBJECTIVE (EXHIBITS)

Communication/speech: Clear:_____ Slurred:_____ Unintelligible:_____ Aphasic:_____

Unusual speech pattern/impairment:_____

Laryngectomy present:_____ Use of speech/ communication aids:_____

Verbal/nonverbal communication with family/ SO(s):_____

Family interaction (behavioral) pattern:_____

Teaching/Learning

SUBJECTIVE REPORTS

Communication: Dominant language (specify): _____ Second language:_____

Literate (reading/writing):_____

Education level:_____ Learning disabilities (specify):_____ Cognitive limitations:_____

Culture/ethnicity:_____ Where born:_____

If immigrant, how long in this country:_____

Health and illness beliefs/practices/customs:____

Which family member makes healthcare decisions/ is spokesperson for client:_____

Presence of Advance Directives:_____

Code status:_____ Durable Medical Power of Attorney:_____ Designee:_____

Health goals:_____

Current health problem:_____

Client understanding of problem:_____

Special healthcare concerns (e.g., impact of religious/cultural practices, healthcare decisions, family involvement):_____

Familial risk factors (indicate relationship): Diabetes:_____ Thyroid (specify):_____ Tuberculosis:_____ Heart disease:_____ Stroke:_____ High BP:_____ Epilepsy/ seizures:_____ Kidney disease:_____ Cancer:___ Mental illness/depression:_____ Other:_____

Prescribed medications (list each separately): Drug:_____ Dose:_____ Times (circle last dose):_____ Take regularly:_____ Purpose:_____ Side effects/problems:_____

Nonprescription drugs/frequency: OTC drugs: _____ Vitamins:_____ Herbals:_____ Street drugs:_____ Alcohol (amount/ frequency):_____ Tobacco:_____ Smokeless tobacco:_____

Admitting diagnosis per provider:_____

Reason for hospitalization (or visit) per client:___ _____

History of current problem/concern:_____

Client expectations of this hospitalization (or visit):_____

Will admission cause any lifestyle changes (describe):_____

Previous illnesses and/or hospitalizations/surgeries:_____

Evidence of failure to improve:_____

Last complete physical examination:_____

Discharge Plan Considerations

Projected length of stay (hours/days):_____

Anticipated date of discharge:_____

Date information obtained:_____ Source:_____

Resources available: Persons:_____ Financial:____ Community supports:_____ Groups:_____

Areas that may require alteration/assistance: Food preparation:_____ Shopping:_____ Transportation:_____ Ambulation:_____ Self-care (specify):_____ Socialization:_____ Medication/IV therapy:_____ Treatments:_____ Wound care:_____ Supplies:_____ Homemaker/maintenance (specify):_____ Physical layout of home (specify):_____

Anticipated changes in living situation after discharge:_____

Living facility other than home (specify):_____

Referrals (date/source/services): Social services: _____ Rehabilitation services:_____ Dietary:_____ Home care:_____ Respiration/Oxygen:_____ Equipment:_____

Supplies: _____

Other:_____

Appendix C

Lunney's Ordinal Scale for Degrees of Accuracy of a Nursing Diagnosis

Value	Criteria
+5	Diagnosis is consistent with all of the cues, supported by highly relevant cues, and precise.
+4	Diagnosis is consistent with most or all of the cues and supported by relevant cues but fails to reflect one or a few highly relevant cues.
+3	Diagnosis is consistent with many of the cues but fails to reflect the specificity of available cues.
+2	Diagnosis is indicated by some of the cues but there are insufficient cues relevant to the diagnosis, and/or the diagnosis is lower priority than other diagnoses.
+1	Diagnosis is suggested by only one or a few cues.
0	Diagnosis is not indicated by any of the cues. No diagnosis is stated when there are sufficient cues to state a diagnosis.
	The diagnosis cannot be rated.
−1	Diagnosis is indicated by more than one cue but should be rejected based on the presence of at least two disconfirming cues.

Reprinted with permission from Lunney, M. (1990). Accuracy of nursing diagnosis: Concepts and developments. *Nursing Diagnosis* 1:12–17.

Self-Monitoring of Accuracy Using the Integrated Model: A Guide

1. Pre-encounter data
   a. What data did I collect before seeing the patient? Did I collect enough (or too much) information at this point?
   b. How did I interpret the data before seeing the patient (e.g., relevance of data, priority of data, nursing responsibilities related to data, health status of patient)? What were my biases?
   c. Did I cluster two or more cues, before contact with the patient, as having specific meaning when occurring together?
   d. Was I naming hypotheses before I saw the patient? Should I have connected the data with hypotheses?
2. Entering the data search field and shaping the direction of data gathering
   a. In what ways did seeing the patient affect my initial assessment?
   b. How did I interpret the data that I initially collected in relation to other data, previous expectations, priorities, my responsibilities, or specific hypotheses? How did the patient interpret my behavior?
   c. Did I rearrange any clusters that existed (in my mind) before seeing the patient?
   d. For which hypotheses was I collecting data? Did I consider hypotheses related to the individuality of the patient? Did the patient express diagnostic hypotheses? Were the diagnoses the same as those that were generated by pre-encounter data, or did seeing the patient revise the names that I was considering?
3. Coalescing the cues into clusters or chunks
   a. To what extent did the clustering of cues make me aware of the need for further data collection?
   b. Did I assign validity and reliability estimates to the data while coalescing them into clusters or chunks?
   c. Did the clusters or chunks of data have meanings that can be validated through the literature?

d. To what extent would other nurses agree with the names that I was considering for the clusters or chunks?

4. Activating possible diagnostic explanations
   a. What data did I collect to support hypotheses? If the answer is none, did I close data collection prematurely? Did limitations in my knowledge prevent me from collecting data for certain diagnoses?
   b. How did I judge the relevance of the data that activated diagnostic hypotheses; for example, were they relevant enough to validate the diagnosis or just predictive? Was my judgment consistent with the judgment of the patient?
   c. Considering the literature on diagnostic concepts, how well did the clusters support the activation of diagnostic hypotheses? Did I consider the unique aspects of this patient when clustering the data for hypotheses?
   d. Did I consider the names of the important hypotheses?

5. Hypothesis- and data-directed searching of the data field
   a. Was my data collection efficient enough to produce highly relevant data for high-priority diagnoses as well as to rule out competitive diagnoses? Was I able to obtain the greatest quantity of relevant data with the least amount of cost to the patient and myself (cost equals time spent, time lost, and effort expended)?
   b. Was I able to interpret the data in relation to many conflicting hypotheses? Was my interpretation specific enough to direct me to precise diagnoses? Was I able to identify the need for further data?
   c. Were previous clusters used, or were they rearranged to produce new clusters?
   d. What diagnostic concepts were considered relevant and valid for testing the goodness of fit after a search of the data field? Were there concepts that I considered briefly during the previous steps but did not pursue?

6. Testing diagnostic hypotheses for goodness of fit
   a. What cues were used to test the goodness of fit?
   b. Were my interpretations of these cues derived from legitimate sources of information: theory, research, norms, and the unique patterns of the patient?
   c. Were the clusters of cues sufficiently well developed for testing the goodness of fit?
   d. Did the diagnostic label fulfill the criteria for goodness of fit?

Reprinted with permission from Lunney, M. (1989). Self-monitoring of accuracy using an integrated model of the diagnostic process. *J Adv Med Surg-Nurs, 1*(3):43–52. Copyright 1989 Aspen Publishers, Inc.

Appendix E

Clinical (Critical) Pathways: A Sample

Clinical pathways may be used as a standardized plan of care or as a guideline for developing an individualized plan for a specific client. Pathways are best used for acute problems for which there are predictable outcomes that must be achieved within a specific time frame. For example, Donald is initially admitted to a medical, or step-down, unit during the acute phase of alcohol withdrawal. Following is a sample clinical pathway for his 5-day length of stay (LOS). After completing this phase, he will be transferred to the behavioral unit for the rehabilitation program; a new clinical pathway will be implemented.

Clinical Pathway: Alcohol Withdrawal—LOS: 5 Days

ND and Categories of Care	Time Dimension	Goals/Actions	Time Dimension	Goals/Actions	Time Dimension	Goals/Actions
risk for Injury R/T CNS agitation	Day 1	Verbalize understanding of unit policies, procedures, and safety concerns relative to individual needs Cooperate with therapeutic regimen	Day 3 Day 4	Vital signs stable I&O balanced Display marked decrease in objective symptoms	Day 5	Be free of injury resulting from ETOH withdrawal Display no objective symptoms of withdrawal

Continued

Clinical Pathway: Alcohol Withdrawal—LOS: 5 Days (*Continued*)

ND and Categories of Care	Time Dimension	Goals/Actions	Time Dimension	Goals/Actions	Time Dimension	Goals/Actions
Referrals	Day 1	CNS/Psychiatrist If indicated: Internist, cardiologist, neurologist				
Diagnostic studies	Day 1	BA level Drug screen (urine and blood) If indicated:CXR, ECG, pulse oximetry	Day 2	Chem panel, serum Mg, amylase RPR UA	Day 4	Repeat of selected studies as indicated
Additional assessments	Day 1	VS, temp, respiratory status/breath sounds q4h	Day 2–3	VS q8h if stable	Day 4–5	VS daily
	Day 1–4	I&O q8h Motor activity, body language, verbalizations, need for/type of restraint				
	Ongoing	Withdrawal symptoms:				
	Stage I	Tremors, N/V, hypertension, tachycardia, diaphoresis, sleeplessness				
	Stage II	Increased hyperactivity, hallucinations, seizure activity				
	Stage III	Extreme autonomic hyperactivity, profound confusion, anxiety, fever				
Medications	Day 1–4	Thiamine 100 mg IM				
	Day 1–5	Serax 15 mg PO tid				
Patient education	Day 1	Orient to room/ unit, schedule, procedures	Day 3	Need for ongoing therapy	Day 5	Schedule follow-up visits if indicated

Clinical Pathway: Alcohol Withdrawal—LOS: 5 Days (*Continued*)

ND and Categories of Care	Time Dimension	Goals/Actions	Time Dimension	Goals/Actions	Time Dimension	Goals/Actions
			Day 3–4	Goals/ availability of AA program		
Additional nursing actions	Day 1	Bed rest 12 hr if in withdrawal Position change, HOB elevated; C, DB exercises if on bedrest Assist with ambulation, self-care as needed	Day 3–5	Activity as tolerated		
	Day 1–2	Encourage fluids if free of N/V				
	Ongoing	Provide environmental safety measures, seizure precautions as indicated Reorient as needed				
ineffective Coping R/T situational crisis, ↓perception of control, evidenced by ETOH abuse, inadequate problem solving	Day 1–5	Participate in development/ evaluation of treatment plan	Day 3	Verbalize under-standing of relationship of ETOH abuse to current situation	Day 5	Plan in place to meet needs post-discharge
	Day 2–5	Interact in group sessions	Day 4	Identify/make contact with potential resources, support groups		
Referrals	Day 1	Psychiatrist	Day 4	Community classes: Assertiveness training Stress management		
	Day 2–5	Group sessions				

Continued

ND and Categories of Care	Time Dimension	Goals/Actions	Time Dimension	Goals/Actions	Time Dimension	Goals/Actions
Clinical Pathway: Alcohol Withdrawal—LOS: 5 Days *(Continued)*						
Additional assessments	Day 1	Understanding of current situation	Day 2–3	Previous coping strategies/consequences		
		Drinking pattern, previous withdrawal, other drug use, attitudes toward substance use		Perception of drug use on life, employment, legal issues		
		History of violence	Day 3–5	Congruency of actions based on insight		
	Day 1–2	Relationships with others: personal, work/school				
		Readiness for group activities				
Medications			Day 5	Naltrexone 50 mg daily, if indicated		
Patient education	Day 1	Physical effects of ETOH abuse	Day 3–5	Human behavior and interactions with others/transactional analysis	Day 5	Medication dose, frequency, side effects
	Day 1–2	Types/use of relaxation techniques				Written instructions for therapeutic program
	Day 2	Consequences of ETOH abuse	Day 4–5	Community resources for self/family Identify goals for change		
Additional nursing actions	Day 1–5	Support patient's taking responsibility for own recovery	Day 2–5	Discuss alternative solutions		
		Provide consistent approach/expectations for behavior		Provide positive feedback for efforts		
		Set limits/confront inappropriate behaviors		Support during confrontation by peer group		
				Encourage verbalization of feelings, personal reflection		

Clinical Pathway: Alcohol Withdrawal—LOS: 5 Days (*Continued*)

ND and Categories of Care	Time Dimension	Goals/Actions	Time Dimension	Goals/Actions	Time Dimension	Goals/Actions
imbalanced Nutrition: less than body requirements R/T biological factors (effects of ETOH on digestive system, hypermetabolic response to withdrawal) as evidenced by food intake <RDA	Day 2–5	Select foods appropriately to meet individual dietary needs	Day 4	Verbalize understanding of effects of ETOH abuse and reduced dietary intake on nutritional status	Day 5	Display stable weight or initial weight gain, as appropriate, and laboratory results WNL
Referrals	Day 1 and prn	Dietitian				
Diagnostic studies	Day 1	CBC, liver function studies Serum albumin, transferrin	Day 2–5	Fingerstick glucose prn		
Additional assessments	Day 1	Weight, skin turgor, condition of mucous membranes, muscle tone			Day 5	Weight
	Day 1–2	Bowel sounds, characteristics of stools				
	Day 1–5	Appetite, dietary intake				
Medications	Day 1–5	Antacid ac and hs Imodium 2 mg prn	Day 2–5	Multivitamin tab daily		
Patient education	Day 1–2	Individual nutritional needs	Day 4	Principles of nutrition, foods for maintenance of wellness		
Additional nursing actions	Day 1	Liquid/bland diet as tolerated	Day 2-5	Advance diet as tolerated		

Continued

Clinical Pathway: Alcohol Withdrawal—LOS: 5 Days (*Continued*)

ND and Categories of Care	Time Dimension	Goals/Actions	Time Dimension	Goals/Actions	Time Dimension	Goals/Actions
	Day 1–5	Encourage small, frequent, nutritious meals/snacks Encourage good oral hygiene pc and hs				

Appendix F

Glossary

ADPIE: Format for charting using the steps of the nursing process—Assessment, Diagnosis (problem), Plan (goals), Implementation (intervention), Evaluation.

Analysis: The process of examining and categorizing information to reach a conclusion about a client's needs.

Assessment: The first step of the nursing process, during which data relating to a client are collected.

Baseline Assessment: Initial data collection done at the time of admission/beginning of shift, with which future assessments are compared.

Charting: The written record of relevant details of the client care and the client's response, including observations and changes in the client's condition.

Client Database: The compilation of data collected about a client; it consists of the nursing history, physical examination, and results of the diagnostic studies.

Client Diagnostic Statement: The outcome of the diagnostic reasoning process; a three-part statement identifying the client's problem/need, etiology of the problem/need, and the associated signs/symptoms.

Collaborative Problem: A need identified by another discipline that will contain a nursing component requiring nursing intervention and/or monitoring.

Concept Mapping: Diagrams of important ideas (client problems and treatments) that are linked together; used to plan nursing care.

Cue(s): A signal that indicates a possible need/direction for care.

DAR: Format for charting—Data, Actions, Response (called FOCUS CHARTING™).

Defining Characteristics: Clinical criteria that represent the presence of a diagnostic category; cluster of signs and symptoms manifesting an actual or wellness nursing diagnosis.

Diagnose: Forming a clinical judgment identifying a disease/condition or human response through scientific evaluation of signs/symptoms, history, and diagnostic studies.

Diagnosis: The second step of the nursing process in which the data collected are analyzed and, through the process of diagnostic reasoning, specific client diagnostic statements are created.

Diagnostic Error: A mistaken assumption leading to a wrong conclusion.

Diagnostic Reasoning: Process of need identification used during the second step of the nursing process: problem sensing, ruling-out process, synthesizing the data, evaluating or confirming the hypothesis, and listing client problems/ needs.

Etiology: Identified causes and/or contributing factors responsible for the presence of a specific client problem/need.

Evaluation: The fifth step of the nursing process during which the client's movement toward specified outcomes is determined and the plan of care is modified or care is terminated, depending on the findings.

Focus Assessment: Gathering of data narrowed to a specific area/topic.

Goal: Broad guidelines indicating the overall direction for movement as a result of the interventions of the healthcare team; divided into long-term and short-term goals.

Implementation: The fourth step of the nursing process in which the plan of care is put into action; performing identified interventions/ activities.

Inference: To conclude/deduce from evidence presented.

Intuition: A sense of something that is not clearly evidenced by known facts.

JCAHO (Joint Commission on Accreditation of Healthcare Organizations): Surveying body that certifies clinical and organizational performance of an institution according to established guidelines.

Long-Term Goals: May not be achieved before discharge from care and may require continued attention by client and /or others.

Measurable Verb: An action/behavior that can be seen or heard used in writing outcomes.

Medical Diagnosis: Illness/condition for which treatment is directed by a licensed physician; focuses on correction/prevention of pathology of specific organs/body systems.

Mind Mapping: A graphic representation of the connections between concepts and ideas that are related to a central subject; used to plan nursing care.

NANDA International (formerly North American Nursing Diagnosis Association): An organization that facilitates the development, refinement, dissemination, use, and evaluation of a standardized nursing diagnosis terminology.

Nurse-Client Relationship: A therapeutic relationship built on a series of interactions, developing over time, and meeting the needs of the client.

Nursing Audit: Procedure to evaluate the quality of nursing care provided, using established criteria/ standards. Concurrent audit is done while nursing care is being performed. Retrospective audit is done after the client is discharged from care.

Nursing Diagnosis: Noun: A label approved by NANDA-I identifying specific client problems/ needs. The means of describing health problems/ life processes amenable to treatment by nurses; may be physical, sociological, or psychological. **Verb:** Process of identifying specific client problems/needs; used by some as the title of the second step of the nursing process.

Nursing Interventions: Prescriptions for specific behaviors expected for the client and/or actions to be carried out by nurses to promote, maintain, or restore health.

Nursing Process: An orderly, logical five-step problem-solving approach to administering nursing care, comprising assessment, diagnosis, planning, implementation, and evaluation.

Nursing Standard: Identified criterion against which nursing care is compared and evaluated; generally reflects the minimum level for nursing care.

Objective Data: What can be observed; for example, vital signs, behaviors, diagnostic studies.

Outcome: The result of actions undertaken to achieve a broader goal; measurable steps to achieve the goals of treatment and to meet discharge criteria.

PES: Format for combining a client Problem (or need) label, Etiology, and Signs/Symptoms to create an individualized diagnostic statement.

Planning: The third step of the nursing process during which goals/outcomes are determined and interventions chosen.

Plan of Care: Written evidence of the second and third steps of the nursing process that identifies the client's problems/needs, goals/outcomes of care, and interventions to treat the problems/needs.

POMR or PORS (Problem-Oriented Medical Record): A method of recording data about the health status of the client relative to specific problems.

Protocol: Written guidelines of steps to be taken for providing client care in a particular situation/condition.

Related Factor: The conditions/circumstances that show some type of patterned relationship/contribute to the development/maintenance of a nursing diagnosis; related to components of the client diagnostic statement.

Risk Factor: The environmental factors and physiological, psychological, genetic, or chemical elements that increase the vulnerability of an individual, family, or community to an unhealthful event.

Risk Nursing Diagnosis: Human response to health conditions/life processes that may develop or recur, particularly if intervention is not undertaken. Because it has not yet occurred, there are no signs/symptoms when the client diagnostic statement is written; instead, the specific risk factors are identified.

Short-Term Goals: Usually must be met before discharge or movement to a less acute level of care.

Sign: Objective or observable evidence or manifestation of a health problem.

SOAP: Format for documentation—Subjective, Objective, Analysis, Plan.

SOAPIER: Format for documentation—Subjective, Objective, Analysis, Plan, Implementation, Evaluation, Revision.

Subjective Data: What the client reports, believes, or feels.

Symptom: Subjectively perceptible change in the body or its functions that indicates disease or the kind or phase of disease.

Synthesize: Viewing all data as a whole to provide a comprehensive picture of the client.

Validating: The process of ensuring that data are factual.

Wellness: A state of optimal health, physical and psychosocial.

Appendix G

NANDA-I Taxonomy II: Definitions of Axes

AXIS 1 DIAGNOSTIC CONCEPT: Defined as the principal element or the fundamental and essential part, the root, of the diagnostic statement.

AXIS 2 SUBJECT OF THE DIAGNOSIS: The person(s) for whom a nursing diagnosis is determined. Values are:

Individual: A single human being distinct from others, a person.

Family: Two or more people having continuous or sustained relationships, perceiving reciprocal obligations, sensing common meaning, and sharing certain obligations toward others; related by blood and/or choice.

Group: A number of people with shared characteristics.

Community: A group of people living in the same locale under the same governance, such as neighborhoods, cities, census tracts. When the unit of care is not explicitly stated, it becomes the individual by default.

AXIS 3 JUDGMENT: A descriptor or modifier that limits or specifies the meaning of the diagnostic concept. Values are:

Anticipatory: Realize beforehand, foresee

Compromised: Damaged, made vulnerable

Decreased: Lessened (in size, amount, or degree)

Defensive: Used or intended to defend or protect

Deficient: Insufficient, inadequate

Delayed: Late, slow, or postponed

Disabled: Limited, handicapped

Disorganized: Not properly arranged or controlled

Disproportionate: Too large or too small in comparison with norm

Disturbed: Agitated, interrupted, interfered with

Dysfunctional: Not operating normally

Effective: Producing the intended or desired effect

Enhanced: Improved in quality, value, or extent

Excessive: Greater than necessary or desirable

Imbalanced: Out of proportion or balance

Impaired: Damaged, weakened

Ineffective: Not producing the intended or desired effect

Interrupted: Having its continuity broken

Low: Below the norm

Organized: Properly arranged or controlled

Perceived: Observed through the senses

Readiness for: In a suitable state for an activity or situation

Situational: Related to a particular circumstance

AXIS 4 LOCATION: Consists of parts/regions of the body and/or their related functions—all tissues, organs, anatomical sites or structures. Values are:

Auditory
Bladder
Cardiopulmonary
Cerebral
Gastrointestinal
Gustatory
Intracranial
Kinesthetic
Mucous membranes
Oral
Olfactory
Peripheral neurovascular
Peripheral vascular
Renal
Skin
Tactile
Visual

AXIS 5 AGE: The age of the person who is the subject of the diagnosis. Values are:

Fetus
Neonate
Infant
Toddler
Preschool child
School-age child
Adolescent
Adult
Older adult

AXIS 6 TIME: The duration of the diagnostic concept. Values are:

Acute: Lasting less than 6 months

Chronic: Lasting more than 6 months

Intermittent: Stopping or starting again at intervals, periodic, cyclic

Continuous: Uninterrupted, going on without stop

AXIS 7 STATUS OF THE DIAGNOSIS: The actuality or potentiality of the problem or the catagorization of the diagnosis as a wellness/ health promotion diagnosis. Values are:

Actual: Existing in fact or reality, existing at the present time

Health Promotion: Behavior motivated by the desire to increase well-being and actualize human health potential (Pender, Murdaugh, & Parsons, 2006)

Risk: Vulnerability, especially as a result of exposure to factors that increase the chance of injury or loss

Wellness: The quality or state of being healthy

Permission from NANDA International (2007). *NANDA-I Nursing Diagnoses: Definitions & Classification 2007–2008.* Philadelphia: NANDA-I. 2007–2008.

NANDA-I Nursing Diagnoses Organized According to Maslow's Hierarchy of Needs and Nursing Framework: A Health Outcome Classification for Nursing Diagnosis

Maslow's Hierarchy of Needs

SELF-ACTUALIZATION

Coping, readiness for enhanced
Coping, readiness for enhanced community
Coping, readiness for enhanced family
Decision Making, readiness for enhanced
Development, risk for delayed
Health-Seeking Behaviors [specify]
Hope, readiness for enhanced
Knowledge, readiness for enhanced
Power, readiness for enhanced
Religiosity, readiness for enhanced
Self-Concept, readiness for enhanced
Spiritual Well-Being, readiness for enhanced

SELF-ESTEEM

Body Image, disturbed
Conflict, decisional (specify)
Coping, defensive
Coping, ineffective
Denial, ineffective
Dignity, risk for compromised human

Distress, moral
Diversional Activity, deficient
Hopelessness
Identity, disturbed personal
Noncompliance [Adherence, ineffective] (specify)
Nutrition: more than body requirements, imbalanced
Nutrition: more than body requirements, risk for imbalanced
Post-Trauma Syndrome
Post-Trauma Syndrome, risk for
Powerlessness
Powerlessness, risk for
Rape-Trauma Syndrome
Rape-Trauma Syndrome: compound reaction
Rape-Trauma Syndrome: silent reaction
Self-Esteem, chronic low
Self-Esteem, situational low
Self-Esteem, risk for situational low
Self-Mutilation
Self-Mutilation, risk for
Suicide, risk for
Violence, [actual/] risk for other-directed
Violence, [actual/] risk for self-directed

LOVE AND BELONGING

Attachment, risk for impaired parent/child
Communication, readiness for enhanced
Conflict, parental role
Coping, compromised family
Coping, disabled family
Development, risk for delayed
Family Processes, interrupted
Family Processes, readiness for enhanced
Family Processes: alcoholism, dysfunctional
Loneliness, risk for
Parenting, impaired
Parenting, risk for impaired
Parenting, readiness for enhanced
Religiosity, impaired
Religiosity, risk for impaired
Relocation Stress Syndrome
Relocation Stress Syndrome, risk for

Role Performance, ineffective
Sexual Dysfunction
Social Interaction, impaired
Social Isolation
Sorrow, chronic
Spiritual Distress
Spiritual Distress, risk for

SAFETY AND SECURITY

Allergy Response, latex
Allergy Response, risk for latex
Autonomic Dysreflexia
Autonomic Dysreflexia, risk for
Anxiety [specify level]
Anxiety, death
Behavior, risk-prone health
Caregiver Role Strain
Caregiver Role Strain, risk for
Contamination
Contamination, risk for
Communication, impaired verbal
Confusion, acute
Confusion, risk for acute
Confusion, chronic
Coping, ineffective community
Death Syndrome, risk for sudden infant
Disuse Syndrome, risk for
Environmental Interpretation Syndrome, impaired
Falls, risk for
Fear
Grieving
Grieving, complicated
Grieving, risk for complicated
Health Maintenance, ineffective
Home Maintenance, impaired
Immunization Status, readiness for enhanced
Infant Behavior, readiness for enhanced organized
Infection, risk for
Injury, risk for
Injury, risk for perioperative-positioning
Knowledge, deficient [Learning Need] (specify)

Lifestyle, sendentary
Memory, impaired
Mobility, impaired bed
Mobility, impaired wheelchair
Peripheral Neurovascular Dysfunction, risk for
Poisoning, risk for
Protection, ineffective
Stress Overload
Therapeutic Regimen Management, effective
Therapeutic Regimen Management, ineffective
Therapeutic Regimen Management, ineffective
   community
Therapeutic Regimen Management, ineffective
   family
Therapeutic Regimen Management, readiness
   for enhanced
Transfer Ability, impaired
Trauma, risk for
Neglect, unilateral
Walking, impaired
Wandering [specify sporadic or continuous]

PHYSIOLOGICAL NEEDS

Activity Intolerance [specify level]
Activity Intolerance, risk for
Intracranial Adaptive Capacity, decreased
Airway Clearance, ineffective
Aspiration, risk for
Body Temperature, risk for imbalanced
Bowel Incontinence
Breastfeeding, effective
Breastfeeding, ineffective
Breastfeeding, interrupted
Breathing Pattern, ineffective
Cardiac Output, decreased
Comfort, readiness for enhanced
Constipation
Constipation, perceived
Constipation, risk for
Dentition, impaired
Diarrhea
Energy Field, disturbed
Failure to Thrive, adult
Fatigue

Fluid Balance, readiness for enhanced
Fluid Volume, deficient
Fluid Volume, excess
Fluid Volume, risk for deficient
Fluid Volume, risk for imbalanced
Gas Exchange, impaired
Glucose, risk for unstable blood
Growth, risk for disproportionate
Growth and Development, delayed
Hyperthermia
Hypothermia
Infant Behavior, disorganized
Infant Behavior, risk for disorganized
Infant Feeding Pattern, ineffective
Insomnia
Liver Function, risk for impaired
Nausea
Nutrition: less than body requirements, im-
   balanced
Nutrition, readiness for enhanced
Oral Mucous Membrane, impaired
Pain, acute
Pain, chronic
Self-Care, readiness for enhanced
Self-Care Deficit (specify): feeding, bathing/
   hygiene, dressing/grooming, toileting
Sensory Perception, disturbed (specify: visual,
   auditory, kinesthetic, gustatory, tactile, olfac-
   tory)
Sexuality Pattern, ineffective
Skin Integrity, impaired
Skin Integrity, risk for impaired
Sleep, readiness for enhanced
Sleep Deprivation
Suffocation, risk for
Surgical Recovery, delayed
Swallowing, impaired
Thermoregulation, ineffective
Thought Processes, disturbed
Tissue Integrity, impaired
Tissue Perfusion, ineffective (specify type: ce-
   rebral, cardiopulmonary, renal, gastrointes-
   tinal, peripheral)
Urinary Elimination, impaired
Urinary Elimination, readiness for enhanced
Urinary Incontinence, functional

Urinary Incontinence, overflow
Urinary Incontinence, reflex
Urinary Incontinence, stress
Urinary Incontinence, total
Urinary Incontinence, urge
Urinary Incontinence, risk for urge
Urinary Retention [acute/chronic]
Ventilation, impaired spontaneous
Ventilatory Weaning Response,
dysfunctional

Nursing Framework: A Health Outcome Classification for Nursing Diagnoses*

SELF-CARE OF NURSING DIAGNOSES

I. Physiological Homeostasis
1.1.0. Alterations in oxygenation
1.1.1. Impaired gas exchange
1.1.2. Ineffective airway clearance
    1.1.2.1. Risk for aspiration
    1.1.2.2. Risk for suffocation
1.1.3. Ineffective breathing pattern
    1.1.3.1. Inability to sustain spontaneous ventilation
    1.1.3.2. Dysfunctional ventilatory weaning response
1.2.0. Alterations in circulation
1.2.1. Altered tissue perfusion
1.2.2. Altered fluid volume
    1.2.2.1. Deficit
    1.2.2.2. Excess
1.2.3. Decreased cardiac output
1.3.0. Alterations in protective mechanisms
1.3.1. Risk for infection
1.3.2. [Bleeding tendency]
1.3.3. Risk for peripheral neurovascular dysfunction
1.3.4. Dysreflexia

1.4.0. Ineffective thermoregulation
1.4.1. Risk for altered body temperature
1.4.1.1. Hypothermia
1.4.1.2. Hyperthermia
1.5.0. Sensory-perceptual alterations
1.5.1. Specific sensory deficit
    1.5.1.1. Impaired vision
    1.5.1.2. Impaired hearing [auditory]
    1.5.1.3. Impaired touch [tactile]
    1.5.1.4. Impaired taste [gustatory]
    1.5.1.5. Impaired smell [olfactory]
    1.5.1.6. Impaired sense of movement [kinesthetic]
    1.5.1.7. [Altered proprioception]
1.5.2. [Altered consciousness]
1.5.3. Discomfort/pain
1.5.3.1. Chronic pain
II. Bodily Comfort
2.1.0. Alterations in nutrition
2.1.1. More than body requirements
2.1.2. Less than body requirements
2.1.3. Effective breastfeeding
2.1.4. Feeding difficulties
    2.1.4.1. Impaired swallowing
    2.1.4.2. Ineffective infant feeding pattern
        2.1.4.2.1. Ineffective breastfeeding
        2.1.4.2.2. Interrupted breastfeeding
2.1.5. Delayed growth
2.2.0. Alterations in elimination
2.2.1. Bowel
    2.2.1.1. Constipation
        2.2.1.1.1. Colonic
        2.2.1.1.2. Perceived
    2.2.1.2. Diarrhea
    2.2.1.3. Incontinence
2.2.2. Bladder
    2.2.2.1. Incontinence
        2.2.2.1.1. Functional
        2.2.2.1.2. Reflex
        2.2.2.1.3. Stress
        2.2.2.1.4. Total
        2.2.2.1.5. Urge

---

*Modified from Jenny, J.: *Classification of Nursing Diagnoses: NANDA Proceedings from the 8th Conference.* Philadelphia: J. B. Lippincott,1989; and Jenny, J.: Classifying nursing diagnoses: A self-care approach. *Nursing and Health Care 10*(2):1983–1988.

2.2.2.2. Retention
2.2.2.3. Altered urination pattern
2.2.3. [Skin]
2.2.4. Toileting difficulties
2.3.0. Impaired tissue integrity
2.3.1. Impaired skin integrity
2.3.2. Impaired oral mucous membrane
2.4.0. Alterations in activity
2.4.1. Impaired physical mobility
    2.4.1.1. [Hyperactivity]
    2.4.1.2. Activity intolerance
    2.4.1.3. Risk for disuse syndrome
2.4.2. Sleep pattern disturbance
2.4.3. Fatigue
2.4.4. Diversional activity/recreation deficit
2.5.0. Altered grooming pattern
2.5.1. Specific grooming difficulties
    2.5.1.1. Bathing/perineal care
    2.5.1.2. [Mouth care]
    2.5.1.3. Dressing
2.5.2. [Self neglect]
    2.5.2.1. Neglect, unilateral
III. Ego Integrity
3.1.0. Altered self concept
3.1.1. Disturbance in body image
3.1.2. Disturbance in self esteem
    3.1.2.1. Chronic low
    3.1.2.2. Situational low
3.1.3. Disturbance in personal identity
3.2.0. Altered thought processes
3.2.1. [Impaired information processing]
3.2.2. [Memory loss]
3.2.3. [Confusion]
3.2.4. [Impaired learning]
3.2.5. [Impaired self-orientation]
3.3.0. [Diminished feelings of personal control]
3.3.1. Anxiety
3.3.2. Fear
3.3.3. Grieving
    3.3.3.1. Anticipatory
    3.3.3.2. Dysfunctional
3.3.4. Risk for violence
    3.3.4.1. Risk for self mutilation
3.3.5. Post-trauma response
    3.3.5.1. Rape-trauma syndrome

      3.3.5.1.1. Compound reaction
      3.3.5.1.2. Silent reaction
3.3.6. Powerlessness
3.3.7. Hopelessness
3.4.0. Spiritual distress
IV. Social Interaction
4.1.0. [Alterations in communication]
4.1.1. Verbal, impaired
4.1.2. [Nonverbal, impaired]
4.2.0. [Alterations in relationships]
4.2.1. Social isolation
4.2.2. [Social withdrawal]
4.2.3. Altered sexuality pattern
    4.2.3.1. Sexual dysfunction
4.3.0. Alterations in role
4.3.1. Impaired parenting
    4.3.1.1. Parental role conflict
4.3.2. [Impaired work functioning]
    4.3.2.1. Caregiver role strain
4.4.0. Alterations in family process
4.4.1. Family coping, potential for growth
4.4.2. Ineffective family coping
    4.4.2.1. Compromised
    4.4.2.2. Disabling
4.5.0. [Risk for abuse]
4.6.0. Developmental delay
V. Health Protection
5.1.0. Health-seeking behaviors
5.2.0. Altered health maintenance
5.2.1. [Inadequate self monitoring]
5.2.2. [Inadequate self protection]
5.2.3. [Reduced use of health services]
5.3.0. [Ineffective stress management]
5.3.1. Ineffective individual coping
    5.3.1.1. Decisional conflict
    5.3.1.2. Ineffective denial
    5.3.1.3. Coping, defensive
5.4.0. Risk for injury
5.4.1. Risk for trauma
5.4.2. [Risk for abuse]
VI. Health Restoration
6.1.0. Ineffective management of therapeutic regimen
6.1.1. Noncompliance [specify]
6.1.2. Impaired adjustment

6.1.3. [Risk for transmitting infection]

VII. Environmental Management

7.1.0. Impaired home maintenance management

7.1.1. [Coping with dysfunctional facilities]

7.1.2. [Inability to perform household tasks]

7.2.0. [Exposure to hazards]

7.3.0. [Separation from community services/ resources]

7.4.0. Relocation stress syndrome

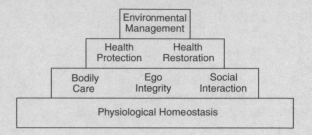

Appendix I

NANDA International Nursing Diagnoses With Definitions, Related/Risk Factors, and Defining Characteristics

Activity Intolerance

DEFINITION: Insufficient physiological or psychological energy to endure or complete required or desired daily activities

RELATED FACTORS: ° Generalized weakness ° Sedentary lifestyle ° Bedrest ° Immobility ° Imbalance between oxygen supply and demand ° [Anemia] ° [Cognitive deficits, extreme stress; depression] ° [Pain, dysrhythmias, vertigo,]

DEFINING CHARACTERISTICS
Subjective: ° Report of fatigue/weakness ° Exertional discomfort/dyspnea ° [Verbalizes no desire and/or lack of interest in activity]
Objective: ° Abnormal heart rate/blood pressure response to activity ° Electrocardiographic changes reflecting arrrhythmias/ischemia ° [Pallor, cyanosis]

FUNCTIONAL LEVEL CLASSIFICATION (GORDON, 1987):

Level I: Walk, regular pace, on level indefinitely; one flight or more but more short of breath than normally
Level II: Walk one city block [or] 500 ft on level; climb one flight slowly without stopping
Level III: Walk no more than 50 ft on level without stopping; unable to climb one flight of stairs without stopping
Level IV: Dyspnea and fatigue at rest

Activity Intolerance, risk for*

DEFINITION: At risk of experiencing insufficient physiological or psychological energy to endure or complete required or desired daily activities

*[Note: A risk diagnosis is not evidenced by signs and symptoms as the problem has not yet occurred; rather, nursing interventions are directed at prevention. Therefore, risk factors present are noted instead.] (s) - sympathetic; (p) = parasympathetic

RISK FACTORS: ° History of previous intolerance ° Presence of circulatory/respiratory problems ° [Dysrhythmias] ° Deconditioned status ° [Aging] ° Inexperience with the activity ° [Diagnosis of progressive disease state/debilitating condition, anemia, extensive surgical procedures] ° [Verbalized reluctance/inability to perform expected activity]

Airway Clearance, ineffective

DEFINITION: Inability to clear secretions or obstructions from the respiratory tract to maintain a clear airway

RELATED FACTORS:
Environmental: ° Smoking ° Second-hand smoke ° Smoke inhalation
Obstructed airway: ° Retained secretions ° Secretions in the bronchi ° Exudate in the alveoli ° Excessive mucus ° Airway spasm ° Foreign body in airway ° Presence of artificial airway
Physiological: ° Chronic obstructive pulmonary disease (COPD) ° Asthma ° Allergic airways ° Hyperplasia of the bronchial walls ° Neuromuscular dysfunction ° Infection

DEFINING CHARACTERISTICS
Subjective: ° Dyspnea
Objective: ° Diminished/adventitious breath sounds [rales, crackles, rhonchi, wheezes] ° Cough, ineffective/absent ° Excessive sputum ° Changes in respiratory rate and rhythm ° Difficulty vocalizing ° Wide-eyed ° Restlessness ° Orthopnea ° Cyanosis

Allergy Response, latex

DEFINITION: An allergic response to natural latex rubber products

RELATED FACTORS: ° Hypersensitivity to natural latex rubber protein

DEFINING CHARACTERISTICS
Subjective: Life-threatening reactions occurring <1 hour after exposure to latex proteins: ° Tightness in chest ° [Feeling breathless]

Gastrointestinal characteristics: Abdominal pain Nausea
Orofacial characteristics: ° Itching of the eyes ° Nasal/facial/oral itching ° Nasal congestion
Generalized characteristics: ° Generalized discomfort ° Increasing complaint of total body warmth
Type IV reactions occurring >1 hour after exposure to latex proteins: ° Discomfort reaction to additives such as thiurams & carbamates
Objective: Life-threatening reactions occurring <1 hour after exposure to latex proteins: ° Contact urticaria progressing to generalized symptoms ° Edema of the lips/tongue/uvula/throat ° Dyspnea ° Wheezing ° Bronchospasm ° Respiratory arrest ° Hypotension ° Syncope ° Cardiac arrest
Orofacial characteristics: ° Edema of sclera/eyelids ° Erythema/tearing of the eyes ° Nasal/facial erythema ° Rhinorrhea
Generalized characteristics: ° Flushing generalized ° Edema ° Restlessness and/or itching of the eyes, and/or erythema
Type IV reactions occurring >1 hour after exposure to latex proteins: ° Eczema ° Irritation ° Redness

Allergy Response, risk for latex

DEFINITION: Risk of hypersensitivity to natural latex rubber products

RISK FACTORS: ° History of reactions to latex ° Allergies to bananas, avocados, tropical fruits, kiwi, chestnuts, poinsettia plants ° History of allergies and asthma ° Professions with daily exposure to latex ° Multiple surgical procedures, especially from infancy

Anxiety [mild, moderate, severe, panic]

DEFINITION: Vague uneasy feeling of discomfort or dread accompanied by an autonomic response (the source often nonspecific or unknown to the individual); a feeling of apprehension caused by anticipation of danger. It is an altering signal that warns of impending danger and enables the individual to take measures to deal with threat

RELATED FACTORS: ° Unconscious conflict about essential [beliefs]/goals/values of life ° Situational/maturational crises ° Stress ° Familial association/heredity ° Interpersonal transmission/contagion ° Threat to self-concept [perceived or actual] ° [Unconscious conflict] ° Threat of death [perceived or actual] ° Threat to or change in health status [progressive/debilitating disease, terminal illness], interaction patterns, role function/status, environment [safety], economic status ° Unmet needs ° Exposure to toxins ° Substance abuse ° [Positive or negative self-talk] ° [Physiological factors, e.g., hyperthyroidism, pheochromocytoma, drug therapy including steroids]

DEFINING CHARACTERISTICS
Subjective: Behavioral: ° Expressed concerns due to change in life events ° Insomnia
Affective: ° Regretful ° Scared ° Rattled ° Distressed ° Apprehensive ° Uncertainty ° Fearful ° Feelings of inadequacy ° Jittery ° Worried ° Painful/persistent increased helplessness ° [Sense of impending doom] ° [Hopelessness]
Cognitive: ° Fear of unspecific consequences ° Awareness of physiological symptoms
Physiological: ° Shakiness
Sympathetic: ° Dry mouth ° Heart pounding ° Weakness ° Respiratory difficulties ° Anorexia ° Diarrhea
Parasympathetic: ° Tingling in extremities ° Nausea ° Abdominal pain ° Diarrhea ° Urinary hesitancy/frequency ° Faintness ° Fatigue ° Sleep disturbance ° [Chest, back, neck pain]
Objective: Behavioral: ° Poor eye contact ° Glancing about ° Scanning ° Vigilance ° Extraneous movement [e.g., foot shuffling, hand/arm movements, rocking motion] ° Fidgeting ° Restlessness ° Diminished productivity ° [Crying/tearfulness] ° [Pacing/purposeless activity] ° [Immobility]
Affective: ° Increased wariness ° Focus on self ° Irritability ° Overexcited ° Anguish

Physiological: ° Voice quivering; trembling/hand tremors ° Increased tension ° Facial tension ° Increased perspiration
Sympathetic: ° Cardiovascular excitation ° Facial flushing ° Superficial vasoconstriction ° Increased pulse/respiration ° Increased blood pressure ° Twitching ° Pupil dilation ° Increased reflexes
Parasympathetic: ° Urinary urgency ° Decreased blood pressure/pulse
Cognitive: ° Preoccupation ° Impaired attention ° Difficulty concentrating ° Forgetfulness ° Diminished ability to problem-solve ° Diminished learning ability ° Rumination ° Tendency to blame others ° Blocking of thought ° Confusion ° Decreased perceptual field

Anxiety, death

DEFINITION: Vague uneasy feeling of discomfort or dread generated by perceptions of a real or imagined threat to one's existance

RELATED FACTORS: ° Anticipating: pain/suffering/adverse consequences of general anesthesia/impact of death on others ° Confornting reality of terminal disease ° Eexperiencing dying process ° Perceived proximity of death ° Discussions on topic of death ° Observations related to death ° Near death experience ° Uncertainty of prognosis ° Nonacceptance of own mortality ° Uncertainty about: the existance of a higher power/life after death/an encounter with a higher power

DEFINING CHARACTERISTICS
Subjective: ° Fear of: Developing a terminal illness/the process of dying/prolonged dying/loss of mental [/physical] abilities when dying/pain or suffering relating to dying/premature death
° Negative thoughts related to death and dying
° Feeling powerlessness over dying ° Worrying about: The impact of one's own death on significant others ° [about meeting one's creator or feeling doubt about the existence of God or higher being]
° Concerns of overworking the caregiver

Aspiration, risk for

DEFINITION: At risk for entry of gastrointestinal secretions, oropharyngeal secretions, or [exogenous food] solids or fluids into tracheobronchial passages [due to dysfunction or absence of normal protective mechanisms]

RISK FACTORS: ° Reduced level of consciousness [sedation/anesthesia] ° Depressed cough/gag reflexes ° Impaired swallowing [inability of the epiglottis and true vocal cords to close off traches] ° Facial/oral/neck surgery or trauma ° Wired jaws ° [Congenital malformations] ° Situation hindering elevation of upper body [weakness, paralysis] ° Incomplete lower esophageal sphincter [hiatal hernia or other esophageal disease affecting stomach valve function] ° Delayed gastric emptying ° Decreased gastrointestinal motility ° Increased intragastric pressure ° Increased gastric residual ° Presence of tracheostomy or endotracheal (ET) tube ° [Inadequate or over-inflation of tracheostomy/ET tube cuff] ° [Presence of] gastrointestinal tubes ° Tube feedings/medication administration

Attachment, risk for impaired parent/child

DEFINITION: Disruption of the interactive process between parent/significant other and child/infant that fosters the development of a protective and nurturing reciprocal relationship

RISK FACTORS: ° Inability of parents to meet personal needs ° Anxiety associated with the parent role ° [Parents who themselves experienced altered attachment] ° Premature infant/ill infant/child who is unable to effectively initiate parental contact due to altered behavioral organization ° Separation ° Physical barriers ° Lack of privacy ° Substance abuse ° [Difficult pregnancy and/or birth (actual or perceived)] ° [Uncertainty of paternity; conception as a result of rape/sexual abuse]

Autonomic Dysreflexia

DEFINITION: Life-threatening, uninhibited sympathetic response of the nervous system to a noxious stimulus after a spinal cord injury (SCI) at T7 or above

RELATED FACTORS: ° Bladder/bowel distention ° [Catheter insertion, obstruction, irrigation] ° Skin irritation ° Deficient patient/caregiver knowledge ° [Sexual excitation, menstruation, pregnancy, labor/delivery] ° [Environmental temperature extremes]

DEFINING CHARACTERISTICS
Subjective: ° *Headache (a diffuse pain in different portions of the head and not confined to any nerve distribution area)* ° *Paresthesia* ° *Chilling* ° *Blurred vision* ° *Chest pain* ° *Metallic taste in mouth* ° Nasal congestion
Objective: ° Paroxysmal hypertension (sudden periodic elevated blood pressure in which systolic pressure >140 mm Hg and diastolic >90 mm Hg) ° Bradycardia or tachycardia (heart rate <60 or >100 beats per minute, respectively) ° Diaphoresis (above the injury) ° Red splotches on skin (above the injury) ° Pallor (below the injury) ° Horner's syndrome [contraction of the pupil, partial ptosis of the eyelid, enophthalmos and sometimes loss of sweating over the affected side of the face] ° Conjunctival congestion ° Pilomotor reflex [gooseflesh formation when skin is cooled]

Autonomic Dysreflexia, risk for

DEFINITION: At risk for life-threatening, uninhibited response of the sympathetic nervous system post spinal shock, in an individual with a spinal cord injury [SCI] or lesion at T6 or above (has been demonstrated in patients with injuries at T7 and T8)

RISK FACTORS:
Musculoskeletal—Integumentary Stimuli: ° Cutaneous stimulations (e.g., pressure ulcer, ingrown

toenail, dressing, burns, rash) ° Sunburns ° Wounds ° Pressure over bony prominences/genitalia ° Range of motion exercises ° Spasms ° Fractures ° Heterotrophic bone

Gastrointestinal Stimuli: ° Constipation ° Difficult passage of feces ° Fecal impaction ° Bowel distention ° Hemorrhoids ° Digital stimulation ° Suppositories ° Enemas ° Gastrointestinal system pathology ° Esophageal reflux ° Gastric ulcers ° Gallstones

Urological Stimuli: ° Bladder distention/spasm ° Detrusor sphincter dyssynergia ° Instrumentation ° Surgery ° Urinary tract infection ° Cystitis ° Urethritis ° Epididymitis ° Calculi

Regulatory Stimuli: ° Temperature fluctuations ° Extreme environmental temperatures

Situational Stimuli: ° Positioning ° Surgical [/diagnostic] procedure ° Constrictive clothing (e.g., straps, stockings, shoes) ° Drug reactions (e.g., decongestants, sympathomimetics, vasoconstrictors) ° Narcotic withdrawal)

Neurological Stimuli: ° Painful/irritating stimuli below the level of injury *Cardiac/pulmonary Problems*: ° Pulmonary emboli ° Deep vein thrombosis

Reproductive [and Sexuality] Stimuli: ° Sexual intercourse ° Ejaculation ° [Vibrator overstimulation ° Scrotal compression] ° Menstruation ° Pregnancy ° Labor and delivery ° Ovarian cyst

Behavior, risk-prone health

DEFINITION: Inability to modify lifestyle/behaviors in a manner consistent with a change in health status

RELATED FACTORS: ° Inadequate comprehension ° Low self-efficacy ° Multiple stressors ° Inadequate social support ° Low socioeconomic status ° Negative attitudes toward health care

DEFINING CHARACTERISTICS
Subjective: ° Minimizes health status change ° Failure to achieve optimal sense of control

Objective: ° Failure to take actions that prevents health problems ° Demonstrates nonacceptance of health status change

Body Image, disturbed

DEFINITION: Confusion [and/or dissatisfaction] in mental picture of one's physical self

RELATED FACTORS: ° Biophysical ° Illness ° Trauma ° Injury ° Surgery ° [Mutilation, pregnancy] ° Illness treatment [change caused by biochemical agents (drugs), dependence on machine] ° Psychosocial ° Cultural ° Spiritual ° Cognitive ° Perceptual ° Developmental changes ° [Maturational changes] ° [Significance of body part or functioning with regard to age, sex, developmental level, or basic human needs]

DEFINING CHARACTERISTICS
Subjective: ° Verbalization of feelings that reflect an altered view of one's body (e.g., appearance, structure, function) ° Verbalization of perceptions that reflect an altered view of one's body in appearance ° Change in lifestyle ° Fear of rejection/reaction by others ° Focus on past strength/function/appearance ° Negative feelings about body (e.g., feelings of helplessness, hopelessness, or powerlessness) ° [Depersonalization/grandiosity] ° Preoccupation with change/loss ° Refusal to verify actual change ° Emphasis on remaining strengths ° Heightened achievement ° Personalization of part/loss by name ° Depersonalization of part or loss by impersonal pronouns

Objective: ° Behaviors of: acknowledgment/monitoring/avoidance of one's body ° Nonverbal response to actual/perceived change in body (e.g., appearance, structure, function) ° Missing body part ° Actual change in structure/function ° Not looking at/not touching body part ° Trauma to nonfunctioning part ° Change in ability to estimate spatial relationship of body to environment ° Extension of body boundary to incorporate environmental objects ° Intentional/unintentional hiding/overexposing body part ° Change in social involvement ° [Aggression; low frustration tolerance level]

Body Temperature, risk for imbalanced

DEFINITION: At risk for failure to maintain body temperature within normal range

RISK FACTORS: ° Extremes of age/weight ° Exposure to cold/cool or warm/hot environments ° Inappropriate clothing for environmental temperature ° Dehydration ° Inactivity ° Vigorous activity ° Medications causing vasoconstriction/vasodilation/sedation ° [Use or overdose of certain drugs or exposure to anesthesia] ° Illness/trauma affecting temperature regulation [e.g., infections, systemic or localized; neoplasms, tumors; collagen/vascular disease] ° Altered metabolic rate

Bowel Incontinence

DEFINITION: Change in normal bowel habits characterized by involuntary passage of stool

RELATED FACTORS: ° Toileting self-care deficit ° Environmental factors (e.g., inaccessible bathroom) ° Impaired cognition ° Immobility ° Dietary habits ° Medications ° Laxative abuse ° Stress ° Colorectal lesions ° Impaired reservoir capacity ° Incomplete emptying of bowel ° Impaction ° Chronic diarrhea ° General decline in muscle tone ° Abnormally high abdominal/intestinal pressure ° Rectal sphincter abnormality ° Loss of rectal sphincter control ° Lower/upper motor nerve damage

DEFINING CHARACTERISTICS
Subjective: ° Recognizes rectal fullness but reports inability to expel formed stool ° Urgency ° Inability to delay defecation ° Self-report of inability to feel rectal fullness
Objective: ° Constant dribbling of soft stool ° Fecal staining of clothing/bedding ° Fecal odor ° Red perianal skin ° Inability to recognize/inattention to urge to defecate

Breastfeeding, effective

DEFINITION: Mother-infant dyad/family exhibits adequate proficiency and satisfaction with breastfeeding process

RELATED FACTORS: ° Basic breastfeeding knowledge ° Normal [maternal] breast structure ° Normal infant oral structure ° Infant gestational age greater than 34 weeks ° Support sources [available] ° Maternal confidence

DEFINING CHARACTERISTICS
Subjective: ° Maternal verbalization of satisfaction with the breastfeeding process
Objective: ° Mother able to position infant at breast to promote a successful latch-on response ° Infant is content after feedings ° Regular and sustained suckling/swallowing at the breast [e.g., 8–10 times/24 h] ° Appropriate infant weight patterns for age ° Effective mother/infant communication pattern [infant cues, maternal interpretation and response] ° Signs/symptoms of oxytocin release (letdown or milk ejection reflex) ° Adequate infant elimination patterns for age; [stools soft; more than 6 wet diapers/day of unconcentrated urine] ° Eagerness of infant to nurse [breastfeed]

Breastfeeding, ineffective

DEFINITION: Dissatisfaction or difficulty a mother, infant, or child experiences with the breastfeeding process

RELATED FACTORS: ° Prematurity ° Infant anomaly ° Poor infant sucking reflex ° Infant receiving [numerous or repeated] supplemental feedings with artificial nipple ° Maternal anxiety/ambivalence ° Knowledge deficit ° Previous history of breastfeeding failure ° Interruption in breastfeeding ° Nonsupportive partner/family ° Maternal breast anomaly ° Previous breast surgery ° [Maternal physical discomfort during feeding]

DEFINING CHARACTERISTICS
Subjective: ° Unsatisfactory breastfeeding process ° Persistence of sore nipples beyond the first week

of breastfeeding ° Insufficient emptying of each breast per feeding ° Inadequate/perceived inadequate milk supply

Objective: ° Observable signs of inadequate infant intake [decrease in number of wet diapers, inappropriate weight loss/inadequate gain] ° Nonsustained/insufficient opportunity for suckling at the breast ° Infant inability [failure] to latch onto maternal breast correctly ° Infant arching/crying at the breast ° Resistant latching on ° Infant exhibiting fussiness/crying within the first hour after breastfeeding ° Unresponsive to other comfort measures ° No observable signs of oxytocin release

Breastfeeding, interrupted

DEFINITION: Break in the continuity of the breastfeeding process as a result of inability or inadvisability to put baby to breast for feeding

RELATED FACTORS: ° Maternal/infant illness ° Prematurity ° Maternal employment ° Contraindications to breastfeeding [e.g., drugs, true breast milk jaundice] ° Need to abruptly wean infant

DEFINING CHARACTERISTICS
Subjective: ° Infant receive no nourishment at the breast for some or all of feedings ° Maternal desire to maintain breastfeeding for infant/child's nutritional needs ° Lack of knowledge regarding expression/storage of breast milk
Objective: ° Separation of mother and infant

Breathing Pattern, ineffective

DEFINITION: Inspiration and/or expiration that does not provide adequate ventilation

RELATED FACTORS: ° Neuromuscular dysfunction ° Spinal cord injury ° Nneurological immaturity ° Musculoskeletal impairment ° Bony/chest wall deformity ° Anxiety[/panic attack] ° Pain ° Perception/cognitive impairment ° Fatigue ° [Deconditioning] ° Respiratory muscle fatigue ° Body position ° Obesity ° Hyperventilation ° Hypoventilation syndrome ° [Alteration of client's normal O_2:CO_2 ratio (e.g., lung diseases, hypertension, airway obstruction, O_2 therapy in COPD)]

DEFINING CHARACTERISTICS
Subjective: ° [Feeling breathless]
Objective: ° Dyspnea ° Orthopnea ° Bradypnea ° Tachypnea ° Alterations in depth of breathing ° Timing ratio ° Prolonged expiration phases ° Pursed-lip breathing ° Decreased minute ventilation/vital capacity ° Decreased inspiratory/expiratory pressure ° Use of accessory muscles to breathe ° Assumption of three-point position ° Altered chest excursion; [Paradoxical breathing patterns] ° Nasal flaring; [grunting] ° Increased anterior-posterior diameter

Cardiac Output, decreased

DEFINITION: Inadequate blood pumped by the heart to meet the metabolic demands of the body. [Note: In a hypermetabolic state, although cardiac output may be within normal range, it may still be inadequate to meet the needs of the body's tissues. Cardiac output and tissue perfusion are interrelated, although there are differences. When cardiac output is decreased, tissue perfusion problems will develop; however, tissue perfusion problems can exist without decreased cardiac output.]

RELATED FACTORS: ° Altered heart rate/rhythm [conduction] ° *Altered stroke volume:* Altered preload [e.g., decreased venous return] ° Altered afterload [e.g., altered systemic vascular resistance] ° Altered contractility [e.g., ventricular-septal rupture, ventricular aneurysm, papillary muscle rupture, valvular disease]

DEFINING CHARACTERISTICS
Subjective: Altered Heart Rate/Rhythm: ° Palpitations
Altered Preload: ° Fatigue
Altered Afterload: [Feeling breathless]

Altered Contractility: ° Orthopnea/paroxysmal nocturnal dyspnea [PND]
Behavioral/Emotional: ° Anxiety
Objective: *Altered Heart Rate/Rhythm:* ° [Dys]arrhythmias (tachycardia, bradycardia) ° EKG [ECG] changes
Altered Preload: ° Jugular vein distention (JVD) ° Edema ° Weight gain ° Increased/decreased central venous pressure (CVP) ° Increased/decreased pulmonary artery wedge pressure (PAWP) ° Murmurs
Altered Afterload: ° Dyspnea ° Clammy skin ° Skin [and mucous membrane] color changes [cyanosis, pallor] ° Prolonged capillary refill ° Decreased peripheral pulses ° Variations in blood pressure readings ° Increased/decreased systemic vascular resistance (SVR) ° Increased/decreased pulmonary vascular resistance (PVR) ° Oliguria ° [Anuria]
Altered Contractility: ° Crackles ° Cough ° Decreased cardiac output/cardiac index ° Decreased ejection fraction ° Decreased stroke volume index (SVI)/left ventricular stroke work index (LVSWI) ° S_3 or S_4 sounds [gallop rhythm]
Behaviorial/Emotional: ° Restlessness

Caregiver Role Strain

DEFINITION: Difficulty in performing caregiver role

RELATED FACTORS:
Care Receiver Health Status: ° Illness severity/chronicity ° Unpredictability of illness course ° Instability of care receiver's health ° Increasing care needs ° Dependency ° Problem behaviors ° Psychological or cognitive problems ° Addiction ° Codependency
Caregiving Activities: ° Discharge of family member to home with significant care needs [e.g., premature bith/congenital defect, frail elder post stroke] ° Unpredictability of care situation ° 24-hour care responsibilities ° Amount/complexity of activities ° Ongoing changes in activities ° Years of caregiving

Caregiver Health Status: ° Physical problems ° Psychological/cognitive problems ° Inability to fulfill one's own/others' expectations ° Unrealistic expectations of self ° Marginal coping patterns ° Addiction ° Codependency
Socioeconomic: ° Competing role commitments ° Alienation/isolation from others ° Insufficient recreation
Caregiver–Care Receiver Relationship: ° Unrealistic expectations of caregiver by care receiver ° History of poor relationship ° Mental status of elder inhibits conversation ° Presence of abuse/violence
Family Processes: ° History of marginal family coping/family dysfunction
Resources: ° Inadequate physical environment for providing care (e.g., housing, temperature, safety) ° Inadequate equipment for providing care ° Inadequate transportation ° Insufficient finances ° Inexperience with caregiving ° Insufficient time ° Physical energy ° Emotional strength ° Lack of support ° Lack of caregiver privacy ° Deficient knowledge about community resources ° Difficulty accessing community resources ° Inadequate community services (e.g., respite services, recreational resources) ° Formal/informal assistance ° Formal/informal support ° Caregiver is not developmentally ready for caregiver role

DEFINING CHARACTERISTICS
Subjective: Caregiving Activities: ° Apprehension about: ° Possible institutionalization of care receiver ° The future regarding care receiver's health/caregiver's ability to provide care ° Care receiver's care if caregiver unable to provide care

CAREGIVER HEALTH STATUS—PHYSICAL: ° GI upset ° Weight change ° Fatigue ° Headaches ° Rash ° Hypertension ° Cardiovascular disease ° Diabetes
CAREGIVER HEALTH STATUS—EMOTIONAL: ° Feeling depressed ° Anger ° Stress ° Frustration ° Increased nervousness ° Disturbed sleep ° Lack of time to meet personal needs
CAREGIVER HEALTH STATUS—SOCIOECONOMIC: ° Changes in leisure activities ° Refuses career advancement

CAREGIVER–CARE RECEIVER RELATIONSHIP: ° Difficulty watching care receiver go through the illness ° Grief/uncertainty regarding changed relationship with care receiver

FAMILY PROCESSES: ° Concern about family members

OBJECTIVE: *Caregiving Activities:* ° Difficulty performing/completing required tasks ° Pre-occupation with care routine ° Dysfunctional change in caregiving activities

CAREGIVER HEALTH STATUS—EMOTIONAL: ° Impatience ° Increased emotional lability ° Somatization ° Impaired individual coping

CAREGIVER HEALTH STATUS—SOCIOECONOMIC: ° Low work productivity ° Withdraws from social life

FAMILY PROCESSES: ° Family conflict

[Authors' note: The presence of this problem may encompass other numerous problems/high-risk concerns such as deficient Diversional Activity, Insomnia, Fatigue, Anxiety, ineffective Coping, compromised/disabled family Coping, decisional Conflict, ineffective Denial, Grieving, Hopelessness, Powerlessness, Spiritual Distress, ineffective Health Maintenance, impaired Home Maintenance, ineffective Sexuality Pattern, readiness for enhanced family Coping, interrupted Family Processes, Social Isolation. Careful attention to data gathering will identify and clarify the client's specific needs, which can then be coordinated under this single diagnostic label.]

Caregiver Role Strain, risk for

DEFINITION: Caregiver is vulnerable for felt difficulty in performing the family caregiver role

RISK FACTORS: ° Illness severity of the care receiver ° Psychological/cognitive problems in care receiver ° Addiction ° Codependency ° Discharge of family member with significant home-care needs ° Premature birth ° Congenital defect ° Unpredictable illness course ° Instability in the care receiver's health ° Duration of caregiving required ° Inexperience with caregiving ° Complexity/amount of caregiving tasks ° Caregiver's competing role commitments ° Caregiver health impairment ° Caregiver is female/spouse ° Caregiver not developmentally ready for caregiver role [e.g., a young adult needing to provide care for middle-aged parent] ° Developmental delay/retardation of the care receiver/caregiver ° Presence of situational stressors that normally affect families (e.g., significant loss, disaster or crisis, economic vulnerability, major life events [such as birth, hospitalization, leaving home, returning home, marriage, divorce, change in employment, retirement, death]) ° Inadequate physical environment for providing care (e.g., housing, transportation, community services, equipment) ° Family/caregiver isolation ° Lack of respite/recreation for caregiver ° Marginal family adaptation ° Family dysfunction prior to the caregiving situation ° Marginal caregiver's coping patterns ° Past history of poor relationship between caregiver and care receiver ° Care receiver exhibits deviant/bizarre behavior ° Presence of abuse/violence

Comfort, readiness for enhanced

DEFINITION: A pattern of ease, relief and transcendence in physical, psychospiritual, environmental, and/or dimensions that can be strengthened

RELATED FACTORS: ° To be developed

DEFINING CHARACTERISTICS
Subjective: ° Expresses desire to enhance: comfort/feeling of contentment ° Relaxation ° Resolution of complaints
Objective: ° [Appears relaxed/calm] ° [Participates in comfort measures of choice]

Communication, impaired verbal

DEFINITION: Decreased, delayed, or absent ability to receive, process, transmit, and use a system of symbols

RELATED FACTORS: ° Decrease in circulation to brain ° Brain tumor ° Anatomic deficit (e.g., cleft palate, alteration of the neurovascular visual

system, auditory system, or phonatory apparatus) °
Difference related to developmental age ° Physical
barrier (tracheostomy, intubation) ° Physiological
conditions [e.g., dyspnea] ° Alteration of central
nervous system (CNS) ° Weakening of the musculoskeletal system ° Psychological barriers (e.g.,
psychosis, lack of stimuli) ° Emotional conditions
[depression, panic, anger] ° Stress ° Environmental
barriers ° Cultural difference ° Lack of information ° Side effects of medication ° Alteration
of self-esteem/self-concept ° Altered perceptions
° Absence of SOs

DEFINING CHARACTERISTICS
Subjective: ° [Reports of difficulty expressing self]
Objective: ° Inability to speak dominant language
° Speaks/verbalizes with difficulty ° Stuttering °
Slurring ° Does not/cannot speak ° Willful refusal
to speak ° Difficulty forming words/sentences (e.g.,
phonia, dyslalia, dysarthria) ° Difficulty expressing
thoughts verbally (e.g., aphasia, dysphasia, apraxia,
dyslexia) ° Inappropriate verbalization, [inces-
sant, loose association of ideas, flight of ideas] °
Difficulty in comprehending/maintaining usual
communicating pattern ° Absence of eye contact
° Difficulty in selective attending ° Partial/total
visual deficit ° Inability/difficulty in use of facial/
body expressions ° Disorientation to person/space/
time ° Dyspnea ° [Inability to modulate speech] °
[Message inappropriate to content] ° [Use of nonverbal cues (e.g., pleading eyes, gestures, turning
away)] ° [Frustration ° Anger ° Hostility]

Communication, readiness for enhanced

DEFINITION: A pattern of exchanging information and ideas with others that is sufficient for
meeting one's needs and life goals, and can be
strengthened

RELATED FACTORS: ° To be developed

DEFINING CHARACTERISTICS
Subjective: ° Expresses willingness to enhance
communication ° Expresses thoughts/feelings °

Expresses satisfaction with ability to share infor-
mation/ideas with others
Objective: ° Able to speak/write a language °
Forms words, phrases, sentences °
Uses/interprets nonverbal cues appropriately

Conflict, decisional (specify)

DEFINITION: Uncertainty about course of
action to be taken when choice among competing actions involves risk, loss, or challenge to
values and beliefs

RELATED FACTORS: ° Unclear personal
values/beliefs ° Perceived threat to value system
° Lack of experience/interference with decision
making ° Lack of relevant information ° Multiple/
divergent sources of information ° Moral obligations require performing/not performing actions
° Moral princples/rules/values support mutually
inconsistent courses of action ° Support system
deficit ° [Age, developmental state] ° [Family
system ° Sociocultural factors] ° [Cognitive/emo-
tional/behavioral level of functioning]

DEFINING CHARACTERISTICS
Subjective: ° Verbalizes: Uuncertainty about
choices ° Undesired consequences of alternative
actions being considered ° Feeling of distress
while attempting a decision ° Questioning moral
principles/rules/values or personal values/beliefs
while attempting a decision
Objective: ° Vacillation between alternative
choices ° Delayed decision making ° Self-focusing
° Physical signs of distress or tension (increased
heart rate; increased muscle tension; restlessness;
etc.)

Conflict, parental role

DEFINITION: Parent experience of role confusion and conflict in response to crisis

RELATED FACTORS: ° Separation from child
due to chronic illness [/disability] ° Intimidation
with invasive modalities (e.g., intubation)/

restrictive modalities (e.g., isolation) ° Specialized care centers ° Home care of a child with special needs [e.g., apnea monitoring, hyperalimentation] ° Change in marital status ° [Conflicts of the role of the single parent] ° Interruptions of family life due to home care regimen (e.g., treatments, caregivers, lack of respite)

DEFINING CHARACTERISTICS
Subjective: ° Parent(s) express(es) concerns/ feeling of inadequacy to provide for child's needs (e.g., physical and emotional) ° Parent(s) express(es) concerns about changes in parental role ° Parent(s) express(es) concern about family (e.g., functioning, communication, health) ° Express(es) concern about perceived loss of control over decisions relating to their child ° Verbalize(s) feelings of frustration/ guilt ° Anxiety ° Fear ° [Verbalizes concern about role conflict of wanting to date while having responsibility of child care]
Objective: ° Demonstrates disruption in caretaking routines ° Reluctant to participate in usual caretaking activities even with encouragement and support

Confusion, acute

DEFINITION: Abrupt onset of reversible disturbances of consciousness, attention, cognition, and perception that develop oaver a short period of time

RELATED FACTORS: ° Alcohol abuse ° Drug abuse ° [Medication reaction/interaction ° Anesthesia/surgery ° Metabolic imbalances] ° Fluctuation in sleep-wake cycle ° Over 60 years of age ° Delirium [including febrile epilepticum— following or instead of an epileptic attack; toxic and traumatic] ° Dementia ° [Exacerbation of a chronic illness, hypoxemia] ° [Severe pain]

DEFINING CHARACTERISTICS
Subjective: ° Hallucinations [visual/auditory] ° [Exaggerated emotional responses]
Objective: ° Fluctuation in cognition/level of consciousness ° Fluctuation in psychomotor

activity, [tremors, body movement] ° Increased agitation/restlessness ° Misperceptions ° [Inappropriate responses] ° Lack of motivation to initiate/follow through with goal-directed/purposeful behavior

Confusion, chronic

DEFINITION: Irreversible, long-standing, and/or progressive deterioration of intellect and personality characterized by decreased ability to interpret environmental stimuli; decreased capacity for intellectual thought processes; and manifested by disturbances of memory, orientation, and behavior

RELATED FACTORS: ° Alzheimer's disease [dementia of the Alzheimer's type] ° Korsakoff's psychosis ° Multi-infarct dementia ° Cerebral vascular attack ° Head injury

DEFINING CHARACTERISTICS
Objective: ° Clinical evidence of organic impairment ° Altered interpretation/response to stimuli ° Progressive/long-standing cognitive impairment ° No change in level of consciousness ° Impaired socialization ° Impaired short-term/long-term memory ° Altered personality

Confusion, risk for acute

DEFINITION: At risk for reversible disturbances of consciousness, attention, cognition, and perception that develop over a short period of time

RISK FACTORS: ° Alcohol abuse ° Substance abuse ° Medication/Drugs: ° anesthesia ° anticholinergics ° diphenhydramine ° opioids ° psychoactive drugs ° multiple medications ° Metabolic abnormalities: ° decreased hemoglobin ° electrolyte imbalances ° dehydration ° increased BUN/creatinine ° azotemia ° malnutrition ° Infection ° Urinary retention ° Pain ° Fluctuation in sleep-wake cycle ° Decreased mobility ° Decreased restraints ° History of stroke ° Impaired cognition ° Dementia ° Sensory deprivation ° Over 60 years of age ° Male gender

Constipation

DEFINITION: Decrease in normal frequency of defecation accompanied by difficult or incomplete passage of stool and/or passage of excessively hard, dry stool

RELATED FACTORS:
Functional: ° Irregular defecation habits ° Inadequate toileting (e.g., timeliness, positioning for defecation, privacy) ° Insufficient physical activity ° Abdominal muscle weakness ° Recent environmental changes ° Habitual denial/ignoring of urge to defecate
Psychological: ° Emotional stress ° Depression ° Mental confusion
Pharmacological: ° Antilipemic agents ° Laxative overdose ° Calcium carbonate ° Aluminum-containing antacids ° Nonsteroidal anti-inflammatory agents ° Opiates ° Anticholinergics ° Diuretics ° Iron salts ° Phenothiazides ° Sedatives ° Bismuth salts ° Sympathomimetics ° Anticonvulsants ° Antidepressants ° Calcium channel blockers
Mechanical: ° Hemorrhoids ° Pregnancy ° Obesity ° Rectal abscess/ulcer/prolapse ° Rectal anal fissures/strictures ° Rectocele ° Prostate enlargement ° Postsurgical obstruction ° Neurological impairment ° Hirschsprung's disease ° Tumors ° Electrolyte imbalance
Physiological: ° Poor eating habits ° Change in usual foods/eating patterns ° Insufficient fiber/fluid intake ° Dehydration ° Inadequate dentition/oral hygiene ° Decreased motility of gastrointestinal tract

DEFINING CHARACTERISTICS
Subjective: ° Change in bowel pattern ° Unable to pass stool ° Decreased volume/frequency of stool ° Increased abdominal pressure ° Feeling of rectal fullness/pressure ° Abdominal pain ° Pain with defecation ° Nausea ° Vomiting ° Headache ° Indigestion ° Generalized fatigue
Objective: ° Hard, formed stool ° Straining with defecation ° Hypoactive/hyperactive bowel sounds ° Borborygmi ° Distended abdomen ° Abdominal tenderness with/without palpable muscle resistance ° Palpable abdominal/rectal mass ° Percussed abdominal dullness ° Presence of soft pastelike stool in rectum ° Oozing liquid stool ° Bright red blood with stool ° Severe flatus ° Anorexia ° Atypical presentations in older adults (e.g., change in mental status, urinary incontinence, unexplained falls, elevated body temperature)

Constipation, perceived

DEFINITION: Self-diagnosis of constipation and abuse of laxatives, enemas, and suppositories to ensure a daily bowel movement

RELATED FACTORS: ° Cultural/family health beliefs ° Faulty appraisal, [long-term expectations/habits] ° Impaired thought processes

DEFINING CHARACTERISTICS
Subjective: ° Expectation of a daily bowel movement ° Expected passage of stool at same time every day ° Overuse of laxatives/enemas/suppositories

Constipation, risk for

DEFINITION: At risk for a decrease in normal frequency of defecation accompanied by difficult or incomplete passage of stool and/or passage of excessively hard, dry stool

RISK FACTORS:
Functional: ° Irregular defecation habits ° Inadequate toileting (e.g., timeliness, positioning for defecation, privacy) ° Insufficient physical activity ° Abdominal muscle weakness ° Recent environmental changes ° Habitual denial/ignoring of urge to defecate
Psychological: ° Emotional stress ° Depression ° Mental confusion
Physiological: ° Change in usual foods/eating patterns ° Insufficient fiber/fluid intake ° Dehydration ° Poor eating habits ° Inadequate dentition

or oral hygiene ° Decreased motility of gastrointestinal tract

Pharmacological: ° Phenothiazines ° Nonsteroidal anti-inflammatory agents ° Sedatives ° Aluminum-containing antacids ° Laxative overuse ° Bismuth salts ° Iron salts ° Anticholinergics ° Antidepressants ° Anticonvulsants ° Antilipemic agents ° Calcium channel blockers ° Calcium carbonate ° Diuretics ° Sympathomimetics ° Opiates

Mechanical: ° Hemorrhoids ° Pregnancy ° Obesity ° Rectal abscess/ulcer ° Rectal anal stricture/fissures ° Rectal prolapse ° Rectocele ° Prostate enlargement ° Postsurgical obstruction ° Neurological impairment ° Hirschsprung's disease ° Tumors ° Electrolyte imbalance

Contamination

DEFINITION: Exposure to environmental contaminants in doses sufficient to cause adverse health effects

RELATED FACTORS:

External: ° Chemical contamination of food/water ° Presence of atmospheric pollutants ° Inadequate municipal services (trash removal, sewage treatment facilities) ° Geographic area (living in area where high level of contaminants exist) ° Playing in outdoor areas where environmental contaminants are used ° Personal/household hygiene practices ° Living in poverty (increases potential for multiple exposure, lack of access to health care, and poor diet) ° Use of environmental contaminants in the home (e.g., pesticides, chemicals, environmental tobacco smoke) ° Lack of breakdown of contaminants once indoors (breakdown is inhibited without sun and rain exposure) ° Flooring surface (carpeted surfaces hold contaminant residue more than hard floor surfaces) ° Flaking, peeling paint/plaster in presence of young children ° Paint, lacquer, etc. in poorly ventilated areas/without effective protection ° Inappropriate use/lack of protective clothing ° Unprotected contact with heavy metals or chemicals (e.g., arsenic, chromium, lead) ° Exposure to radiation (occupation in radi-

ography, employment in nuclear industries and lectrical generating plants, living near nuclear industries and electrical generation plants) ° Exposure to disaster (natural or man-made); exposure to bioterrorism

Internal: ° Age (children less than 5 years, older adults) ° Gestational age during exposure ° Developmental characteristics of children ° Female gender ° Pregnancy ° Nutritional factors (e.g., obesity, vitamin and mineral deficiencies) ° Pre-existing disease states ° Smoking ° Concomitant exposure ° Previous exposures

DEFINING CHARACTERISTICS

(Defining characteristics are dependent on the causative agent. Agents cause a variety of individual organ responses as well as systemic responses.)

Subjective/Objective:

Pesticides: ° (Major categories of pesticides: Insecticides, herbicides, fungicides, antimicrobials, rodenticides) ° (Major pesticides: organophosphates, carbamates, organochlorines, pyrethrium, arsenic, glycophosphates, bipyridyis, chlorophenoxy) ° Dermatological/gastrointestinal/neurological/ pulmonary/renal effects of pesticide exposure

Chemicals: ° (Major chemical agents: petroleum based agents, anticholinesterases; Type I agents act on proximal tracheobronchial portion of the respiratory tract, Type II agents act on alveoli, Type III agents produce systemic effects) ° Dermatological/ gastrointestinal/immunologic/neurological/pulmonary/renal effects of chemical exposure

Biologics: ° Dermatological/gastrointestinal/neurological/pulmonary/renal effects of exposure to biologicals (toxins from living organisms [bacteria, viruses, fungi])

Pollution: ° (Major locations: Air, water, soil) ° (Major agents: Asbestos, radon, tobacco [smoke], heavy metal, lead, noise, exhaust) ° Neurological/ pulmonary effects of pollution exposure

Waste: ° (Categories of waste: trash, raw sewage, industrial waste) ° Dermatological/gastrointestinal/hepatic/pulmonary effects of waste exposure

Radiation: ° (Categories: Internal—ingestion of radioactive material (e.g., food/water contamination),

External—exposure through direct contact with radioactive material) ° Immunologic/genetic/neurological/oncologic effects of radiation exposure

Contamination, risk for

DEFINITION: Accentuated risk of exposure to environmental contaminants in doses sufficient to cause adverse health effects

RISK FACTORS:
External: ° Chemical contamination of food/water ° Presence of atmospheric pollutants ° Inadequate municipal services (trash removal, sewage treatment facilities) ° Geographic area (living in area where high level of contaminants exist) ° Playing in outdoor areas where environmental contaminants are used ° Personal/household hygiene practices ° Living in poverty (increases potential for multiple exposure, lack of access to health care, and poor diet) ° Use of environmental contaminants in the home (e.g., pesticides, chemicals, environmental tobacco smoke) ° Lack of breakdown of contaminants once indoors (breakdown is inhibited without sun and rain exposure) ° Flooring surface (carpeted surfaces hold contaminant residue more than hard floor surfaces) ° Flaking, peeling paint/plaster in presence of young children ° Paint, lacquer, etc. in poorly ventilated areas/without effective protection ° Inappropriate use/lack of protective clothing ° Unprotected contact with heavy metals or chemicals (e.g., arsenic, chromium, lead) ° Exposure to radiation (occupation in radiography, employment in nuclear industries and electrical generating plants, living near nuclear industries and electrical generation plants) ° Exposure to disaster (natural or manmade); exposure to bioterrorism
Internal: ° Age (children less than 5 years, older adults) ° Gestational age during exposure ° Developmental characteristics of children ° Female gender ° Pregnancy ° Nutritional factors (e.g., obesity, vitamin and mineral deficiencies) ° Pre-existing disease states ° Smoking ° Concomitant exposure ° Previous exposures

Coping, compromised family

DEFINITION: Usually supportive primary person (family member or close friend [significant other]) provides insufficient, ineffective, or compromised support, comfort, assistance, or encouragement that may be needed by the client to manage or master adaptive tasks related to his/her health challenge

RELATED FACTORS: ° Coexisting situations affecting the significant person ° Situational/developmental crises the significant person may be facing ° Prolonged disease [/disability progression] that exhausts the supportive capacity of SO(s) ° Exhaustion of supportive capacity of significant people ° Inadequate/incorrect information or understanding by a primary person ° Temporary preoccupation by a significant person ° Temporary family disorganization/role changes ° [Lack of mutual decision-making skills] ° [Diverse coalitions of family members]

DEFINING CHARACTERISTICS
Subjective: ° Client expresses a complaint/concern about significant other's response to health problem ° SO expresses an inadequate understanding/knowledge base, which interferes with effective supportive behaviors ° SO describes preoccupation with personal reaction (e.g., fear, anticipatory grief, guilt, anxiety) to client's need
Objective: ° Significant person attempts assistive/supportive behaviors with unsatisfactory results ° SO displays protective behavior disproportionate to the client's abilities/need for autonomy ° SO enters into limited personal communication with client ° SO withdraws from client ° [SO displays sudden outbursts of emotions/emotional lability or interferes with necessary nursing/medical interventions]

Coping, defensive

DEFINITION: Repeated projection of falsely positive self-evaluation based on a self-protective pattern that defends against underlying perceived threats to positive self-regard

RELATED FACTORS: ° To be developed by NANDA ° [Refer to ND ineffective Coping.]

DEFINING CHARACTERISTICS
Subjective: ° Denial of obvious problems/weaknesses ° Projection of blame/responsibility ° Hypersensitive to slight/criticism ° Grandiosity ° Rationalizes failures ° [Refuses/rejects assistance]
Objective: ° Superior attitude toward others ° Difficulty establishing/maintaining relationships ° [Avoidance of intimacy] ° Hostile laughter ° Ridicule of others ° [Aggressive behavior] ° Difficulty in perception of reality/reality testing ° Lack of follow-through or participation in treatment/therapy ° [Attention-seeking behavior]

Coping, disabled family

DEFINITION: Behavior of significant person (family member or primary person) that disables his/her capacities and the client's capacity to effectively address tasks essential to either person's adaptation to the health challenge

RELATED FACTORS: ° Significant person with chronically unexpressed feelings (e.g., guilt, anxiety, hostility, despair) ° Dissonant coping styles for dealing with adaptive tasks by the significant person and client/among significant people ° Highly ambivalent family relationships ° Arbitrary handling of a family's resistance to treatment [that tends to solidify defensiveness as it fails to deal adequately with underlying anxiety] ° [High-risk family situations, such as single or adolescent parent, abusive relationship, substance abuse, acute/chronic disabilities, member with terminal illness]

DEFINING CHARACTERISTICS
Subjective: ° [Expresses despair regarding family reactions/lack of involvement]
Objective: ° Psychosomaticism ° Intolerance ° Rejection ° Abandonment ° Desertion ° Agitation ° Aggression ° Hostility ° Depression ° Carrying on usual routines without regard for client's needs ° Disregarding client's needs ° Neglectful care of the client in regard to basic human needs/

illness treatment ° Neglectful relationships with other family members ° family behaviors that are detrimental to well-being ° Distortion of reality regarding the client's health problem ° Impaired restructuring of a meaningful life for self ° Impaired individualization ° Prolonged overconcern for client ° Taking on illness signs of client ° Client's development of dependence

Coping, ineffective

DEFINITION: Inability to form a valid appraisal of the stressors, inadequate choices of practiced responses, and/or inability to use available resources

RELATED FACTORS: ° Situational/maturational crises ° High degree of threat ° Inadequate opportunity to prepare for stressor ° Disturbance in pattern of appraisal of threat ° Inadequate level of confidence in ability to cope ° Inadequate level of perception of control ° Uncertainty ° Inadequate resources available ° Inadequate social support created by characteristics of relationships ° Disturbance in pattern of tension release ° Inability to conserve adaptive energies ° Gender differences in coping strategies ° [Work overload ° No vacations ° Too many deadlines] ° [Impairment of nervous system ° Cognitive/sensory/perceptual impairment ° Memory loss] ° [Severe/chronic pain]

DEFINING CHARACTERISTICS
Subjective: ° Verbalization of inability to cope or inability/ask for help ° Sleep disturbance ° Fatigue ° Abuse of chemical agents ° [Reports of muscular/emotional tension] ° [Lack of appetite]
Objective: ° Lack of goal-directed behavior/resolution of problem, including inability to attend to and difficulty with organizing information ° [Lack of assertive behavior] ° Use of forms of coping that impede adaptive behavior [including inappropriate use of defense mechanisms, verbal manipulation] ° Inadequate problem-solving ° Inability to meet role expectations/basic needs [e.g., skipping meals, little/no exercise] ° Decreased use of

social support ° Poor concentration ° Change in usual communication patterns ° High illness rate [e.g., high blood pressure, ulcers, irritable bowel, frequent headaches/neckaches] ° Risk taking ° Destructive behavior toward self [including overeating, excessive smoking/drinking, overuse of prescribed/OTC medications, illicit drug use] ° [Behavioral changes, e.g., impatience, frustration, irritability, discouragement]

Coping, ineffective community

DEFINITION: Pattern of community activities for adaptation and problem solving that is unsatisfactory for meeting the demands or needs of the community

RELATED FACTORS: ° Deficits in social support services/resources ° Inadequate resources for problem solving ° Ineffective/nonexistent community systems (e.g., lack of emergency medical system, transportation system, or disaster planning systems) ° Natural or man-made disasters

DEFINING CHARACTERISTICS
Subjective: ° Community does not meet its own expectations ° Expressed vulnerability ° Expressed community powerlessness ° Stressors perceived as excessive
Objective: ° Deficits of community participation ° Excessive community conflicts ° High illness rates ° Increased social problems (e.g., homicide, vandalism, arson, terrorism, robbery, infanticide, abuse, divorce, unemployment, poverty, militancy, mental illness)

Coping, readiness for enhanced

DEFINITION: A pattern of cognitive and behavioral efforts to manage demands that is sufficient for well-being and can be strengthened

RELATED FACTORS: ° To be developed

DEFINING CHARACTERISTICS
Subjective: ° Defines stressors as manageable ° Seeks social support/knowledge of new strategies ° Acknowledges power

Objective: ° Uses a broad range of problem-oriented/emotion-oriented strategies ° Uses spiritual resources

Coping, readiness for enhanced community

DEFINITION: Pattern of community activities for adaptation and problem-solving that is satisfactory for meeting the demands or needs of the community but can be improved for management of current and future problems/stressors

RELATED FACTORS: ° Social supports available ° Resources available for problem-solving ° Community has a sense of power to manage stressors

DEFINING CHARACTERISTICS

One or more characteristics that indicate effective coping:
Subjective: ° Agreement that community is responsible for stress management
Objective: ° Active planning by community for predicted stressors ° Active problem-solving by community when faced with issues ° Positive communication among community members ° Positive communication between community/aggregates and larger community ° Programs available for recreation/relaxation ° Resources sufficient for managing stressors

Coping, readiness for enhanced family

DEFINITION: Effective managing of adaptive tasks by family member involved with the client's health challenge, who now exhibits desire and readiness for enhanced health and growth in regard to self and in relation to the client

RELATED FACTORS: ° Needs sufficiently gratified to enable goals of self-actualization to surface ° Adaptive tasks effectively addressed to enable goals of self-actualization to surface ° [Developmental stage, situational crises/supports]

DEFINING CHARACTERISTICS
Subjective: ° Family member attempts to describe growth impact of crisis [on his or her own values, priorities, goals, or relationships] ° Individual expresses interest in making contact with others who has experienced a similar situation
Objective: ° Family member moves in direction of health-promoting/enriching ° Chooses experiences that optimize wellness

Death Syndrome, risk for sudden infant

DEFINITION: Presence of risk factors for sudden death of and infant under 1 year of age [Sudden Infant Death Syndrome (SIDS) is the sudden death of an infant under 1 year of age, which remains unexplained after a thorough case investigation, including performance of a complete autopsy, examination of the death scene, and review of the clinical history. SIDS is a subset of Sudden Unexpected Death in Infancy (SUDI) that is the sudden and unexpected death of an infant due to natural or unnatural causes.]

RISK FACTORS:
Modifiable: ° Delayed/lack of prenatal care ° Infants placed to sleep in the prone/side-lying position ° Soft underlayment (loose articles in the sleep environment) ° Infant overheating/overwrapping ° Prenatal/postnatal smoke exposure
Potentially modifiable: ° Young maternal age ° Low birth weight ° Prematurity *Nonmodifiable:* ° Male gender ° Ethnicity (e.g., African American, Native American) ° Seasonality of SIDS deaths (higher in winter and fall months) ° Infant age of 2 to 4 months

Decision Making, readiness for enhanced

DEFINITION: A pattern of choosing courses of action that is sufficient for meeting short and long term health-related goals and can be strengthened

RELATED FACTORS: ° To be developed

DEFINING CHARACTERISTICS
Subjective: ° Expresses desire to enhance: Decision making ° Congruency of decisions with personal values and goals ° Congruency of decisions with sociocultural values and goals ° Risk benefit analysis of decisions ° Understanding of choices for decision making ° Understanding of the meaning of choices ° Use of reliable evidence for decisions

Denial, ineffective

DEFINITION: Conscious or unconscious attempt to disavow the knowledge or meaning of an event to reduce anxiety/fear, but leading to the detriment of health

RELATED FACTORS: ° Anxiety ° Threat of inadequacy in dealing with strong emotions ° Lack of control of life situation ° Fear of loss of autonomy ° Overwhelming stress ° Lack of competency in using effective coping mechanisms ° Threat of unpleasant reality ° Fear of separation/death ° Lack of emotional support from others

DEFINING CHARACTERISTICS
Subjective: ° Minimizes symptoms ° Displaces source of symptoms to other organs ° Unable to admit impact of disease on life pattern ° Displaces fear of impact of the condition ° Does not admit fear of death or invalidism
Objective: ° Delays seeking healthcare attention to the detriment of health ° Does not perceive personal relevance of symptoms or danger ° Unable to admit impact of disease on life pattern ° Does not perceive personal relevance of danger ° Makes dismissive gestures/comments when speaking of distressing events ° Displays inappropriate affect ° Uses self-treatment

Dentition, impaired

DEFINITION: Disruption in tooth development/eruption patterns or structural integrity of individual teeth

RELATED FACTORS: ° Dietary habits ° Nutritional deficits ° Selected prescription medications ° Chronic use of tobacco/coffee/tea/red wine ° Ineffective oral hygiene ° Sensitivity to heat or cold ° Chronic vomiting ° Deficient knowledge regarding dental health ° Excessive use of abrasive cleaning agents/intake of fluorides ° Barriers to self-care ° Lack of access/economic barriers to professional care ° Genetic predisposition ° Bruxism ° [Traumatic injury/surgical intervention]

DEFINING CHARACTERISTICS
Subjective: ° Toothache
Objective: ° Halitosis ° Tooth enamel discoloration ° Erosion of enamel ° Excessive plaque ° Worn down/abraded teeth ° Crown/root caries ° Tooth fracture(s) ° Loose teeth ° Missing teeth ° Absence of teeth ° Premature loss of primary teeth ° Incomplete eruption for age (may be primary or permanent teeth) ° Excessive calculus ° Malocclusion/tooth misalignment ° Asymmetrical facial expression

Development, risk for delayed

DEFINITION: At risk for delay of 25% or more in one or more of the areas of social or self-regulatory behavior, or cognitive, language, gross or fine motor skills

RISK FACTORS
Prenatal: ° Maternal age <15 or >35 years ° Unplanned/unwanted pregnancy ° Lack of/ate/poor prenatal care ° Inadequate nutrition ° Poverty ° Illiteracy ° Genetic/endocrine disorders ° Infections ° Substance abuse
Individual: ° Prematurity ° Congenital/genetic disorders ° Vision/hearing impairment ° Frequent otitis media ° Inadequate nutrition ° Failure to thrive ° Chronic illness ° Chemotherapy ° Radiation therapy ° Brain damage (e.g., hemorrhage in postnatal period, shaken baby, abuse, accident) ° Seizures ° Positive drug screening(s) ° Substance abuse ° Lead poisoning ° Foster/adopted child ° Behavior disorders ° Technology-dependent ° Natural disaster

Environmental: ° Poverty ° Violence
Caregiver: ° Mental retardation ° Severe learning disability ° Abuse ° Mental illness

Diarrhea

DEFINITION: Passage of loose, unformed stools

RELATED FACTORS:
Psychological: ° High stress levels ° Anxiety
Situational: ° Laxative/alcohol abuse ° Toxins ° Contaminants ° Adverse effects of medications ° Radiation ° Tube feedings ° Travel
Physiological: ° Inflammation ° Irritation ° Infectious processes ° Parasites ° Malabsorption

DEFINING CHARACTERISTICS
Subjective: ° Abdominal pain ° Urgency ° Cramping
Objective: ° Hyperactive bowel sounds ° At least three loose liquid stools per day

Dignity, risk for compromised human

DEFINITION: At risk for perceived loss of respect and honor

RISK FACTORS:

° Loss of control of body functions; exposure of the body ° Perceived humiliation/invasion of privacy ° Disclosure of confidential information ° Stigmatizing label ° Use of undefined medical terms ° Perceived dehumanizing treatment/intrusion by clinicians ° Inadequate participation in decision making ° Cultural incongruity

Distress, moral

DEFINITION: Response to the inability to carry out one's chosen ethical/moral decision/action

RELATED FACTORS:

° Conflict among decision-makers, [e.g., patient/family, health care providers, insurance payers, regulatory agencies] ° Conflicting information guiding moral/ethical decision-making ° Cultural conflicts ° Treatment decisions ° End of life decisions ° Loss of autonomy ° Time constraints for decision-making ° Physical distance of decision maker

DEFINING CHARACTERISTICS
Subjective: ° Expresses anguish (e.g., powerlessness, guilt, frustration, anxiety, self-doubt, fear) over difficulty acting on one's moral choice

Disuse Syndrome, risk for

DEFINITION: At risk for deterioration of body systems as the result of prescribed or unavoidable musculoskeletal inactivity

(Note: Complications from immobility can include pressure ulcer, constipation, stasis of pulmonary secretions, thrombosis, urinary tract infection and/or retention, decreased strength or endurance, orthostatic hypotension, decreased range of joint motion, disorientation, body image disturbance, and powerlessness.)

RISK FACTORS: ° Severe pain ° [Chronic pain] ° Paralysis ° [Other neuromuscular impairment] ° Mechanical/prescribed immobilization ° Altered level of consciousness ° [Chronic physical/mental illness]

Diversional Activity, deficient

DEFINITION: Decreased stimulation from (or interest or engagement in) recreational or leisure activities [Note: Internal/external factors may or may not be beyond the individual's control.]

RELATED FACTORS: ° Environmental lack of diversional activity [e.g., long-term hospitalization; frequent, lengthy treatments, homebound] ° [Physical/developmental limitations] ° [Bedridden] ° [Fatigue] ° [Pain] ° [Situational crisis] ° [Lack of resources] ° [Psychological condition/depression]

DEFINING CHARACTERISTICS
Subjective: ° Patient's statement regarding boredom (e.g., wish there were something to do, to read, etc.) ° Usual hobbies cannot be undertaken

in hospital [home or other care setting] ° [Changes in abilities/physical limitations]
Objective: ° [Flat affect; disinterest, inattentiveness] ° [Lethargy] ° [Withdrawal] ° [Restlessness] ° [Crying] ° [Hostility] ° [Overeating or lack of interest in eating] ° [Weight loss or gain]

Energy Field, disturbed

DEFINITION: Disruption of the flow of energy [aura] surrounding a person's being that results in a disharmony of the body, mind and/or spirit

RELATED FACTORS: Slowing or blocking of energy flow secondary to: *Pathological factors:* ° Illness ° Pregnancy ° *Injury*
Treatment related factors: ° Immbolility ° Labor and delivery ° Perioperative experience ° Chemotherapy
Situational factors: ° Pain ° Fear ° Anxiety ° Grieving
Maturational factors: ° Age-related developmental difficulties/crisis

DEFINING CHARACTERISTICS
Objective: Perception of changes in patterns of energy flow, such as: ° Movement wave/spike/tingling/dense/flowing) ° Sounds (tone/words)° Temperature change (warmth/coolness) ° Visual changes (image/color) ° Disruption of the field (deficient, hole, spike, bulge, obstruction, congestion, diminished flow in energy field)

Environmental Interpretation Syndrome, impaired

DEFINITION: Consistent lack of orientation to person, place, time, or circumstances over more than 3 to 6 months, necessitating a protective environment

RELATED FACTORS: ° Dementia [e.g., Alzheimer's disease, multi-infarct, Pick's disease, AIDS dementia] ° Huntington's disease ° Depression

DEFINING CHARACTERISTICS
Objective: ° Consistent disorientation ° Chronic confusional states ° Inability to follow simple

directions ° Inability to reason/concentrate ° Slow in responding to questions ° Loss of occupation/social functioning

Failure to Thrive, adult

DEFINITION: Progressive functional deterioration of a physical and cognitive nature. The individual's ability to live with multisystem diseases, cope with ensuing problems, and manage his/her care is remarkably diminished

RELATED FACTORS: ° Depression ° [Major disease/degenerative condition] ° [Aging process]

DEFINING CHARACTERISTICS
Subjective: ° Expresses loss of interest in pleasurable outlets ° Altered mood state ° Verbalizes desire for death
Objective: ° Inadequate nutritional intake ° Consumption of minimal to no food at most meals (i.e., consumes less than 75% of normal requirements) ° Anorexia ° Unintentional weight loss (e.g., 5% in 1 month, 10% in 6 months) ° Physical decline (e.g., fatigue, dehydration, incontinence of bowel and bladder) ° Cognitive decline: problems with responding to environmental stimuli; demonstrated difficulty in reasoning, decision making, judgment, memory, concentration, decreased perception ° Apathy ° Decreased participation in activities of daily living [ADLs] ° Self-care deficit ° Neglect of home environment/financial responsibilities ° Decreased social skills/social withdrawal ° Frequent exacerbations of chronic health problems

Falls, risk for

DEFINITION: Increased susceptibility to falling that may cause physical harm

RISK FACTORS:
Adults: ° History of falls ° Wheelchair use ° Use of assistive devices (e.g., walker, cane) ° Age 65 or over ° Lives alone ° Lower limb prosthesis
Physiological: ° Presence of acute illness ° Postoperative conditions ° Visual/hearing difficulties °

Arthritis ° Orthostatic hypotension ° Faintness when turning/extending neck ° Sleeplessness ° Anemias ° Vascular disease ° Neoplasms (i.e., fatigue/limited mobility) ° Urgency ° Incontinence ° Diarrhea ° Postprandial blood sugar changes ° [Hypoglycemia] ° Impaired physical mobility ° Foot problems ° Decreased lower extremity strength ° Impaired balance ° Difficulty with gait ° Proprioceptive deficits [e.g., unilateral neglect] ° Neuropathy
Cognitive: ° Diminished mental status [e.g., confusion, delirium, dementia, impaired reality testing]
Medications: ° Antihypertensive agents ° ACE inhibitors ° Diuretics ° Tricyclic antidepressants ° Antianxiety agents ° Hypnotics ° Tranquilizers° Narcotics ° Alcohol use
Environment: ° Restraints ° Weather conditions (e.g., wet floors/ice) ° Cluttered environment ° Throw/scatter rugs ° No antislip material in bath/shower ° Unfamiliar, dimly lit room
Children: ° <2 years of age ° Male gender when <1 year of age ° Lack of: gate on stairs; window guards; auto restraints ° Unattended infant on elevated surface ° Bed located near window ° Lack of parental supervision

Family Processes: alcoholism, dysfunctional

DEFINITION: Psychosocial, spiritual, and physiological functions of the family unit are chronically disorganized, which leads to conflict, denial of problems, resistance to change, ineffective problem solving, and a series of self-perpetuating crises

RELATED FACTORS: ° Abuse of alcohol [/addictive substances] ° Family history of alcoholism/resistance to treatment ° Inadequate coping skills ° Addictive personality ° Lack of problem-solving skills ° Biochemical influences ° Genetic predisposition

DEFINING CHARACTERISTICS
SUBJECTIVE: *Feelings:* ° Anxiety ° Tension ° Distress ° Decreased self-esteem ° Worthlessness ° Lingering resentment ° Anger

° Suppressed rage ° Frustration ° Shame ° Embarrassment ° Hurt ° Unhappiness ° Guilt ° Emotional isolation ° Loneliness ° Powerlessness ° Insecurity ° Hopelessness ° Rejection ° Responsibility for alcoholic's behavior ° Vulnerability ° Mistrust ° Depression ° Hostility ° Fear ° Confusion ° Dissatisfaction ° Loss ° Being different from other people ° Misunderstood ° Emotional control by others ° Being unloved ° Lack of identity ° Abandonment ° Confused love and pity ° Moodiness ° Failure

Roles and Relationships: ° Family denial ° Deterioration in family relationships ° Disturbed family dynamics ° Ineffective spouse communication ° Marital problems ° Intimacy dysfunction ° Altered role function ° Disrupted family roles/rituals ° Inconsistent parenting ° Low perception of parental support ° Chronic family problems ° Lack of skills necessary for relationships ° Lack of cohesiveness ° Pattern of rejection ° Economic problems ° Neglected obligations

OBJECTIVE: *Feelings:* ° Repressed emotions

Roles and Relationships: ° Closed communication systems ° Triangulating family relationships ° Reduced ability of family members to relate to each other for mutual growth and maturation ° Family does not demonstrate respect for individuality/autonomy of its members

Behaviors: ° Alcohol abuse ° Substance abuse other than alcohol ° Nicotine addiction ° Enabling to maintain drinking [/substance use] ° Inadequate understanding/deficient knowledge about alcoholism [/substance abuse] ° Family special occasions are alcohol-centered ° Rationalization/denial of problems ° Refusal to get help ° Inability to accept/receive help appropriately ° Inappropiate expression of anger ° Blaming ° Criticizing ° Verbal abuse of children/spouse/parent ° Lying ° Broken promises ° Lack of reliability ° Manipulation ° Dependency ° Inability to express/accept wide range of feelings ° Difficulty with intimate relationships ° Diminished physical contact ° Harsh self-judgment ° Difficulty having fun ° Self-blaming ° Isolation ° Unresolved grief ° Seeking approval/affirmation °

Impaired/contradictory/paradoxical/controlling communication ° Power struggles ° Ineffective problem-solving skills ° Lack of dealing with conflict ° Orientation toward tension relief rather than achievement of goals ° Agitation ° Escalating conflict ° Chaos ° Disturbances in concentration ° Disturbances in academic performance in children ° Failure to accomplish developmental tasks ° Difficulty with life-cycle transitions ° Inability to meet emotional/security/spiritual needs of its members ° Inability to adapt to change ° Immaturity ° Stress-related physical illnesses ° Inability to accept health ° Inability to deal with traumatic experiences constructively

Family Processes, interrupted

DEFINITION: Change in family relationships and/or functioning

RELATED FACTORS: ° Situational transition/crises ° Developmental transition/crises [e.g., loss or gain of a family member, adolescence, leaving home for college] ° Shift in health status of a family member ° Family roles shift ° Power shift of family members ° Modification in family finances/social status ° Interaction with community

DEFINING CHARACTERISTICS
Subjective: ° *Changes in:* ° Power alliances ° Satisfaction with family ° Expressions of conflict within family ° Effectiveness in completing assigned tasks ° Stress-reduction behaviors ° Expressions of conflict with/isolation from community resources ° Somatic complaints ° [Family expresses confusion about what to do; verbalizes they are having difficulty responding to change]

Objective: ° *Changes in:* ° Assigned tasks ° Participation in problem solving/decision making ° Communication patterns ° Mutual support ° Availability for emotional support/affective responsiveness ° Intimacy ° Patterns ° Rituals

Family Processes, readiness for enhanced

DEFINITION: A pattern of family functioning that is sufficient to support the well-being of family members and can be strengthened

RELATED FACTORS: ° To be developed

DEFINING CHARACTERISTICS
Subjective: ° Expresses willingness to enhance family dynamics ° Communication is adequate ° Relationships are generally positive ° Interdependent with community ° Family tasks are accomplished ° Energy level of family supports activities of daily living ° Family adapts to change
Objective: ° Family functioning meets needs of family members ° Activities support the safety/growth of family members ° Family roles are appropriate/flexable for developmental stages ° Respect for family members is evident ° Boundaries of family members are maintained ° Family resilience is evident ° Balance exists between autonomy and cohesiveness

Fatigue

DEFINITION: An overwhelming sustained sense of exhaustion and decreased capacity for physical and mental work at usual level

RELATED FACTORS
Psychological: ° Stress ° Anxiety ° Boring lifestyle ° Depression
Environmental: ° Noise ° Lights ° Humidity ° Temperature
Situational: ° Occupation ° Negative life events
Physiological: ° Increased physical exertion ° Sleep deprivation ° Pregnancy ° Disease states ° Malnutrition ° Anemia ° Poor physical condition ° [Altered body chemistry (e.g., medications, drug withdrawal, chemotherapy)]

DEFINING CHARACTERISTICS
Subjective: ° Verbalization of an unremitting/overwhelming lack of energy ° Inability to maintain usual routines/level of physical activity ° Perceived need for additional energy to accomplish routine tasks ° Increase in rest requirements ° Tired ° Inability to restore energy even after sleep ° Feelings of guilt for not keeping up with responsibilities ° Compromised libido ° Increase in physical complaints
Objective: ° Lethargic ° Listless ° Drowsy ° Lack of energy ° Compromised concentration ° Disinterest in surroundings ° Introspection ° Decreased performance ° [Accident-prone]

Fear [specify focus]

DEFINITION: Response to perceived threat [real or imagined] that is consciously recognized as a danger

RELATED FACTORS: ° Innate origin (e.g., sudden noise, height, pain, loss of physical support) ° Innate releasers (neurotransmitters) ° Phobic stimulus ° Learned response (e.g., conditioning, modeling from or identification with others) ° Unfamiliarity with environmental experience(s) ° Separation from support system in potentially stressful situation (e.g., hospitalization, hospital procedures [/treatments]) ° Language barrier ° Sensory impairment

DEFINING CHARACTERISTICS
Subjective: ° Report of: ° Apprehension ° Excitement ° Being scared ° Alarm ° Panic ° Terror ° Dread ° Decreased self-assurance ° Increased tension ° Jitteriness
Cognitive: ° Identifies object of fear ° Stimulus believed to be a threat
Physiological: ° Anorexia ° Nausea ° Fatigue ° Dry mouth ° [Palpitations]
Objective: Cognitive: ° Diminished productivity/learning ability/problem solving
Behaviors: ° Increased alertness ° Avoidance [/flight] ° Attack behaviors ° Impulsiveness ° Narrowed focus on the source of the fear
Physiological: ° Increased pulse ° Vomiting ° Diarrhea ° Muscle tightness ° Increased respiratory rate ° Dyspnea ° Increased systolic blood pressure ° Pallor ° Increased perspiration ° Pupil dilation

Fluid Balance, readiness for enhanced

DEFINITION: A pattern of equilibrium between fluid volume and chemical composition of body fluids that is sufficient for meeting physical needs and can be strengthened

RELATED FACTORS: ° To be developed

DEFINING CHARACTERISTICS
Subjective: ° Expresses willingness to enhance fluid balance ° No excessive thirst
Objective: ° Stable weight; no evidence of edema ° Moist mucous membranes ° Intake adequate for daily needs ° Straw-colored urine ° Specific gravity within normal limits ° Urine output appropriate for intake ° Good tissue turgor ° [No signs of] dehydration

[Fluid Volume, deficient (hyper/hypotonic)]

[NOTE: NANDA has restricted Fluid Volume deficit to address only isotonic dehydration. For patient needs related to dehydration associated with alterations in sodium, the authors have provided this second diagnostic category.]

DEFINITION: [Decreased intravascular, interstitial, and/or intracellular fluid. This refers to dehydration with changes in sodium.]

RELATED FACTORS: ° [Hypertonic dehydration: uncontrolled diabetes mellitus/insipidus, HHNC, increased intake of hypertonic fluids/IV therapy, inability to respond to thirst reflex/inadequate free water supplementation (high-osmolarity enteral feeding formulas), renal insufficiency/failure] ° [Hypotonic dehydration: chronic illness/malnutrition, excessive use of hypotonic IV solutions (e.g., D5W), renal insufficiency]

DEFINING CHARACTERISTICS
Subjective: ° [Fatigue] ° [Nervousness] ° [Exhaustion] ° [Thirst]

Objective: ° [Increased urine output, dilute urine (initially)] ° [Decreased output/oliguria] ° [Weight loss] ° [Decreased venous filling] ° [Hypotension (postural)] ° [Increased pulse rate] ° [Decreased pulse volume/pressure] ° [Decreased skin turgor] ° [Dry skin/mucous membranes] ° [Increased body temperature] ° [Change in mental status (e.g., confusion)] ° [Hemoconcentration] ° [Altered serum sodium]

Fluid Volume, deficient [isotonic]

[Note: This diagnosis has been structured to address isotonic dehydration (hypovolemia) when fluids and electrolytes are lost in even amounts and excluding states in which changes in sodium occur. For client needs related to dehydration associated with alterations in sodium, refer to [deficient Fluid Volume: hyper/hypotonic]

DEFINITION: Decreased intravascular, interstitial and/or intracellular fluid. This refers to dehydration, water loss alone without change in sodium.

RELATED FACTORS: ° Active fluid volume loss [e.g., hemorrhage, gastric intubation, diarrhea, wounds; abdominal cancer; burns, fistulas, ascites (third spacing); use of hyperosmotic radiopaque contrast agents] ° Failure of regulatory mechanisms [e.g., fever/thermoregulatory response, renal tubule damage] ° [Impaired access/intake/absorption of fluids]

DEFINING CHARACTERISTICS
Subjective: ° Thirst ° Weakness
Objective: ° Decreased urine output ° Increased urine concentration ° Decreased venous filling ° Decreased pulse volume/pressure ° Sudden weight loss (except in third spacing) ° Decreased BP ° Increased pulse rate ° Increased body temperature ° Decreased skin/tongue turgor ° Dry skin/mucous membranes ° Change in mental state ° Elevated hematocrit

Fluid Volume, excess

DEFINITION: Increased isotonic fluid retention

RELATED FACTORS: ° Compromised regulatory mechanism [e.g., syndrome of inappropriate antidiuretic hormone (SIADH), or decreased plasma proteins as found in conditions such as malnutrition, draining fistulas, burns, organ failure] ° Excess fluid intake ° Excess sodium intake ° [Drug therapies such as chlorpropamide, tolbutamide, vincristine, triptylines, carbamazepine]

DEFINING CHARACTERISTICS
Subjective: ° Anxiety ° [Difficulty breathing]
Objective: ° Edema ° Anasarca ° Weight gain over short period of time ° Intake exceeds output ° Oliguria ° Specific gravity changes ° Adventitious breath sounds [rales or crackles] ° Changes in respiratory pattern ° Dyspnea ° Orthopnea ° Pulmonary congestion ° Pleural effusion ° Pulmonary artery pressure changes ° BP changes ° Increased central venous pressure ° Jugular vein distention ° Positive hepatojugular reflex ° S_3 heart sound ° Change in mental status ° Restlessness ° Decreased Hb/Hct ° Altered electrolytes ° Azotemia

Fluid Volume, risk for deficient

DEFINITION: At risk for experiencing vascular, cellular, or intracellular dehydration

RISK FACTORS: ° Extremes of age/weight ° Loss of fluid through abnormal routes (e.g., indwelling tubes) ° Knowledge deficiency ° Factors influencing fluid needs (e.g., hypermetabolic states) ° Medications (e.g., diuretics) ° Excessive losses through normal routes (e.g., diarrhea) ° Deviations affecting access/intake/absorption of fluids

Fluid Volume, risk for imbalanced

DEFINITION: At risk for a decrease, an increase, or a rapid shift from one to the other of intravascular, interstitial, and/or intracellular fluid. This refers to body fluid loss, gain, or both.

RISK FACTORS: ° Scheduled for major invasive procedures ° [Rapid/sustained loss, e.g., hemorrhage, burns, fistulas] ° [Rapid fluid replacement]

Gas Exchange, impaired

DEFINITION: Excess or deficit in oxygenation and/or carbon dioxide elimination at the alveoli-capillary membrane [This may be an entity of its own but also may be an end result of other pathology with an interrelatedness between airway clearance and/or breathing pattern problems.]

RELATED FACTORS: ° Ventilation-perfusion imbalance [as in altered blood flow (e.g., pulmonary embolus, increased vascular resistance), vasospasm, heart failure, hypovolemic shock] ° Alveolar-capillary membrane changes [e.g., acute adult respiratory distress syndrome); chronic conditions such as restrictive/obstructive lung disease, pneumoconiosis, respiratory depressant drugs, brain injury, asbestosis/silicosis] ° [Altered oxygen supply (e.g., altitude sickness)] ° [Altered oxygen-carrying capacity of blood (e.g., sickle cell/other anemia, carbon monoxide poisoning)]

DEFINING CHARACTERISTICS
Subjective: ° Dyspnea ° Visual disturbances ° Headache upon awakening ° [Sense of impending doom]
Objective: ° Confusion ° [Decreased mental acuity] ° Restlessness ° Irritability ° [Agitation] ° Somnolence ° [Lethargy] ° Abnormal ABGs/arterial pH ° Hypoxia ° Hypoxemia ° Hypercapnia ° Hypercarbia ° Decreased carbon dioxide ° Cyanosis (in neonates only) ° Abnormal skin color (e.g., pale, dusky) ° Abnormal breathing (e.g., rate, rhythm, depth) ° Nasal flaring ° Tachycardia ° [Dysrhythmias] ° Diaphoresis ° [Polycythemia]

Glucose, risk for unstable blood

DEFINITION: Risk for variation of blood glucose/sugar levels from the normal range

RISK FACTORS:
° Lack of acceptance of diagnosis; deficient knowledge of diabetes management (e.g., action plan) ° Lack of diabetes management/adherence to diabetes management (e.g., action plan) ° Inadequate blood glucose monitoring ° Medication management ° Dietary intake ° Weight gain/loss ° Rapid growth periods ° Pregnancy ° Physical health status/activity level ° Stress ° Mental health status ° Developmental level

Grieving

DEFINITION: A normal complex process that includes emotional, physical, spiritual, social, and intellectual responses and behaviors by which individuals, families, and communities incorporate an actual, anticipated, or perceived loss into their daily lives

RELATED FACTORS: ° Anticipatory loss of significant other/significant object (e.g., possessions, job, status, home, parts and processes of body) ° Death of significant other ° Loss of significant object

DEFINING CHARACTERISTICS
Subjective: ° Anger ° Pain ° Suffering ° Dispair ° Blame ° Alteration in: activity level, sleep/dream patterns ° Making meaning of the loss ° Personal growth ° Experiencing relief
Objective: ° Detachment ° Disorganization ° Psychological distress ° Panic behavior ° Maintaining the connection to the deceased ° Alterations in immune/neuroendocrine function

Grieving, complicated

DEFINITION: A disorder that occurs after the death of a significant other [/object], in which the experience of distress accompanying bereavement fails to follow normative expectations and manifests in functional impairment

RELATED FACTORS: ° Death/sudden death of a significant other ° Emotional instability °

Lack of social support ° [Loss of significant object (e.g., possessions, job, status, home, ideals, parts and processes of the body—amputation, paralysis, chronic/terminal illness]

DEFINING CHARACTERISTICS
Subjective: ° Verbalizes: ° Anxiety ° Lack of acceptance of the death ° Persistant painful memories ° Distressful feelings about the deceased° Self-blame Verbalizes feelings of: ° Anger ° Disbelief ° Detachment from others ° Verbalizes feeling: ° Dazed ° Empty ° Stunned ° In shock ° Decreased sense of wellbeing ° Fatigue ° Low levels of intimacy ° Depression ° Yearning
Objective: ° Decreased functioning in life roles ° Persistant emotional distress ° Separation/traumatic distress ° Preoccupation with thoughts of the deceased ° Longing/searching for the deceased ° Self-blame ° Experiencing somatic symptoms of the deceased ° Rumination ° Grief avoidance

Grieving, risk for complicated

DEFINITION: At risk for a disorder that occurs after the death of a significant other, in which the experience of distress accompanying bereavement fails to follow normative expectations and manifests in functional impairment

RISK FACTORS:
° Death of a significant other ° Emotional instability ° Lack of social support ° [Loss of significant object (e.g., possessions, job, status, home, parts and processes of body)]

Growth, risk for disproportionate

DEFINITION: At risk for growth above the 97th percentile or below the third percentile for age, crossing two percentile channels; disproportionate growth

RISK FACTORS:
Prenatal: ° Maternal nutrition ° Maternal infection ° Multiple gestation ° Substance use/abuse ° Teratogen exposure ° Congenital/genetic disorders [e.g., dysfunction of endocrine gland, tumors]

Individual: ° Prematurity ° Malnutrition ° Caregiver/individual maladaptive feeding behaviors ° Insatiable appetite ° Anorexia ° [Impaired metabolism, greater-than-normal energy requirements] ° Infection ° Chronic illness [e.g., chronic inflammatory diseases] ° Substance [use]/abuse [including anabolic steroids]
Environmental: ° Deprivation ° Poverty ° Violence ° Natural disasters ° Teratogen ° Lead poisoning
Caregiver: ° Abuse ° Mental illness/retardation ° Severe learning disability

Growth and Development, delayed

DEFINITION: Deviations from age-group norms

RELATED FACTORS: ° Inadequate caretaking ° [Physical/emotional neglect or abuse] ° Indifference ° Inconsistent responsiveness ° Multiple caretakers ° Separation from significant others ° Environmental/stimulation deficiences ° Effects of physical disability [handicapping condition] ° Prescribed dependence [insufficient expectations for self-care] ° [Physical/emotional illness (chronic, traumatic), e.g., chronic inflammatory disease, pituitary tumors, impaired nutrition/metabolism, greater-than-normal energy requirements; prolonged/painful treatments; prolonged/repeated hospitalizations] ° [Sexual abuse] ° [Substance use/abuse]

DEFINING CHARACTERISTICS
Subjective: ° Inability to perform self-care/self-control activities appropriate for age
Objective: ° Delay/difficulty in performing skills typical of age group ° [Loss of previously acquired skills, precocious/accelerated skill attainment] ° Altered physical growth ° Flat affect, listlessness, decreased responses ° [Sleep disturbances, negative mood/response]

Health Maintenance, ineffective

DEFINITION: Inability to identify, manage, and/or seek out help to maintain health

[This diagnosis contains components of other NDs. We recommend subsuming health maintenance interventions under the "basic" nursing diagnosis when a single causative factor is identified (e.g., deficient Knowledge (specify); ineffective Therapeutic Regimen Management, chronic Confusion, impaired verbal Communication, disturbed Thought Process, ineffective Coping, compromised family Coping, delayed Growth and Development).]

RELATED FACTORS: ° Deficient communication skills [written, verbal, gestural] ° Unachieved developmental tasks ° Inability to make appropriate judgments ° Perceptual/cognitive impairment ° Diminished/lack of gross skills ° Diminished/lack of fine motor skills ° Ineffective individual/family coping ° Complicated grieving ° Spiritual distress ° Insufficient resource (e.g., equipment, finances) ° [Lack of psychosocial supports]

DEFINING CHARACTERISTICS
Subjective: ° Lack of expressed interest in improving health behaviors ° [Reported compulsive behaviors]
Objective: ° Demonstrated lack of knowledge regarding basic health practices ° Inability to take the responsibility for meeting basic health practices ° History of lack of health-seeking behavior ° Demonstrated lack of adaptive behaviors to environmental changes ° Impairment of personal support system ° [Observed compulsive behaviors]

Health-Seeking Behaviors (specify)

DEFINITION: Active seeking (by a person in stable health) of ways to alter personal health habits and/or the environment in order to move toward a higher level of health (Note: Stable health is defined as achievement of age-appropriate illness-prevention measures; client reports good or excellent health, and signs and symptoms of disease, if present, are controlled.)

RELATED FACTORS: ° To be developed ° [Situational/maturational occurrence precipitating concern about current health status]

DEFINING CHARACTERISTICS
Subjective: ° Expressed desire to seek a higher level of wellness ° Expressed desire for increased control of health practice ° Expressed concern about current environmental conditions on health status ° Stated unfamiliarity with wellness community resources ° [Expressed desire to modify codependent behaviors]
Objective: ° Demonstrated lack of knowledge in health promotion behaviors ° Observed unfamiliarity with wellness community resources

Home Maintenance, impaired

DEFINITION: Inability to independently maintain a safe growth-promoting immediate environment

RELATED FACTORS: ° Disease ° Injury ° Insufficient family organization/planning ° Insufficient finances ° Impaired functioning ° Lack of role modeling ° Unfamiliarity with neighborhood resources ° Deficient knowledge ° Inadequate support systems

DEFINING CHARACTERISTICS
Subjective: ° Household members express difficulty in maintaining their home in a comfortable [safe] fashion ° Household members request assistance with home maintenance ° Household members describe outstanding debts/financial crises
Objective: ° Disorderly/unclean surroundings ° Offensive odors ° Inappropriate household temperature ° Presence of vermin ° Repeated hygienic disorders/infections ° Lack of necessary equipment ° Unavailable cooking equipment ° Insufficient/lack of clothes/linen ° Overtaxed family members

Hope, readiness for enhanced

DEFINITION: A pattern of expectations and desires that is sufficient for mobilizing energy on one's own behalf and can be strengthened

RELATED FACTORS: ° To be developed

DEFINING CHARACTERISTICS
Subjective: ° Expresses desire to enhance: ° Hope ° Belief in possibilities ° Congruency of expectations with desires ° Ability to set achievable goals ° Problem-solving to meet goals ° Expresses desire to enhance: ° Sense of meaning to life ° Interconnectedness with others ° Spirituality

Hopelessness

DEFINITION: Subjective state in which an individual sees limited or no alternatives or personal choices available and is unable to mobilize energy on own behalf

RELATED FACTORS: ° Prolonged activity restriction creating isolation ° Deteriorating physiological condition ° Long-term stress ° Abandonment ° Lost belief in spiritual power/transcendent values[/God]

DEFINING CHARACTERISTICS
Subjective: ° Verbal cues (despondent content, "I can't," sighing) ° [Believes things will not change/problems will always be there]
Objective: ° Passivity ° Decreased verbalization ° Decreased affect ° Decreased appetite ° Decreased response to stimuli ° [Depressed cognitive functions, problems with decisions, thought processes; regression] ° Lack of initiative/involvement in care ° Sleep pattern disturbance ° Turning away from speaker ° Shrugging in response to speaker ° [Withdrawal from environs] ° [Closing eyes] ° [Lack of involvement/interest in significant others] ° [Angry outbursts] ° [Substance abuse]

Hyperthermia

DEFINITION: Body temperature elevated above normal range

RELATED FACTORS: ° Exposure to hot environment ° Inappropriate clothing ° Vigorous activity ° Dehydration ° Decreased perspiration °

Medications ° Anesthesia ° Increased metabolic rate ° Illness ° Trauma

DEFINING CHARACTERISTICS
Subjective: ° [Headache]
Objective: ° Increase in body temperature above normal range ° Flushed skin ° Warm to touch ° Increased respiratory rate ° Tachycardia ° [Unstable BP] ° Seizures ° [Muscle rigidity/fasciculations] ° [Confusion]

Hypothermia

DEFINITION: Body temperature below normal range

RELATED FACTORS: ° Exposure to cool or cold environment [prolonged exposure, e.g., homeless, immersion in cold water/near-drowning; induced hypothermia/cardiopulmonary bypass] ° Inadequate clothing ° Evaporation from skin in cool environment ° Decreased ability to shiver ° Aging [or very young] ° [Debilitating] illness ° Trauma ° Damage to hypothalamus ° Malnutrition ° Decreased metabolic rate ° Inactivity ° Consumption of alcohol ° Medications ° [Drug overdose]

DEFINING CHARACTERISTICS
Objective: ° Body temperature below normal range ° Shivering ° Piloerection ° Cool skin ° Pallor ° Slow capillary refill ° Cyanotic nailbeds ° Hypertension ° Tachycardia ° [Core temperature 95°F/35°C: increased respirations, poor judgment, shivering] ° [Core temperature 95° to 93.2° F/35° to 34°C: bradycardia or tachycardia, myocardial irritability/dysrhythmias, muscle rigidity, shivering, lethargic/confused, decreased coordination] ° [Core temperature 93.2° to 86° F/34° to 30°C: hypoventilation, bradycardia, generalized rigidity, metabolic acidosis, coma] ° [Core temperature below 86° F/30°C: no apparent vital signs, heart rate unresponsive to drug therapy, comatose, cyanotic, dilated pupils, apneic, areflexic, no shivering (appears dead)]

Identity, disturbed personal

DEFINITION: Inability to distinguish between self and nonself

RELATED FACTORS: ° To be developed ° [Organic brain syndrome] ° [Poor ego differentiation, as in schizophrenia] ° [Panic/dissociative states] ° [Biochemical body change]

DEFINING CHARACTERISTICS: ° To be developed
Subjective: ° [Confusion about sense of self, purpose or direction in life, sexual identification/preference]
Objective: ° [Difficulty in making decisions] ° [Poorly differentiated ego boundaries] ° [See ND Anxiety, panic, for additional characteristics]

Immunization Status, readiness for enhanced

DEFINITION: A pattern of conforming to local, national, and/or international standards of immunization to prevent infectious disease(s) that is sufficient to protect a person, family, or community and can be strengthened

RELATED FACTORS: ° To be developed

DEFINING CHARACTERISTICS
Subjective: ° Expresses desire to enhance: ° Knowledge of immunization standards ° Immunization status ° Identification of providers of immunizations ° Record-keeping of immunizations ° Identification of possible problems associated with immunizations ° Behavior to prevent infectious diseases

Infant Behavior, disorganized

DEFINITION: Disintegrated physiological and neurobehavioral responses of infant to the environment

RELATED FACTORS
Prenatal: ° Congenital/genetic disorders ° Teratogenic exposure ° [Exposure to drugs/substances]
Postnatal: ° Prematurity ° Oral/motor problems ° Feeding intolerance ° Malnutrition ° Invasive procedures ° Pain
Individual: ° Gestational/postconceptual age ° Immature neurological system ° Illness ° [Infection] ° [Hypoxia/birth asphyxia]

Environmental: ° Physical environment inappropriateness ° Sensory inappropriateness/overstimulation/deprivation ° Lack of containment within environment

Caregiver: ° Cue misreading ° Cue knowledge deficit ° Environmental stimulation contribution

DEFINING CHARACTERISTICS

Objective: Regulatory Problems: ° Inability to inhibit startle ° Irritability

State-Organization System: ° Active-awake (fussy, worried gaze) ° Quiet-awake (staring, gaze aversion) ° Diffuse sleep ° State-oscillation ° Irritable crying

Attention-Interaction System: ° Abnormal response to sensory stimuli (e.g., difficult to soothe, inability to sustain alert status)

Motor System: ° Finger splay ° Fisting ° Hands to face ° Hyperextension of extremities ° Tremors ° Startles ° Twitches ° Jittery ° Uncoordinated movement ° Changes to motor tone ° Altered primitive reflexes

Physiological: ° Bradycardia ° Tachycardia ° Arrhythmias ° Skin color changes ° "Time-out signals" (e.g., gaze, grasp, hiccough, cough, sneeze, sigh, slack jaw, open mouth, tongue thrust) ° Feeding intolerances

Infant Behavior, risk for disorganized

DEFINITION: Risk for alteration in integration and modulation of the physiological and behavioral systems of functioning (i.e., autonomic, motor, state, organizational, self-regulatory, and attentional-interactional systems)

RISK FACTORS: ° Pain ° Oral/motor problems ° Environmental overstimulation ° Lack of containment within environment ° Invasive/painful procedures ° Prematurity ° [Immaturity of the CNS] ° [Genetic problems that alter neurological and/or physiological functioning] ° [Conditions resulting in hypoxia and/or birth asphyxia] ° [Malnutrition] ° [Infection] ° [Maternal substance use/abuse] ° [Environmental events/conditions e.g., separation from parents, exposure to loud noise, excessive handling, bright lights]

Infant Behavior, readiness for enhanced organized

DEFINITION: A pattern of modulation of the physiological and behavioral systems of functioning (i.e., autonomic, motor, state-organizational, self-regulators, and attentional-interactional systems) in an infant that is satisfactory but that can be improved

RELATED FACTORS: ° Prematurity ° Pain

DEFINING CHARACTERISTICS

Objective: ° Stable physiological measures ° Definite sleep-wake states ° Use of some self-regulatory behaviors ° Response to stimuli (e.g., visual, auditory)

Infant Feeding Pattern, ineffective

DEFINITION: Impaired ability of an infant to suck or coordinate the suck/swallow response resulting in inadequate oral nutrition for metabolic needs

RELATED FACTORS: ° Prematurity ° Neurological impairment/delay ° Oral hypersensitivity ° Prolonged NPO ° Anatomic abnormality

DEFINING CHARACTERISTICS

Subjective: ° [Caregiver reports infant is unable to initiate or sustain an effective suck]

Objective: ° Inability to initiate/sustain an effective suck ° Inability to coordinate sucking, swallowing, and breathing

Infection, risk for

DEFINITION: At increased risk for being invaded by pathogenic organisms

RISK FACTORS: ° Inadequate primary defenses (broken skin, traumatized tissue, decrease in ciliary action, stasis of body fluids, change in pH secretions, altered peristalsis) ° Inadequate secondary defenses (e.g., decreased hemoglobin, leukopenia, suppressed inflammatory response) °

Inadequate acquired immunity ° Immunosuppression ° Tissue destruction ° Increased environmental exposure ° Invasive procedures ° Chronic disease ° Malnutrition ° Trauma ° Pharmaceutical agents (e.g., immunosuppressants, [antibiotic therapy]) ° Rupture of amniotic membranes ° Insufficient knowledge to avoid exposure to pathogens

Injury, risk for

DEFINITION: At risk of injury as a result of environmental conditions interacting with the individual's adaptive and defensive resources
[Author's note: The potential for injury differs from individual to individual/situation to situation. It is our belief that the environment is not safe and there is no way to list everything that might present a danger to someone. Rather, we believe nurses have the responsibility to educate people throughout their life cycles to live safely in their environment.]

RISK FACTORS:
Internal: ° Physical (e.g., broken skin, altered mobility) ° Tissue hypoxia ° Malnutrition ° Abnormal blood profile (e.g., leukocytosis/leukopenia, altered clotting factors, thrombocytopenia, sickle cell, thalassemia, decreased hemoglobin) ° Biochemical dysfunction ° Sensory dysfunction ° Integrative/effector dysfunction ° Immune/autoimmune dysfunction ° Developmental age (physiological, psychosocial) ° Psychological (affective, orientation)
External: ° Biological (e.g., immunization level of community, microorganism) ° Chemical (e.g., pollutants, poisons, drugs, pharmaceutical agents, alcohol, nicotine, preservatives, cosmetics, dyes) ° Nutritional (e.g., vitamins, food types) ° Physical (e.g., design, structure, and arrangement of community, building, and/or equipment), mode of transport or transportation ° Human (e.g., nosocomial agents, staffing patterns; cognitive, affective, and psychomotor factors)

Injury, risk for perioperative positioning

DEFINITION: At risk for injury as a result of the environmental conditions found in the perioperative setting

RISK FACTORS: ° Disorientation ° Sensory/perceptual disturbances due to anesthesia ° Immobilization ° Muscle weakness ° [Preexisting musculoskeletal conditions] ° Obesity ° Emaciation ° Edema ° [Elderly]

Insomnia

DEFINITION: A sustained disruption in amount and quality of sleep that impairs functioning

RELATED FACTORS:
° Intake of stimulants/alcohol ° Medications ° Gender-related hormonal shifts ° Stress (e.g., ruminative pre-sleep pattern) ° Depression ° Fear ° Anxiety ° Grief ° Impairment of normal sleep pattern (e.g., travel, shift work, parental responsibilities, interruptions for interventions) ° Inadequate sleep hygiene (current) ° Activity pattern (e.g., timing, amount) ° Physical discomfort (e.g., body temperature, pain, shortness of breath, cough, gastroesophageal reflux, nausea, incontinence/urgency) ° Environmental factors (e.g., ambient noise, daylight/darkness exposure, ambient temperature/humidity, unfamiliar setting)

DEFINING CHARACTERISTICS
Subjective: Patient reports: ° Difficulty falling/staying asleep ° Waking up too early ° Dissatisfaction with sleep (current) ° Non-restorative sleep ° Sleep disturbances that produce next-day consequences ° Lack of energy ° Difficulty concentrating ° Changes in mood ° Decreased health status/quality of life ° Increased accidents

Objective: ° Observed lack of energy ° Observed changes in affect ° Increased work/school absenteeism

Intracranial adaptive capacity, decreased

DEFINITION: Intracranial fluid dynamic mechanisms that normally compensate for increases in intracranial volume are compromised, resulting in repeated disproportionate increases in intracranial pressure (ICP) in response to a variety of noxious and non-noxious stimuli

RELATED FACTORS: ° Brain injuries ° Sustained increase in ICP = 10 to 15 mm Hg ° Decreased cerebral perfusion pressure ≤50 to 60 mm Hg ° Systemic hypotension with intracranial hypertension

DEFINING CHARACTERISTICS
Objective: ° Repeated increases in ICP of >10 mm Hg for more than 5 minutes following a variety of external stimuli ° Disproportionate increase in ICP following stimulus ° Elevated P_2 ICP waveform ° Volume pressure response test variation (volume-pressure ratio 2, pressure-volume index <10) ° Baseline ICP ≤10 mm Hg ° Wide amplitude ICP waveform ° [Altered level of consciousness—coma] ° [Changes in vital signs, cardiac rhythm]

Knowledge, deficient [Learning Need] (specify)

DEFINITION: Absence or deficiency of cognitive information related to specific topic [Lack of specific information necessary for client/SO(s) to make informed choices regarding condition/treatment/lifestyle changes]

RELATED FACTORS: ° Lack of exposure ° Information misinterpretation ° Unfamiliarity with information resources ° Lack of recall ° Cognitive limitation ° Lack of interest in learning °

[Request for no information] ° [Inaccurate/incomplete information presented]

DEFINING CHARACTERISTICS
Subjective: ° Verbalization of the problem ° [Request for information] ° [Statements reflecting misconceptions]
Objective: ° Inaccurate follow-through of instruction ° Inadequate performance of test ° Exaggerated/inappropriate behaviors (e.g., hysterical, hostile, agitated, apathetic) ° [Development of preventable complication]

Knowledge (specify), readiness for enhanced

DEFINITION: The presence or acquisition of cognitive information related to a specific topic is sufficient for meeting health-related goals and can be strengthened

RELATED FACTORS: ° To be developed

DEFINING CHARACTERISTICS
Subjective: ° Expresses an interest in learning ° Explains knowledge of the topic ° Describes previous experiences pertaining to the topic
Objective: ° Behaviors congruent with expressed knowledge

Lifestyle, sedentary

DEFINITION: Reports a habit of life that is characterized by a low physical activity level

RELATED FACTORS: ° Lack of interest/motivation/resources (time, money, companionship, facilities) ° Lack of training for accomplishment of physical exercise ° Deficient knowledge of health benefits of physical exercise

DEFINING CHARACTERISTICS
Subjective: ° Verbalizes preference for activities low in physical activity

Objective: ° Chooses a daily routine lacking physical exercise ° Demonstrates physical deconditioning

Liver Function, risk for impaired

DEFINITION: At risk for liver dysfunction

RISK FACTORS: ° Viral infection (e.g., Hepatitis A, Hepatitis B. Hepatitis C, Esptein-Barr) ° HIV co-infection ° Hepatotoxic medications (e.g., acetaminophen, statins) ° Substance abuse (e.g., alcohol, cocaine)

Loneliness, risk for

DEFINITION: At risk for experiencing discomfort associated with a desire or need for more contact with others

RISK FACTORS: ° Affectional deprivation ° Physical isolation ° Cathectic deprivation ° Social isolation ° [Problems of attachment for children] ° [Chaotic family relationships]

Memory, impaired

DEFINITION: Inability to remember or recall bits of information or behavioral skills [Impaired memory may be attributed to physiopathological or situational causes that are either temporary or permanent.]

RELATED FACTORS: ° Hypoxia ° Anemia ° Fluid and electrolyte imbalance ° Decreased cardiac output ° Neurological disturbances [e.g., brain injury/concussion] ° Excessive environmental disturbances ° [Manic state, fugue, traumatic event] ° [Substance use/abuse] ° [Effects of medications] ° [Age]

DEFINING CHARACTERISTICS
Subjective: ° [Reported] experiences of forgetting ° Inability to recall recent or past events/factual information [/familiar persons, places, items]

Objective: ° [Observed] experiences of forgetting ° Inability to determine if a behavior was performed ° Inability to learn/retain new skills/information ° Inability to perform a previously learned skill ° Forgetting to perform a behavior at a scheduled time

Mobility, impaired bed

DEFINITION: Limitation of independent movement from one bed position to another

RELATED FACTORS: ° Neuromuscular/musculoskeletal impairment ° Insufficient muscle strength ° Deconditioning ° Obesity ° Environmental contraints (i.e., bed size/type, treatment equipment, restraints) ° Pain ° Sedating medications ° Deficient knowledge ° Cognitive impairment

DEFINING CHARACTERISTICS
Subjective: ° [Reported difficulty performing activities]
Objective: ° *Impaired ability to:* Turn from side to side ° Move from supine to sitting or sitting to supine ° "Scoot" or reposition self in bed ° Move from supine to prone or prone to supine ° Move from supine to long-sitting or long-sitting to supine

Mobility, impaired physical [specify level]

DEFINITION: Limitation in independent, purposeful physical movement of the body or of one or more extremities

RELATED FACTORS: ° Sedentary lifestyle ° Activity intolerance ° Disuse ° Deconditioning ° Decreased endurance ° Limited cardiovascular endurance ° Decreased muscle strength/control/mass ° Joint stiffness ° Contracture ° Loss of integrity of bone structures ° Pain/discomfort ° Neuromuscular/musculoskeletal impairment ° Sensoriperceptual/cognitive impairment ° Developmental delay ° Depressive mood state ° Anxiety ° Malnutrition ° Altered cellular metabolism ° Body mass index above 75th age-appropriate percentile ° Deficient knowledge regarding value of physical activity ° Cultural beliefs regarding age-appropriate activity ° Lack of environmental supports (e.g., physical or social) ° Prescribed movement restrictions ° Medications ° Reluctance to initiate movement

DEFINING CHARACTERISTICS

Subjective: ° [Report of pain/discomfort on movement] ° [Unwillingness to move]

Objective: ° Limited range of motion ° Limited ability to perform gross fine/motor skills ° Difficulty turning ° Slowed movement ° Uncoordinated/jerky movements ° Movement-induced tremor ° Decreased [slower] reaction time ° Postural instability ° Gait changes ° Engages in substitutions for movement (e.g., increased attention to other's activity, controlling behavior, focus on preillness disability/activity)

- *Suggested Functional Level Classification:*

0—Completely independent

1—Requires use of equipment or device

2—Requires help from another person for assistance, supervision, or teaching

3—Requires help from another person and equipment device

4—Dependent, does not participate in activity

Mobility, impaired wheelchair

DEFINITION: Limitation of independent operation of wheelchair within environment

RELATED FACTORS: ° Neuromuscular/musculosketal impairments (e.g., contractures) ° Insufficient muscle strength ° Limited endurance ° Deconditioning ° Obesity ° Impaired vision ° Pain ° Depressed mood ° Cognitive impairment ° Deficient knowledge ° Environmental constraints (e.g., stairs, inclines, uneven surfaces, unsafe obstacles, distances, lack of assistive devices or persons, wheelchair type)

DEFINING CHARACTERISTICS

Subjective/Objective: ° Inability to operate manual/power wheelchair on: ° Even/uneven surface ° An incline/decline ° Curbs

Note: Specify level of independence (Refer to ND Mobility, impaired physical)

Nausea

DEFINITION: A subjective unpleasant, wave-like sensation in the back of the throat, epigastrium, or abdomen that may lead to the urge or need to vomit

RELATED FACTORS: *Treatment:* ° Gastric irritation ° Gastric distention Pharmaceuticals [e.g., analgesics—aspirin/nonsterodial anti-inflammatory drugs/opioids, anesthesia, antivirals for HIV, steroids, antibiotics, chemotherapeutic agents] ° [Radiation therapy/exposure]

Biophysical: ° Biochemical disorders (e.g., uremia, diabetic ketoacidosis, pregnancy) ° Localized tumors (e.g., acoustic neuroma, primary or secondary brain tumors, bone metastases at base of skull) ° Intra-abdominal tumors ° Toxins (e.g., tumor-produced peptides, abnormal metabolites due to cancer) ° Esophageal/pancreatic disease ° Liver/splenetic capsule stretch ° Gastric distention [e.g., delayed gastric emptying, pyloric intestinal obstruction, external compression of the stomach, other organ enlargement that slows stomach functioning (squashed stomach syndrome)] ° Gastric irritation [e.g., pharyngeal and/or peritoneal inflammation] ° Motion sickness ° Meniere's disease ° Labyrinthitis ° Increased intracranial pressure ° Meningitis

Situational: ° Noxious odors/taste ° Unpleasant visual stimulation ° Pain ° Psychological factors ° Anxiety ° Fear

DEFINING CHARACTERISTICS

Subjective: ° Reports nausea ["sick to stomach"]

Objective: ° Aversion toward food ° Increased salivation ° Sour taste in mouth ° Increased swallowing ° Gagging sensation

Neglect, unilateral

DEFINITION: Impairment in sensory and motor response, mental representation, and spatial attention to body and the corresponding environment characterized by inattention to one side and overattention to the opposite side. Left side neglect is more severe and persistent than right side neglect.

RELATED FACTORS: ° *Brain injury from:* ° Cerebrovascular problems ° Neurological illness ° Trauma ° Tumor Left hemiplegia from CVA of the right hemisphere ° Hemianopsia

DEFINING CHARACTERISTICS
Subjective: ° *[Reports feeling that part does not belong to own self]*
Objective: ° Marked deviation of the eyes/head/trunk (as if drawn magnetically) to the non-neglected side to stimuli and activities on that side ° Failure to move eyes/head/limbs/trunk in the neglected hemisphere despite being aware of a stimulus in that space ° Failure to notice people approaching from the neglected side ° Displacement of sounds to the non-neglected side ° Appears unaware of positioning of neglected limb ° Lack of safety precautions with regard to the neglected side ° Failure to: eat food from portion of the plate on the neglected side; dress/groom neglected side ° Difficulty remembering details of internally represented familiar scenes that are on the neglected side ° Use of only vertical half of page when writing ° Failure to cancel lines on the half of the page on the neglected side° Substitution of letters to form alternative words that are similar to the original in length when reading ° Distortion/omission of drawing on the half of the page on the neglected side ° Perseveration of visual motor tasks on non-neglected side ° Transfer of pain sensation to the non-neglected side

Noncompliance [Adherence, ineffective] (specify)

DEFINITION: Behavior of person and/or caregiver that fails to coincide with a health-promoting or therapeutic plan agreed on by the person (and/or family and/or community) and healthcare professional. In the presence of an agreed-on health-promoting or therapeutic plan, person's or caregiver's behavior is fully or partially nonadherent and may lead to clinically ineffective or partially ineffective outcomes.

[Author's note: When the plan of care is reviewed with the client/SO, use of the term *noncompliance* may create a negative response and sense of conflict between healthcare providers and client. Labeling the client noncompliant may also lead to problems with third-party reimbursement. Where possible, use of the ND: ineffective Therapeutic Regimen Management is recommended.]

RELATED FACTORS:
Healthcare Plan: ° Duration ° Cost ° Intensity ° Complexity ° Financial flexibility of plan
Individual Factors: ° Personal/developmental abilities ° Knowledge/skill relevant to the regimen behavior ° Motivational forces ° Individual's value system ° Health beliefs ° Cultural influences ° Spiritual values ° Significant others ° [Altered thought processes such as depression, paranoia] ° [Difficulty changing behavior, as in addictions] ° [Denial] ° [Issues of secondary gain]
Health System: ° Individual health coverage ° Credibility of provider ° Client-provider relationships ° Provider continuity/regular follow-up ° Provider reimbursement ° Communication/teaching skills of the provider ° Access/convenience of care ° Satisfaction with care
Network: ° Involvement of members in health plan ° Social value regarding plan ° Perceived beliefs of significant others

DEFINING CHARACTERISTICS
Subjective: ° [Does not perceive illness/risk to be serious, does not believe in efficacy of therapy, unwilling to follow treatment regimen or accept side effects/limitations]
Objective: ° Behavior indicative of failure to adhere ° Objective tests (e.g., physiological measures, detection of physiological markers) ° Failure to progress ° Evidence of development of complications/exacerbation of symptoms ° Failure to keep appointments ° [Inability to set or attain mutual goals]

Nutrition: less than body requirements, imbalanced

DEFINITION: Intake of nutrients insufficient to meet metabolic needs

RELATED FACTORS: ° Inability to ingest/digest food ° Inability to absorb nutrients ° Biological/psychological/economic factors ° [Increased metabolic demands, e.g., burns] ° [Lack of information, misinformation, misconceptions]

DEFINING CHARACTERISTICS
Subjective: ° Reported food intake less than RDA (recommended daily allowances) ° Lack of food ° Lack of interest in food ° Aversion to eating ° Reported altered taste sensation ° Perceived inability to digest food ° Satiety immediately after ingesting food ° Abdominal pain/cramping ° Lack of information, misinformation, misconceptions
Objective: ° Body weight 20% or more under ideal [for height and frame] [Decreased subcutaneous fat/muscle mass] ° Loss of weight with adequate food intake ° Hyperactive bowel sounds ° Diarrhea ° Steatorrhea ° Weakness of muscles required for swallowing or mastication ° Poor muscle tone ° Sore buccal cavity ° Pale mucous membranes ° Capillary fragility ° Excessive loss of hair [or increased growth of hair on body (lanugo)] ° [Cessation of menses] ° [Abnormal laboratory studies (e.g., decreased albumin, total proteins; iron deficiency; electrolyte imbalances)]

Nutrition: more than body requirements, imbalanced

DEFINITION: Intake of nutrients that exceeds metabolic needs

RELATED FACTORS: ° Excessive intake in relationship to metabolic need
[Note: Underlying cause is often complex and may be difficult to diagnose/treat.]

DEFINING CHARACTERISTICS
Subjective: ° Dysfunctional eating patterns (e.g., pairing food with other activities) ° Eating in response to external cues (e.g., time of day, social situation) ° Concentrating food intake at end of day ° Eating in response to internal cues other than hunger (e.g., anxiety) ° Sedentary activity level
Objective: ° Weight 20% over ideal for height and frame [obese] ° Triceps skin fold >15 mm in men, >25 mm in women ° [Percentage of body fat greater than 22% for trim women and 15% for trim men]

Nutrition, readiness for enhanced

DEFINITION: A pattern of nutrient intake that is sufficient for meeting metabolic needs and can be strengthened

RELATED FACTORS: ° To be developed

DEFINING CHARACTERISTICS
Subjective: ° Expresses knowledge of healthy food and fluid choices/willingness to enhance nutrition ° Eats regularly ° Attitude toward eating/drinking is congruent with health goals
Objective: ° Consumes adequate food/fluid ° Follows an appropriate standard for intake (e.g., the food pyramid or American Diabetic Association Guidelines)
° Safe preparation/storage for food/fluids

Nutrition: risk for more than body requirements, imbalanced

DEFINITION: At risk for intake of nutrients that exceeds metabolic needs.

RISK FACTORS: ° Dysfunctional eating patterns ° Pairing food with other activities ° Eating in response to external cues other than hunger (e.g., time of day, social situation) ° Eating in response to internal cues other than hunger (such as anxiety) ° Concentrating food intake at end of day ° Parental obesity ° Rapid transition across growth percentiles in children ° Reported use of solid food as major food source before 5 months of age ° Higher baseline weight at beginning of each pregnancy ° Observed use of food as reward/comfort measure ° [Frequent/repeated dieting] ° [Alteration in usual activity patterns/sedentary lifestyle] ° [Majority of foods consumed are concentrated, high-calorie/fat sources] ° [Lower socioeconomic status]

Oral Mucous Membrane, impaired

DEFINITION: Disruption of the lips and/or soft tissue of the oral cavity

RELATED FACTORS: ° Dehydration ° NPO for more than 24 hours ° Malnutrition ° Decreased salivation ° Medication side effects ° Diminished hormone levels (women) ° Mouth breathing ° Deficient knowledge of appropriate oral hygiene ° Ineffective oral hygiene ° Barriers to oral self-care/professional care ° Mechanical factors (e.g., ill-fitting dentures; braces; tubes [ET, nasogastric], surgery in oral cavity) ° Loss of supportive structures ° Trauma ° Cleft lip or palate ° Chemical irritants (e.g., alcohol, tobacco, acidic foods, regular use of inhalers or other noxious agents) ° Chemotherapy ° Immunosuppression ° Immunocompromised ° Decreased platelets ° Infection ° Radiation therapy ° Stress ° Depression

DEFINING CHARACTERISTICS
Subjective: ° Xerostomia [dry mouth] ° Oral pain/discomfort ° Reports bad taste in mouth ° Diminished taste ° Difficulty eating/swallowing
Objective: ° Coated tongue ° Smooth atrophic tongue ° Geographic tongue ° Gingival/mucosal pallor ° Stomatitis ° Hyperemia ° Gingival hyperplasia ° Macroplasia ° Vesicles ° Nodules ° Papules ° White patches/plaques ° Spongy patches ° White curdlike exudate ° Oral lesions/ulcers ° Fissures ° Bleeding ° Chelitis ° Desquamation ° Mucosal denudation ° Purulent drainage/exudates ° Presence of pathogens ° Enlarged tonsils ° Edema ° Halitosis ° Gingival recession, pockets deeper than 4 mm ° [Carious teeth] ° Red or bluish masses (e.g., hemangiomas) ° Difficult speech

Pain, acute

DEFINITION: Unpleasant sensory and emotional experience arising from actual or potential tissue damage or described in terms of such damage (International Association for the Study of Pain); sudden or slow onset of any intensity from mild to severe with an anticipated or predictable end and a duration of less than 6 months

RELATED FACTORS: ° Injuring agents (biological, chemical, physical, psychological)

DEFINING CHARACTERISTICS
Subjective: ° Verbal/coded report [may be less from patients younger than age 40, men, and some cultural groups] ° Changes in appetite ° [Pain unrelieved and/or increased beyond tolerance]
Objective: ° Observed evidence of pain ° Guarded behavior ° Protective gestures ° Positioning to avoid pain ° Facial mask ° Sleep disturbance (eyes lack luster, beaten look, fixed or scattered movement, grimace) ° Expressive behavior (e.g., restlessness, moaning, crying, vigilance, irritability, sighing) ° Distraction behavior (e.g., pacing, seeking out other people and/or activities, repetitive activities) ° Changes in muscle tone (may span from listless [flaccid] to rigid) ° Diaphoresis ° Changes in blood pressure/heart rate/respiration rate ° Pupillary dilation ° Self-focusing ° Narrowed focus (altered time perception, impaired thought process, reduced interaction with people and environment)

Pain, chronic

DEFINITION: Unpleasant sensory and emotional experience arising from actual or potential tissue damage or described in terms of such damage (International Association for the Study of Pain); sudden or slow onset of any intensity from mild to severe, constant or recurring without an anticipated or predictable end and a duration of greater than 6 months

[Pain is a signal that something is wrong. Chronic pain can be recurrent and periodically disabling (e.g., migraine headaches) or may be unremitting. Although chronic pain syndrome includes various learned behaviors, psychological factors become the primary contribution to impairment. It is a complex entity, combining elements from other NDs (e.g., Powerlessness; deficit Diversional Activity; interrupted Family Processes; Self-Care Deficit; and risk for Disuse Syndrome).]

RELATED FACTORS: ° Chronic physical/psychosocial disability

DEFINING CHARACTERISTICS
Subjective: ° Verbal/coded report ° Fear of reinjury ° Altered ability to continue previous activities ° Changes in sleep patterns ° Fatigue ° Anorexia ° [Preoccupation with pain] ° [Desperately seeks alternative solutions/therapies for relief/control of pain]
Objective: ° Observed protective behavior ° Guarding behavior ° Irritability ° Restlessness ° Facial mask ° Self-focusing ° Reduced interaction with people ° Depression ° Atrophy of involved muscle group ° Sympathetic mediated responses (temperature, cold, changes of body position, hypersensitivity)

Parenting, readiness for enhanced

DEFINITION: A pattern of providing an environment for children or other dependent person(s) that is sufficient to nurture growth and development and can be strengthened

RELATED FACTORS: ° To be developed

DEFINING CHARACTERISTICS
Subjective: ° Expresses willingness to enhance parenting ° Children or other dependent person(s) express(es) satisfaction with home environment
Objective: ° Emotional support of children [/dependent person(s)] ° Evidence of attachment ° Needs of children [/dependent person(s)] are met (e.g., physical and emotional) ° Exhibits realistic expectations of children [/dependent person(s)]

Parenting, impaired

DEFINITION: Inability of the primary caretaker to create, maintain, or regain an environment that promotes the optimum growth and development of the child

RELATED FACTORS:
Infant or Child: ° Premature birth ° Multiple births ° Not gender desired ° Illness ° Separation from parent ° Difficult temperament ° Temperamental conflicts with parental expectations ° Handicapping condition ° Developmental delay ° Altered perceptual abilities ° Attention-deficit hyperactivity disorder
Knowledge: ° Deficient knowledge about child development/health maintenance, parenting skills ° Inability to respond to infant cues ° Unrealistic expectation [for self, infant, partner] ° Lack of educational ° Limited cognitive functioning ° Lack of cognitive readiness for parenthood ° Poor communication skills ° Preference for physical punishment
Physiological: ° Physical illness
Psychological: ° Young parental age ° Lack of prenatal care ° Difficult birthing process ° High number of/closely spaced pregnancies ° Sleep disruption/ deprivation ° Depression ° History of substance abuse ° Disability ° History of mental illness
Social: ° Presence of stress (e.g., financial, legal, recent crisis, cultural move [e.g., from another country/cultural group within same country]) ° Job problems ° Unemployment ° Financial difficulties ° Relocations ° Poor home environment ° Situational/chronic low self-esteem ° Lack of family cohesiveness ° Marital conflict ° Change in

family unit ° Inadequate child-care arrangements ° Role strain ° Single parents ° Father/mother of child not involved ° Lack of/or poor parental role model ° Lack of valuing of parenthood ° Inability to put child's needs before own ° Unplanned or unwanted pregnancy ° Low socioeconomic class ° Poverty ° Lack of resources ° Lack of transportation ° Poor problem-solving skills ° Maladaptive coping strategies ° Lack of social support networks ° Social isolation ° History of being abusive/being abused ° Legal difficulties

DEFINING CHARACTERISTICS

SUBJECTIVE: *Parental:* ° Statements of inability to meet child's needs ° Verbalization of inability to control child ° Negative statements about child ° Verbalization of frustration/role inadequacy

OBJECTIVE: *Infant or Child:* ° Frequent accidents/illness ° Failure to thrive ° Poor academic performance/cognitive development ° Poor social competence ° Behavior disorders ° Incidence of trauma (e.g., physical and psychological)/abuse ° Lack of attachment ° Lack of separation anxiety ° Runaway

PARENTAL: ° Maternal-child interaction deficit ° Poor parent-child interaction ° Little cuddling ° Inadequate attachment ° Inadequate child health maintenance ° Unsafe home environment ° Inappropriate child-care arrangements ° Inappropriate stimulation (e.g., visual, tactile, auditory) ° Inappropriate caretaking skills ° Inconsistent care/behavior management ° Inflexibility to meet needs of child ° Frequently punitive ° Rejection of/hostility to child ° Child abuse/neglect ° Abandonment

Parenting, risk for impaired

DEFINITION: Risk for inability of the primary caretaker to create, maintain, or regain an environment that promotes the optimum growth and development of the child

RISK FACTORS:

Infant or Child: ° Altered perceptual abilities ° Attention-deficit hyperactivity disorder ° Difficult temperament ° Temperamental conflicts with parental expectation ° Premature birth ° Multiple births ° Not gender desired ° Illness ° Prolonged separation from parent ° Handicapping condition/developmental delay

Knowledge: ° Unrealistic expectation of child ° Deficient knowledge about child development/ health maintenance, parenting skills ° Low educational level or attainment ° Lack of cognitive readiness for parenthood ° Low cognitive functioning ° Poor communication skills ° Inability to respond to infant cues ° Preference for physical punishment

Physiological: ° Physical illness

Psychological: ° Young parental age ° Closely spaced pregnancies ° High number of pregnancies ° Difficult birthing process ° Sleep disruption/ deprivation ° Depression ° History of substance abuse ° Disability ° History of mental illness

Social: ° Stress ° Unemployment ° Financial difficulties ° Poor home environments ° Relocation [including cultural move (e.g., from another country/cultural group within same country)] ° Situational/chronic low self-esteem ° Lack of family cohesiveness ° Marital conflict ° Change in family unit ° Inadequate child-care arrangements ° Role strain ° Single parent ° Father/mother of child not involved ° Parent-child separation ° Poor/lack of parental role model ° Lack of valuing of parenthood ° Unplanned/unwanted pregnancy ° Late/ lack of prenatal care ° Low socioeconomic class ° Poverty ° Lack of resources/access to resources ° Lack of transportation ° Poor problem-solving skills ° Maladaptive coping strategies ° Lack of social support network ° Social isolation ° History of being abused/ being abusive ° Legal difficulties

Peripheral Neurovascular Dysfunction, risk for

DEFINITION: At risk for disruption in circulation, sensation, or motion of an extremity

RISK FACTORS: ° Fractures ° Trauma ° Vascular obstruction ° Mechanical compression (e.g., tourniquet, cane, cast, brace, dressing, restraint) ° Orthopedic surgery ° Immobilization

Poisoning, risk for

DEFINITION: Accentuated risk of accidental exposure to, or ingestion of, drugs or dangerous products in doses sufficient to cause poisoning [or the adverse effects of prescribed medication/drug use]

RISK FACTORS:
Internal: ° Reduced vision ° Lack of safety/drug education ° Lack of proper precaution ° [Unsafe habits] ° [Disregard for safety measures] ° [Lack of supervision] ° Verbalization of occupational is setting without adequate safeguards ° Cognitive/emotional difficulties ° [Age, e.g., young child, elderly person] ° [Chronic disease state/disability] ° [Cultural or religious beliefs/practices]
External: ° Large supplies of drugs in house ° Medicines stored in unlocked cabinets accessible to children/ confused individuals ° Availability of illicit drugs potentially contaminated by poisonous additives ° Dangerous products placed within reach of children/confused individuals ° [Therapeutic margin of safety of specific drugs (e.g., therapeutic versus toxic level, half-life, method of uptake and degradation in body, adequacy of organ function)] ° [Use of multiple herbal supplements or megadosing]

Post-Trauma Syndrome [specify stage]

DEFINITION: Sustained maladaptive response to a traumatic, overwhelming event

RELATED FACTORS: ° Events outside the range of usual human experience ° Serious threat to self/loved ones ° Serious injury to self/loved ones ° Serious accidents (e.g., industrial, motor-vehicle) ° Abuse (physical and psychosocial) ° Criminal victimization ° Rape ° Witnessing muti-lation/violent death ° Tragic occurrence involving multiple deaths ° Disasters ° Sudden destruction of one's home/community ° Epidemics ° Wars ° Being held prisoner of war ° Torture

DEFINING CHARACTERISTICS
Subjective: ° Intrusive thoughts/dreams ° Nightmares ° Flashbacks ° Palpitations ° Headaches ° [Loss of interest in usual activities] ° [Loss of feeling of intimacy/sexuality] ° Hopelessness ° Shame ° [Excessive verbalization of the traumatic event] ° [Verbalization of survival guilt/guilt about behavior required for survival] ° Anxiety ° Fear ° Grieving ° Reports feeling numb ° Depression ° Difficulty in concentrating ° Gastric irritability ° [Changes in appetite/sleep pattern] ° [Chronic fatigue/easy fatigability]
Objective: ° Hypervigilance ° Exaggerated startle response ° Irritability ° Neurosensory irritability ° Denial ° Repression ° Avoidance ° Alienation ° Detachment ° Psychogenic amnesia ° Altered mood states ° Aggression ° [Poor impulse control/explosiveness] ° Rage ° Panic attacks ° Horror ° Substance abuse ° Compulsive behavior ° Enuresis (in children) ° [Difficulty with interpersonal relationships] ° [Dependence on others] ° [Work/school failure]
[Stages:
Acute subtype: Begins within 6 months and does not last longer than 6 months
Chronic subtype: Lasts longer than 6 months
Delayed subtype: Period of latency of 6 months or longer before onset of symptoms]

Post-Trauma Syndrome, risk for

DEFINITION: At risk for sustained maladaptive response to a traumatic, overwhelming event

RISK FACTORS: ° Occupation (e.g., police, fire, rescue, corrections, emergency room staff, mental health worker, [responder family members]) ° Perception of event ° Exaggerated sense of responsibility ° Diminished ego strength ° Survivor's role in the event ° Inadequate social support ° Nonsupportive environment ° Displacement from home ° Duration of the event

Power, readiness for enhanced

DEFINITION: A pattern of participating knowingly in change that is sufficient for well-being and can be strengthened

RELATED FACTORS: ° To be developed

DEFINING CHARACTERISTICS
Subjective: ° *Expresses readiness to enhance*: ° Power ° Knowledge for participation in change ° Awareness of possible changes to be made ° Identification of choices that can be made for change *Expresses readiness to enhance:* ° Freedom to perform actions for change ° Involvement in creating change ° Participation in choices for daily living and health

Powerlessness [specify level]

DEFINITION: Perception that one's own action will not significantly affect an outcome; a perceived lack of control over a current situation or immediate happening

RELATED FACTORS: ° Health-care environment [e.g., loss of privacy, personal possessions, control over therapies] ° Interpersonal interaction [e.g., misuse of power, force; abusive relationships] ° Illness-related regimen [e.g., chronic/debilitating conditions] ° Lifestyle of helplessness [e.g., repeated failures, dependency]

DEFINING CHARACTERISTICS
  SUBJECTIVE: *Low:* ° Expressions of uncertainty about fluctuating energy levels
  MODERATE: ° Expressions of dissatisfaction/frustration over inability to perform previous tasks/activities ° Expression of doubt regarding role performance ° Fear of alienation from caregivers ° Reluctance to express true feelings ° Resentment ° Anger ° Guilt
  SEVERE: ° Verbal expressions of having no control (e.g., over self-care, situation, outcome) ° Depression over physical deterioration
  OBJECTIVE: *Low:* ° Passivity

MODERATE: ° Dependence on others that may result in irritability ° Inability to seek information regarding care ° Passivity ° Nonparticipation in care/decision making when opportunities are provided ° Does not monitor progress ° Does not defend self-care practices when challenged
  SEVERE: ° Apathy° [Withdrawal] ° [Resignation] ° [Crying]

Powerlessness, risk for

DEFINITION: At risk for perceived lack of control over a situation and/or one's ability to significantly affect an outcome

RISK FACTORS:
Physiological: ° Illness [hospitalization, intubation, ventilator, suctioning] ° Dying ° Acute injury ° Progressive debilitating disease process (e.g., spinal cord injury, multiple sclerosis) ° Aging [e.g., decreased physical strength, decreased mobility]
Psychosocial: ° Deficient knowledge (e.g., illness or healthcare system) ° Lifestyle of dependency° Inadequate coping patterns ° Absence of integrality (e.g., essence of power) ° Situational/chronic low self-esteem ° Disturbed body image

Protection, ineffective

DEFINITION: Decrease in ability to guard self from internal or external threats such as illness or injury

RELATED FACTORS: ° Extremes of age ° Inadequate nutrition ° Alcohol abuse ° Abnormal blood profiles (e.g., leukopenia, thrombocytopenia, anemia, coagulation) ° Drug therapies (e.g., antineoplastic, corticosteroid, immune, anticoagulant, thrombolytic) ° Treatments (e.g., surgery, radiation) ° Cancer ° Immune disorders

DEFINING CHARACTERISTICS
Subjective: ° Neurosensory alterations ° Chilling ° Itching ° Insomnia ° Fatigue ° Weakness ° Anorexia

Objective: ° Deficient immunity ° Impaired healing ° Altered clotting ° Maladaptive stress response ° Perspiring [inappropriate] ° Dyspnea ° Cough ° Restlessness ° Immobility ° Disorientation ° Pressure sores

Rape-Trauma Syndrome

DEFINITION: Sustained maladaptive response to a forced, violent sexual penetration against the victim's will and consent. [Rape is not a sexual crime, but a crime of violence and identified as sexual assault. Although attacks are most often directed toward women, men also may be victims.]

Note: This syndrome includes the following three subcomponents: Rape-Trauma, Compound reaction, and Silent reaction. In this text each appears as a separate diagnosis.

RELATED FACTORS: ° Rape [actual/attempted forced sexual penetration]

DEFINING CHARACTERISTICS
Subjective: ° Embarrassment ° Humiliation ° Shame ° Guilt ° Self-blame ° Loss of self-esteem ° Helplessness ° Powerlessness ° Shock ° Fear ° Anxiety ° Anger ° Revenge ° Nightmares ° Sleep disturbances ° Change in relationships ° Sexual dysfunction
Objective: ° Physical trauma [e.g., bruising, tissue irritation] ° Muscle tension/spasms ° Confusion ° Disorganization ° Inability to make decisions ° Agitation ° Hyperalertness ° Aggression ° Mood swings ° Vulnerability ° Dependence ° Depression ° Substance abuse ° Suicide attempts ° Denial ° Phobias ° Paranoia ° Dissociative disorders

Rape-Trauma Syndrome: compound reaction

DEFINITION: Forced violent sexual penetration against the victim's will and consent. The trauma syndrome that develops from this attack or attempted attack includes an acute phase of disorganization of the victim's lifestyle and a long-term process of reorganization of lifestyle.

RELATED FACTORS: ° To be developed

DEFINING CHARACTERISTICS
Subjective: *Acute phase:* ° Multiple physical symptoms (e.g., gastrointestinal irritability, genitourinary discomfort, muscle tension, sleep pattern disturbance) ° Reactivated symptoms of such previous conditions (i.e., physical/psychiatric illness) ° Substance abuse
Objective: *Acute phase:* ° Emotional reactions (e.g., anger, embarrassment, fear of physical violence and death, humiliation, self-blame, revenge)
Long-term phase: ° Changes in lifestyle (e.g., changes in residence, dealing with repetitive nightmares and phobias, seeking family/social network support)

Rape-Trauma Syndrome: silent reaction

DEFINITION: Forced violent sexual penetration against the victim's will and consent. The trauma syndrome that develops from this attack or attempted attack includes an acute phase of disorganization of the victim's lifestyle and a long-term process of reorganization of lifestyle.

RELATED FACTORS: ° To be developed

DEFINING CHARACTERISTICS
Subjective: ° Increase in nightmares ° Abrupt changes in relationships with men ° Pronounced changes in sexual behavior
Objective: ° Increasing anxiety during interview (e.g., blocking of associations, long periods of silence; minor stuttering, physical distress) ° No verbalization of the occurrence of rape ° Sudden onset of phobic reactions

Religiosity, impaired

DEFINITION: Impaired ability to exercise reliance on beliefs and/or participate in rituals of a particular faith tradition

[NANDA-I] recognizes that the term 'religiosity" may be culture specific; however, the term is useful in the U.S. and is well-supported in the U.S. literature.

RELATED FACTORS:
Developmental and Situational: ° Life transitons ° Aging ° End-stage life crises
Physical: ° Illness ° Pain
Psychological Factors: ° Ineffective support/coping ° Anxiety ° Fear of death ° Personal crisis [/disaster] ° Lack of security ° Use of religion to manipulate
Sociocultural: ° Cultural/environmental barriers to practicing religion ° Lack of social integration ° Lack of sociocultural interaction
Spiritual: ° Spiritual crises ° Suffering

DEFINING CHARACTERISTICS
Subjective: ° Expresses emotional distress because of separation from faith community ° Expresses a need to reconnect with previous belief patterns/customs ° Questions religious belief patterns/customs ° Difficulty adhering to prescribed religious beliefs and rituals (e.g., religious ceremonies, dietary regulations, clothing, prayer, worship/religious services, private religious behaviors/reading religious materials/media, holiday observances, meetings with religious leaders)

Religiosity, readiness for enhanced

DEFINITION: Ability to increase reliance on religious beliefs and/or participate in rituals of a particular faith tradition
[NANDA-I] recognizes that the term "religiosity" may be culture specific; however, the term is useful in the U.S. and is well-supported in the U.S. literature.

RELATED FACTORS: ° To be developed

DEFINING CHARACTERISTICS
Subjective: ° Expresses desire to strengthen religious belief patterns/customs that had provided comfort/religion in the past ° Request for

assistance to increase participation in prescribed religious beliefs (e.g., religious ceremonies, dietary regulations/rituals, clothing, prayer, worship/religious services, private religious behaviors, reading religious materials/media, holiday observances) ° Requests assistance expanding religious options/religious materials/experiences ° Requests meeting with religious leaders/facilitators ° Requests forgiveness/reconciliation ° Questions/rejects belief patterns/customs that are harmful

Religiosity, risk for impaired

DEFINITION: At risk for an impaired ability to exercise reliance on religious beliefs and/or participate in rituals of a particular faith tradition
[NANDA-I] recognizes that the term "religiosity" may be culture specific; however, the term is useful in the U.S. and is well-supported in the U.S. literature.

RISK FACTORS:
Developmental: ° Life transitions
Environmental: ° Lack of transportation ° Barriers to practicing religion
Physical: ° Illness ° Hospitalization ° Pain
Psychological: ° Inadequate coping/caregiving ° Ineffective support ° Depression ° Lack of security
Sociocultural: ° Lack of social interaction ° Social isolation ° Cultural barrier to practicing religion
Spiritual: ° Suffering

Relocation Stress Syndrome

DEFINITION: Physiological and/or psychosocial disturbance following transfer from one environment to another

RELATED FACTORS: ° Losses ° Feeling of powerlessness ° Lack of adequate support system ° Lack of predeparture counseling ° Unpredictability of experience ° Isolation ° Language barrier ° Impaired psychosocial health ° Passive coping ° Decreased health status

DEFINING CHARACTERISTICS

Subjective: ° Anxiety (e.g., separation) ° Anger ° Insecurity ° Worry ° Fear ° Loneliness ° Depression ° Unwillingness to move° Concern over relocation ° Sleep disturbance

Objective: ° Move from one environment to another ° Increased [frequency of] verbalization of needs ° Pessimism ° Frustration ° Increased physical symptoms/illness ° Withdrawal ° Aloneness ° Alienation ° [Hostile behavior/outbursts] ° Loss of identity ° Loss of self-worth/self-esteem ° Dependency ° [Increased confusion] ° [Cognitive impairment]

Relocation Stress Syndrome, risk for

DEFINITION: At risk for physiological and/or psychosocial disturbance following transfer from one environment to another

RISK FACTORS: ° Move from one environment to another ° Moderate to high degree of environmental change [e.g., physical, ethnic, cultural] ° Lack of adequate support system/group ° Lack of predeparture counseling ° Passive coping ° Feelings of powerlessness ° Losses ° Moderate mental competence ° Unpredictability of experiences

Role Performance, ineffective

DEFINITION: Patterns of behavior and self-expression that do not match the environmental context, norms, and expectations [Note: There is a typology of roles: Sociopersonal (friendship, family, marital, parenting, community), home management, intimacy (sexuality, relationship building), leisure/exercise/recreation, self-management, socialization (developmental transitions), community contributor, and religious.]

RELATED FACTORS:

Knowledge: ° Inadequate/lack of role model ° Inadequate role preparation (e.g., role transition, skill, rehearsal, validation) ° Lack of education ° [Developmental transitions] ° Unrealistic role expectations

Physiological: ° Body image alteration ° Cognitive deficits ° Neurological deficits ° Physical illness ° Mental illness ° Depression ° Low self-esteem ° Fatigue ° Pain ° Substance abuse

Social: ° Inadequate role socialization [e.g., role model, expectations, responsibilities] ° Young age ° Developmental level ° Lack of resources ° Low socioeconomic status ° Stress ° Conflict ° Job schedule demands ° Domestic violence ° Inadequate support system ° Lack of rewards ° Inappropriate linkage with the healthcare system

DEFINING CHARACTERISTICS

Subjective: ° Altered role perceptions ° Change in self-/other'sperception of role ° Change in usual patterns of responsibility/capacity to resume ° Inadequate opportunities for role enactment ° Role dissatisfaction ° Role overload ° Role denial ° Discrimination [by others] ° Powerlessness

Objective: ° Deficient knowledge ° Inadequate role competency/skills ° Inadequate adaptation to change ° Inappropriate developmental expectations ° Inadequate confidence ° Inadequate motivation ° Inadequate self-management/coping ° Inadequate external support for role enactment ° Role strain ° Role conflict/ confusion ° Role ambivalence ° [Failure to assume role] ° Uncertainty ° Anxiety ° Depression ° Pessimistic ° Domestic violence ° Harassment ° System conflict

Self-Care, readiness for enhanced

DEFINITION: A pattern of performing activities for oneself that helps to meet health-related goals and can be strengthened

RELATED FACTORS:° To be developed

DEFINING CHARACTERISTICS

Subjective: ° Expresses desire to enhance independence in maintaining: life/health/personal development/well-being ° *Expresses desire to*

enhance: ° Self-care ° Knowledge for strategies for self-care ° Responsibility for self-care

[Note: Based on the definition and defining characteristics of this ND, the focus appears to be broader than simply meeting routine basic ADLs and addresses independence in maintaining overall health, personal development, and general well-being.]

Self-Care Deficit [specify level] feeding, bathing/hygiene, dressing/grooming, toileting

DEFINITION: Impaired ability to perform or complete feeding, bathing/hygiene, dressing and grooming, or toileting activities for oneself [on a temporary, permanent, or progressing basis] (Specify level of independence using a standardized functional scale)

[Note: Self-Care also may be expanded to include the practices used by the client to promote health, the individual responsibility for self, a way of thinking. Refer to NDs impaired Home Maintenance, ineffective Health Maintenance.]

RELATED FACTORS:
° Weakness ° Fatigue ° Decreased motivation ° Neuromuscular/musculoskeletal impairment ° Environmental barriers ° Severe anxiety ° Pain ° Discomfort ° Perceptual/cognitive impairment ° [Mechanical restrictions such as cast, splint, traction, ventilator] ° Inability to perceive body part/spatial relationship [bathing/hygiene] ° Impaired transfer ability [self-toileting] ° Impaired mobility status [self-toileting]

DEFINING CHARACTERISTICS
a. bathing/hygiene Self-Care Deficit (levels 0–4)
Inability to: ° Get bath supplies ° Wash body ° Obtain water source ° Regulate bath water ° Access bathroom [tub] ° Dry body
b. dressing/grooming Self-Care Deficit (levels 0–4)
Inability to: ° Choose clothing ° Pick up clothing ° Put clothing on upper/lower body ° Put on socks/shoes ° Use zippers/assistive devices ° Remove clothes ° Maintain appearance at a satisfactory level
Impaired ability to: ° Obtain clothing ° Put on/take off necessary items of clothing ° Fasten clothing
c. feeding Self-Care Deficit (levels 0–4)
Inability to: ° Prepare food for ingestion ° Open containers ° Handle utensils ° Get food onto utensil ° Bring food from a receptacle to the mouth ° Ingest food safely ° Manipulate food in mouth ° Chew/swallow food ° Pick up cup or glass ° Use assistive device ° Ingest sufficient food ° Complete a meal ° Ingest food in a socially acceptable manner
d. toileting Self-Care Deficit (levels 0–4)
Inability to: ° Get to toilet or commode ° Manipulate clothing for toileting ° Sit on/rise from toilet or commode ° Carry out proper toilet hygiene ° Flush toilet or [empty] commode

Self-Concept, readiness for enhanced

DEFINITION: A pattern of perceptions or ideas about the self that is sufficient for well-being and can be strengthened

RELATED FACTORS: ° To be developed

DEFINING CHARACTERISTICS
Subjective: ° Expresses willingness to enhance self-concept ° Accepts strengths/limitations ° Expresses confidence in abilities ° Expresses satisfaction with thoughts about self/sense of worthiness ° Expresses satisfaction with body image/personal identity/role performance
Objective: ° Actions are congruent with expressed feelings and thoughts

Self-Esteem, chronic low

DEFINITION: Long-standing negative self-evaluation/feelings about self or self-capabilities

RELATED FACTORS: ° To be developed ° [Fixation in earlier level of development] ° [Continual negative evaluation of self/capabilities from childhood] ° [Personal vulnerability] ° [Life choices perpetuating failure] ° [Ineffective social/ occupational functioning] ° [Feelings of abandonment by significant other] ° [Willingness to tolerate possibly life-threatening domestic violence] ° [Chronic physical/psychiatric conditions]° [Antisocial behaviors]

DEFINING CHARACTERISTICS

Subjective: ° Self-negating verbalization ° Expressions of shame/guilt ° Evaluates self as unable to deal with events ° Rejects positive feedback/exaggerates negative feedback about self
Objective: ° Hesitant to try new things/situations ° Frequent lack of success in life events ° Overly conforming ° Dependent on others' opinions ° Excessively seeks reassurance ° Lack of eye contact ° Nonassertive ° Passive ° Indecisive

Self-Esteem, situational low

DEFINITION: Development of a negative perception of self-worth in response to a current situation (specify)

RELATED FACTORS: ° Developmental changes [e.g., maturational transitions, adolescence, aging] ° Functional impairments ° Disturbed body image ° Loss [e.g., loss of health status, body part, independent functioning; memory deficit/cognitive impairment] ° Social role changes ° Failures/rejections ° Lack of recognition [/rewards] ° [Feelings of abandonment by SO] ° Behavior inconsistent with values

DEFINING CHARACTERISTICS

Subjective: ° Verbally reports current situational challenge to self-worth ° Expressions of helplessness/uselessness ° Evaluation of self as unable to deal with situations or events
Objective: ° Self-negating verbalizations ° Indecisive/nonassertive behavior

Self-Esteem, risk for situational low

DEFINITION: At risk for developing negative perception of self-worth in response to a current situation (specify)

RISK FACTORS: ° Developmental changes ° Disturbed body image ° Functional impairment ° Loss [e.g., loss of health status, body part, independent functioning, memory deficit/cognitive impairment] ° Social role changes ° Unrealistic self-expectations ° History of learned helplessness ° History of neglect/abuse/abandonment ° Behavior inconsistent with values ° Lack of recognition [/rewards] ° Failures ° Rejections ° Decreased control over environment ° Physical illness

Self-Mutilation

DEFINITION: Deliberate self-injurious behavior causing tissue damage with the intent of causing nonfatal injury to attain relief of tension

RELATED FACTORS: ° Adolescence ° Peers who self-mutilate ° Isolation from peers ° Dissociation ° Depersonalization ° Psychotic state (e.g., command hallucinations) ° Character disorder ° Borderline personality disorders ° Emotionally disturbed ° Developmentally delayed/autistic individuals ° History of self-injurious behavior ° History of inability to plan solutions/see long-term consequences ° Childhood illness/surgery ° Childhood sexual abuse ° Battered child ° Disturbed/unstable body image ° Eating disorders ° Inadequate coping ° Perfectionism ° Negative feelings (e.g., depression, rejection, self-hatred, separation anxiety, guilt) ° Low/unstable self-esteem ° Poor communication between parent and adolescent ° Lack of family confidante ° Feels threatened with loss of significant relationship [e.g., loss of parent/parental relationship] ° Disturbed interpersonal relationships ° Use of manipulation to obtain nurturing relationship with others ° Family alcoholism/divorce ° Violence between parental figures ° Family history of self-destructive behaviors ° Living in nontraditional settings (e.g., foster, group, or institutional care) ° Incarceration ° Inability to express tension verbally ° Mounting tension that is intolerable ° Needs quick reduction of stress ° Irresistible urge to cut/damage self ° Impulsivity ° Labile behavior ° Sexual identity crisis ° Substance abuse

DEFINING CHARACTERISTICS

Subjective: ° Self-inflicted burns (e.g., eraser, cigarette) ° Ingestion/inhalation of harmful substances/objects

Objective: ° Cuts/scratches on body ° Picking at wounds ° Biting ° Abrading ° Severing ° Insertion of object(s) into body orifice(s) ° Hitting ° Constricting a body part

Self-Mutilation, risk for

DEFINITION: At risk for deliberate self-injurious behavior causing tissue damage with the intent of causing nonfatal injury to attain relief of tension

RISK FACTORS: ° Adolescence ° Peers who self-mutilate ° Isolation from peers ° Dissociation ° Depersonalization ° Psychotic state (e.g., command hallucinations) ° Character disorders ° Borderline personality disorders ° Emotionally disturbed child ° Developmentally delayed/autistic individuals ° History of self-injurious behavior ° History of inability to plan solutions/see long-term consequences ° Childhood illness/surgery ° Childhood sexual abuse ° Battered child ° Disturbed/unstable body image ° Eating disorders ° Ineffective coping ° Loss of control over problem-solving situations ° Perfectionism ° Negative feelings (e.g., depression, rejection, self-hatred, separation anxiety, guilt) ° Low/unstable self-esteem ° Feels threatened with loss of significant relationship [e.g., loss of parent/parental relationship] ° Loss of siginificant relationship ° Lack of family confidante ° Disturbed interpersonal relationships ° Use of manipulation to obtain nurturing relationship with others ° Family alcoholism/divorce ° Violence between parental figures ° Family history of self-destructive behaviors ° Living in nontraditional settings (e.g., foster, group, or institutional care) ° Incarceration ° Inability to express tension verbally ° Mounting tension that is intolerable ° Needs quick reduction of stress ° Irresistible urge to damage self ° Impulsivity ° Sexual identity crisis ° Substance abuse

Sensory Perception, disturbed (specify: visual, auditory, kinesthetic, gustatory, tactile, olfactory)

DEFINITION: Change in the quantity or patterning of incoming stimuli accompanied by a diminished, exaggerated, distorted, or impaired response to such stimuli

RELATED FACTORS: ° Insufficient environmental stimuli [e.g., therapeutically restricted environments—isolation, intensive care, bedrest, traction, confining illnesses, incubator; socially restricted environment—institutionalization, homebound, aging, chronic/terminal illness, infant deprivation; stigmatized—mentally ill/developmentally delayed/handicapped] ° Excessive environmental stimuli [e.g., excessive noise level, such as work environment, client's immediate environment (ICU with support machinery and the like)] ° Altered sensory reception/transmission/integration [e.g., neurological disease, trauma, or deficit; altered status of sense organs] ° Biochemical imbalances [e.g., elevated BUN, elevated ammonia, hypoxia] ° Electrolyte imbalance ° [Drugs, e.g., stimulants or depressants, mind-altering drugs] ° Psychological stress; [sleep deprivation]

DEFINING CHARACTERISTICS

Subjective: ° [Reported] change in sensory acuity [e.g., photosensitivity, hypoesthesias/hyperesthesias, diminished/altered sense of taste, inability to tell position of body parts (proprioception)] ° Sensory distortions

Objective: ° [Measured] change in sensory acuity ° Change in usual response to stimuli [e.g., rapid mood swings, exaggerated emotional responses, anxiety/panic state ° Change in behavior pattern ° Restlessness ° Irritability ° Change in problem-solving abilities ° Poor concentration ° Disorientation ° Hallucinations ° [Illusions] ° [Bizarre thinking] ° Impaired communication ° [Motor incoordination, altered sense of balance/falls (e.g., Ménière's syndrome)]

Sexuality Dysfunction

DEFINITION: The state in which an individual experiences a change in sexual function during the sexual response phases of desire, excitation, and/or orgasm which is viewed as unsatisfying, unrewarding, inadequate.

RELATED FACTORS: ° Ineffectual/ absent role models ° Lack of significant other ° Lack of privacy ° Misinformation or lack of knowledge ° Vulnerability ° Physical abuse ° Psychosocial abuse (e.g., harmful relationships) ° Altered body function/structure (e.g., pregnancy, recent childbirth, drugs, surgery, anomalies, disease process, trauma, [paraplegia/quadriplegia], radiation, [effects of aging]) ° Biopsychosocial alteration of sexuality ° Values conflict

DEFINING CHARACTERISTICS
Subjective: ° Verbalization of problem [e.g., loss of sexual desire, premature ejaculation, dyspareunia, vaginismus] ° Actual/perceived limitation imposed by disease/therapy ° Perceived deficiency of sexual desire ° Perceived alteration in sexual excitation ° Alterations in achieving sexual satisfaction ° Inability to achieve desired satisfaction ° Alterations in achieving perceived sex role ° Seeking confirmation of desirability [concern about body image] ° Change on interest in self/others

Sexuality Patterns, ineffective

DEFINITION: Expressions of concern regarding own sexuality

RELATED FACTORS: ° Knowledge/skill deficit about alternative responses to health-related transitions, altered body function or structure, illness, or medical treatment ° Lack of privacy ° Impaired relationship with a significant other ° Lack of SO ° Ineffective/absent role models ° Conflicts with sexual orientation or variant preferences ° Fear of pregnancy/acquiring a sexually transmitted disease

DEFINING CHARACTERISTICS
Subjective: ° Reported: ° Difficulties in sexual behaviors/activities ° Changes in sexual behaviors/activities ° Limitations in sexual behaviors/ activities ° Alteration in relationship with SO ° Alterations in achieving perceived sex role ° Conflicts involving values ° [Expressions of feeling alienated, lonely, loss, powerless, angry]

Skin Integrity, impaired

DEFINITION: Altered epidermis and/or dermis

RELATED FACTORS:
External: ° Hyperthermia ° Hypothermia ° Chemical substance ° Radiation ° Medications ° Physical immobilization ° Humidity ° Moisture ° [Excretions/secretions] ° Mechanical factors (e.g., shearing forces, pressure, restraint) ° [Trauma/ injury] ° [Surgery] ° Extremes in age
Internal: ° Imbalanced nutritional state (e.g., obesity, emaciation) ° Impaired metabolic state ° Changes in fluid status ° Skeletal prominence ° Changes in turgor (change in elasticity) ° [Presence of edema] ° Impaired circulation/sensation ° Changes in pigmentation ° Developmental factors ° Immunological deficit ° [Psychogenic factors e.g., obsessive compulsive behaviors]

DEFINING CHARACTERISTICS
Subjective: ° [Reports of itching, pain, numbness of affected/surrounding area]
Objective: ° Disruption of skin surface [epidermis] ° Destruction of skin layers [dermis] ° Invasion of body structures

Skin Integrity, risk for impaired

DEFINITION: At risk for skin being adversely altered. Note: Risk should be determined by the use of a standardized risk assessment tool [e.g., Braden, Norton, or similar scale].

RISK FACTORS:
External: ° Chemical substance ° Radiation ° Hypothermia ° Hyperthermia ° Physical immobilization ° Humidity ° Moisture ° Excretions °

Secretions ° Mechanical factors (e.g., shearing forces, pressure, restraint) ° Extremes of age *Internal*: ° Imbalanced nutritional state (e.g., obesity, emaciation) ° Impaired metabolic state ° [Presence of edema] ° Skeletal prominence ° Changes in skin turgor [/elasticity] ° Impaired circulation/sensation ° Changes in pigmentation ° Developmental factors ° Immunologic factors ° Medications ° Psychogenetic factors

Sleep, readiness for enhanced

DEFINITION: A pattern of natural, periodic suspension of consciousness that provides adequate rest, sustains a desired lifestyle, and can be strengthened

RELATED FACTORS: ° To be developed

DEFINING CHARACTERISTICS
Subjective: ° Expresses willingness to enhance sleep ° Expresses a feeling of being rested after sleep ° Follows sleep routines that promote sleep habits
Objective: ° Amount of sleep and REM sleep is congruent with developmental needs ° Occasional or infrequent use of medications to induce sleep

Sleep Deprivation

DEFINITION: Prolonged periods of time without sleep (sustained natural, periodic suspension of relative consciousness)

RELATED FACTORS: ° Sustained environmental stimulation ° Sustained uncomfortable sleep environment ° Inadequate daytime activity ° Sustained circadian asynchrony ° Aging-related sleep stage shifts ° Non–sleep-inducing parenting practices ° Sustained inadequate sleep hygiene ° Prolonged use of pharmacological or dietary antisoporifics ° Prolonged discomfort (e.g., physical, psychological ° Periodic limb movement (e.g., restless leg syndrome, nocturnal myoclonus) ° Sleep-related: enuresis ° Sleep-related painful erections ° Nightmares ° Sleepwalking ° Sleep terror ° Sleep apnea ° Sundowner's syndrome ° Dementia ° Idiopathic CNS hypersomnolence ° Narcolepsy ° Familial sleep paralysis

DEFINING CHARACTERISTICS
Subjective: ° Daytime drowsiness ° Decreased ability to function ° Malaise ° Lethargy ° Fatigue ° Anxiety ° Perceptual disorders (e.g., disturbed body sensation, delusions, feeling afloat) ° Heightened sensitivity to pain
Objective: ° Restlessness ° Irritability ° Inability to concentrate ° Slowed reaction ° Listlessness ° Apathy ° Fleeting nystagmus ° Hand tremors ° Acute confusion ° Transient paranoia ° Agitation ° Combativeness ° Hallucinations

Social Interaction, impaired

DEFINITION: Insufficient or excessive quantity or ineffective quality of social exchange

RELATED FACTORS: ° Deficit about ways to enhance mutuality (e.g., knowledge, skill) ° Communication barriers [including head injury, stroke, other neurological conditions affecting ability to communicate] ° Self-concept disturbance ° Absence of significant others ° Limited physical mobility [e.g., neuromuscular disease] ° Therapeutic isolation ° Sociocultural dissonance ° Environmental barriers ° Disturbed thought processes

DEFINING CHARACTERISTICS
Subjective: ° Discomfort in social situations ° Inability to receive/communicate a satisfying sense of social engagement (e.g., belonging, caring, interest, or shared history) ° Family report of changes in interaction (e.g., style, pattern)
Objective: ° Use of unsuccessful social interaction behaviors ° Dysfunctional interaction with others

Social Isolation

DEFINITION: Aloneness experienced by the individual and perceived as imposed by others and as a negative or threatened state

RELATED FACTORS: ° Factors contributing to the absence of satisfying personal relationships (e.g., delay in accomplishing developmental tasks) ° Immature interests ° Alterations in physical appearance ° Altered state of wellness ° Alterations in mental status ° Unaccepted social behavior/values ° Inadequate personal resources ° Inability to engage in satisfying personal relationships ° [Traumatic incidents or events causing physical and/or emotional pain]

DEFINING CHARACTERISTICS
Subjective: ° Expresses feelings of aloneness imposed by others ° Expresses feelings of rejection ° Insecurity in public ° Inability to meet expectations of others ° Inadequate purpose in life ° Developmentally inappropriate interests ° Experiences feelings of difference from others ° Expresses values unacceptable to the dominant cultural group
Objective: ° Absence of supportive SO(s) [family, friends, group] ° Sad/dull affect ° Uncommunicative ° Withdrawn ° No eye contact ° Evidence of handicap (e.g., physical, mental) ° Illness ° Developmentally inappropriate behaviors ° Repetitive meaningless actions ° Seeks to be alone ° Preoccupation with own thoughts ° Shows behavior unaccepted by dominant cultural group ° Exists in a subculture ° Projects hostility

Sorrow, chronic

DEFINITION: Cyclical, recurring, and potentially progressive pattern of pervasive sadness experienced (by a parent or caregiver, individual with chronic illness or disability) in response to continual loss, throughout the trajectory of an illness or disability

RELATED FACTORS: ° Death of a loved one ° Experiences chronic illness/disability (e.g., physical or mental) ° Crises in management of the illness ° Crises related to developmental stages ° Missed opportunities/milestones ° Unending caregiving

DEFINING CHARACTERISTICS
Subjective: ° Expresses negative feelings (e.g., anger, being misunderstood, confusion, depression, disappointment, emptiness, fear, frustration, guilt, self-blame, helplessness, hopelessness, loneliness, low self-esteem, recurring loss, overwhelmed) ° Expresses feelings of sadness (e.g., periodic, recurrent) ° Expresses feelings that may interfere with ability to reach highest level of personal/social well-being

Spiritual Distress

DEFINITION: Impaired ability to experience and integrate meaning and purpose in life through a person's connectedness with self, others, art, music, literature, nature, and/or a power greater than oneself

RELATED FACTORS: ° Active dying ° Loneliness ° Social alienation ° Self-alienation ° Sociocultural deprivation ° Anxiety ° Pain ° Life change ° Chronic illness [of self or others] ° Death ° [Challenged belief/ value system (e.g., moral/ethical implications of therapy]

DEFINING CHARACTERISTICS
SUBJECTIVE: *Connections to self:* ° Expresses lack of: Hope ° Meaning/purpose in life ° Serenity (e.g., peace) ° Love ° Acceptance ° Forgiveness of self ° Courage ° [Expresses:] Anger ° Guilt
CONNECTIONS WITH OTHERS: ° Refuses interactions with significant other(s)/spiritual leaders ° Verbalizes being separated from support system ° Expresses alienation ° Connections with Art, Music, Literature, Nature: ° Inability to express previous state of creativity (e.g., singing/listening to music/writing) ° Disinterested in nature/ reading spiritual literature
CONNECTIONS WITH POWER GREATER THAN SELF: ° Sudden changes in spiritual practices ° Inability to pray/participate in religious activities ° Inability to experience the transcendent ° Expresses being

abandoned ° Expresses hopelessness/suffering/having anger toward God ° Request to see a religious leader

OBJECTIVE: Connections to Self: ° Poor coping **CONNECTIONS WITH POWER GREATER THAN SELF:** ° Inability to be introspective

Spiritual Distress, risk for

DEFINITION: At risk for an impaired ability to experience and integrate meaning and purpose in life through connectedness with self, others, art, music, literature, nature, and/or a power greater than oneself

RISK FACTORS: *Physical:* ° Physical/chronic illness ° Substance abuse
Psychosocial: ° Stress ° Anxiety ° Depression ° Low self-esteem ° Poor relationships ° Blocks to experiencing love ° Inability to forgive ° Loss ° Separated support sytem ° Racial/cultural conflict ° Changes in religious rituals/spiritual practices
Developmental: ° Life changes
Environmental: Environmental changes ° Natural disasters

Spiritual Well-Being, readiness for enhanced

DEFINITION: Ability to experience and integrate meaning and purpose in life through connectedness with self, others, art, music, literature, nature, and/or a power greater than oneself that can be strengthened

RELATED FACTORS: ° To be developed

DEFINING CHARACTERISTICS

SUBJECTIVE: *Connections to Self:* Expresses desire for enhanced: ° Acceptance ° Coping ° Courage ° Forgiveness of self ° Hope ° Joy ° Love ° Meaning/purpose in life ° Satisfying philosophy of life ° Surrender ° Expresses lack of serenity (e.g., peace) ° Meditation

Connections with Others: ° Requests interactions with significant others/spiritual leaders ° Requests forgiveness of others
Connections with Powers Greater Than Self: ° Participates in religious activities ° Prays ° Expresses reverence/awe ° Reports mystical experiences

OBJECTIVE: *Connections with Others:* ° Provides service to others
Connections with Art, Music, Literature, Nature: ° Displays creative energy (e.g., writing, poetry, singing) ° Listens to music ° Reads spiritual literature ° Spends time outdoors

Stress Overload

DEFINITION: Excessive amounts and types of demands that require action

RELATED FACTORS:
Inadequate resources (e.g., financial, social, education/knowledge level) Intense, repeated stressors (e.g., family violence, chronic illness, terminal illness) Multiple coexisting stressors (e.g., environmental threats/demands; physical threats/demands; social threats/demands)

DEFINING CHARACTERISTICS
Subjective: ° Expresses difficulty in functioning/problems with decision making ° Expresses a feeling of pressure/tension/increased feelings of impatience/anger ° Reports negative impact from stress (e.g., physical symptoms, psychological distress, feeling of "being sick" or of "going to get sick") ° Reports situational stress as excessive (e.g., rates stress level as a seven or above on a 10-point scale)
Objective: ° Demonstrates increased feelings of impatience/anger

Suffocation, risk for

DEFINITION: Accentuated risk of accidental suffocation (inadequate air available for inhalation)

RISK FACTORS:
Internal: ° Reduced olfactory sensation ° Reduced motor abilities ° Lack of safety education/

precautions ° Cognitive/emotional difficulties [e.g., altered consciousness/mentation] ° Disease/ injury process

External: ° Pillow/propped bottle placed in an infant's crib ° Hanging a pacifier around infant's neck ° Playing with plastic bags ° Inserting small objects into airway ° Leaving children unattended in water ° Discarded refrigerators without removed doors ° Vehicle warming in closed garage [/faulty exhaust system] ° Use of fuel-burning heaters not vented to outside ° Household gas leaks ° Smoking in bed ° Low-strung clothesline ° Eating large mouthfuls [or pieces] of food

Suicide, risk for

DEFINITION: At risk for self-inflicted, life-threatening injury

RISK FACTORS:
Behavioral: ° History of prior suicide attempt ° Buying a gun ° Stockpiling medicines ° Making/ changing a will ° Giving away possessions ° Sudden euphoric recovery from major depression ° Impulsiveness ° Marked changes in behavior/ attitude/school performance
Demographic: ° Age (e.g., elderly, young adult males, adolescents) ° Race (e.g., Caucasian, Native American) ° Male gender ° Divorced ° Widowed
Physical: ° Physical/terminal illness ° Chronic pain
Psychological: ° Family history of suicide ° Abuse in childhood ° Substance use/abuse ° Psychiatric illness/disorder (e.g., depression, schizophrenia, bipolar disorder) ° Guilt ° Gay or lesbian youth
Situational: ° Living alone ° Retired ° Economic instability ° Relocation ° Institutionalization ° Loss of autonomy/independence ° Presence of gun in home ° Adolescents living in nontraditional settings (e.g., juvenile detention center, prison, halfway house, group home)
Social: ° Loss of important relationship ° Disrupted family life ° Poor support systems ° Social isolation ° Grief ° Loneliness ° Hopelessness

° Helplessness ° Legal/disciplinary problems ° Cluster suicides
Verbal: ° Threats of killing oneself ° States desire to die [/end it all]

Surgical Recovery, delayed

DEFINITION: Extension of the number of postoperative days required to initiate and perform activities that maintain life, health, and well-being

RELATED FACTORS: ° Extensive/prolonged surgical procedure ° Pain ° Obesity ° Preoperative expectations ° Postoperative surgical site care

DEFINING CHARACTERISTICS
Subjective: ° Perception that more time is needed to recover ° Report of pain/discomfort ° Fatigue ° Loss of appetite with or without nausea ° Postpones resumption of work/employment activities
Objective: ° Evidence of interrupted healing of surgical area (e.g., red, indurated, draining, immobilized) ° Difficulty in moving about ° Requires help to complete self-care

Swallowing, impaired

DEFINITION: Abnormal functioning of the swallowing mechanism associated with deficits in oral, pharyngeal, or esophageal structure or function

RELATED FACTORS:
Congenital Deficits: ° Upper airway anomalies ° Mechanical obstruction (e.g., edema, tracheostomy tube, tumor) ° History of tube feeding ° Neuromuscular impairment (e.g., decreased or absent gag reflex, decreased strength or excursion of muscles involved in mastication, perceptual impairment, facial paralysis) ° Conditions with significant hypotonia ° Respiratory disorders ° Congenital heart disease ° Behavioral feeding problems ° Self-injurious behavior ° Failure to thrive ° Protein energy malnutrition
Neurological Problems: ° Nasal/nasopharyngeal cavity defects ° Upper airway anomalies ° Oropharyngeal/laryngeal abnormalities °

Tracheal/laryngeal/esophageal defects ° Gastro-esophageal reflux disease ° Achalasia ° Traumas ° Acquired anatomic defects ° Cranial nerve involvement ° Traumatic head injury ° Prematurity ° Developmental delay ° Cerebral palsy

DEFINING CHARACTERISTICS

Subjective: ° *Esophageal Phase Impairment:* ° Complaints [reports] of "something stuck" ° Odynophagia ° Food refusal ° Volume limiting ° Heartburn ° Epigastric pain ° Nighttime coughing/awakening

Objective: ° *Oral Phase Impairment:* ° Weak suck resulting in inefficient nippling ° Slow bolus formation ° Lack of tongue action to form bolus ° Premature entry of bolus ° Incomplete lip closure ° Food pushed out of/falls from mouth ° Lack of chewing ° Coughing/choking/gagging before a swallow ° Piecemeal deglutition ° Abnormality in oral phase of swallow study ° Inability to clear oral cavity ° Pooling in lateral sulci ° Nasal reflux ° Sialorrhea or drooling ° Long meals with little consumption

Pharyngeal Phase Impairment: ° Food refusal ° Altered head positions ° Delayed/multiple swallows ° Inadequate laryngeal elevation ° Abnormality in pharyngeal phase by swallow study ° Choking ° Coughing ° Gagging ° Nasal reflux ° Gurgly voice quality ° Unexplained fevers ° Recurrent pulmonary infections

Esophageal Phase Impairment: ° Observed evidence of difficulty in swallowing (e.g., stasis of food in oral cavity, coughing/choking) ° Abnormality in esophageal phase by swallow study ° Hyperextension of head (e.g., arching during or after meals) ° Repetitive swallowing ° Bruxism ° Unexplained irritability surrounding mealtime ° Acidic smelling breath ° Regurgitation of gastric contents (wet burps) ° Vomitus on pillow ° Vomiting ° Hematemesis

Therapeutic Regimen Management, effective

DEFINITION: Pattern of regulating and integrating into daily living a program for treatment of illness and its sequelae that is satisfactory for meeting specific health goals

RELATED FACTORS: ° To be developed ° [Complexity of healthcare management; therapeutic regimen] ° [Added demands made on individual or family] ° [Adequate social supports]

DEFINING CHARACTERISTICS

Subjective: ° Verbalizes desire to manage the treatment of illness/prevention of sequelae ° Verbalizes intent to reduce risk factors for progression of illness and sequelae

Objective: ° Appropriate choices of daily activities for meeting the goals of a treatment or prevention program ° Illness symptoms are within a normal range of expectation

Therapeutic Regimen Management, ineffective

DEFINITION: Pattern of regulating and integrating into daily living a program for treatment of illness and the sequelae of illness that is unsatisfactory for meeting specific health goals

RELATED FACTORS: ° Complexity of healthcare system/therapeutic regimen ° Decisional conflicts ° Economic difficulties ° Excessive demands made (e.g., individual or family) ° Family conflict ° Family patterns of health care ° Inadequate number of cues to action ° Knowledge deficits ° Mistrust of regimen/healthcare personnel ° Perceived seriousness/susceptibility/barriers/benefits ° Powerlessness ° Social support deficits

DEFINING CHARACTERISTICS

Subjective: ° Verbalized desire to manage the illness ° Verbalized difficulty with prescribed regimens

Objective: ° Failure to include treatment regimens in daily routines/take action to reduce risk factors ° Makes choices in daily living ineffective for meeting the health goals ° [Unexpected acceleration of illness symptoms]

Therapeutic Regimen Management, ineffective community

DEFINITION: Pattern of regulating and integrating into community processes programs for treatment of illness and the sequelae of illness that are unsatisfactory for meeting health-related goals

RELATED FACTORS: ° To be developed ° [Lack of safety for community members] ° [Economic insecurity] ° [Healthcare not available] ° [Unhealthy environment] ° [Education not available for all community members] ° [Lack of means to meet human needs for recognition, fellowship, security, and membership]

DEFINING CHARACTERISTICS
Subjective: ° [Community members/agencies verbalize overburdening of resources for meeting therapeutic needs of all members]
Objective: ° Deficits in advocates for aggregates ° Deficits in community activities for prevention ° Illness symptoms above the norm expected for the population ° Unexpected acceleration of illness ° Insufficient healthcare resources (e.g., people, programs) ° Unavailable healthcare resources for illness care ° [Deficits in community for collaboration and development of coalitions to address needs]

Therapeutic Regimen Management, ineffective family

DEFINITION: Pattern of regulating and integrating into family processes a program for treatment of illness and the sequelae of illness that is unsatisfactory for meeting specific health goals

RELATED FACTORS: ° Complexity of healthcare system/therapeutic regimen ° Decisional conflicts ° Economic difficulties ° Excessive demands ° Family conflicts

DEFINING CHARACTERISTICS
Subjective: ° Verbalizes difficulty with therapeutic regimen ° Verbalizes desire to manage the illness

Objective: ° Inappropriate family activities for meeting health goals ° Acceleration of illness symptoms of a family member ° Failure to take action to reduce risk factors ° Lack of attention to illness

Therapeutic Regimen management, readiness for enhanced

DEFINITION: A pattern of regulating and integrating into daily living a program for treatment of illness and its sequelae that is sufficient for meeting health-related goals and can be strengthened

RELATED FACTORS: ° To be developed

DEFINING CHARACTERISTICS
Subjective: ° Expresses desire to manage the illness (e.g., treatment, prevention) ° Expresses little difficulty with prescribed regimens ° Describes reduction of risk factors
Objective: Choices of daily living are appropriate for meeting goals (e.g., treatment, prevention) ° No unexpected accleration of illness symptoms

Thermoregulation, ineffective

DEFINITION: Temperature fluctuation between hypothermia and hyperthermia

RELATED FACTORS: ° Trauma [e.g., intracranial surgery, or head injury] ° Illness [e.g., cerebral edema, CVA] ° Immaturity ° Aging [e.g., loss/absence of brown adipose tissue] ° Fluctuating environmental temperature ° [Changes in hypothalamic tissue causing alterations in emission of thermosensitive cells and regulation of heat loss/production] ° [Changes in metabolic rate/activity] ° [Changes in level/action of thyroxine and catecholamines] ° [Chemical reactions in contracting muscles]

DEFINING CHARACTERISTICS

Objective: ° Fluctuations in body temperature above and below the normal range ° Tachycardia

° Reduction in body temperature below normal range ° Cool skin ° Moderate pallor ° Mild shivering ° Piloerection ° Cyanotic nail beds ° Slow capillary refill ° Hypertension ° Warm to touch ° Flushed skin ° Increased respiratory rate ° Seizures

Thought Processes, disturbed

DEFINITION: Disruption in cognitive operations and activities

RELATED FACTORS: ° To be developed ° [Physiological changes] ° [Aging] [Hypoxia] ° [Head injury] ° [Malnutrition] ° [Infections] ° [Biochemical changes] ° [Medications] ° [Substance abuse] ° [Sleep deprivation] ° [Psychological conflicts] ° [Emotional changes] ° [Mental disorders]

DEFINING CHARACTERISTICS
Subjective: ° [Ideas of reference] ° [Hallucinations] ° [Delusions]
Objective: ° Inaccurate interpretation of environment ° Inappropriate/nonreality-based thinking ° Egocentricity ° Memory deficit ° [Confabulation] ° Hypervigilance ° Hypovigilance ° Cognitive dissonance, [decreased ability to grasp ideas, make decisions, problem-solve, use abstract reasoning or conceptualize, calculate; disordered thought sequencing] ° Distractibility ° [Altered attention span] ° [Inappropriate social behavior]

Tissue Integrity, impaired

DEFINITION: Damage to mucous membrane, corneal, integumentary, or subcutaneous tissues

RELATED FACTORS: ° Altered circulation ° Nutritional factors (e.g., deficit or excess) ° [Metabolic/endocrine dysfunction] ° Fluid deficit/excess ° Knowledge deficit ° Impaired physical mobility ° Chemical irritants [e.g., body excretions, secretions, medications] ° Radiation ° Temperature extremes ° Mechanical (e.g., pressure, shear, friction) ° [Surgery] ° Knowledge deficit ° [Infection]

DEFINING CHARACTERISTICS
Objective: ° Damaged tissue (e.g., cornea, mucous membrane, integumentary, subcutaneous ° Destroyed tissue)

Tissue Perfusion, ineffective (specify): renal, cerebral, cardiopulmonary, gastrointestinal, peripheral

DEFINITION: Decrease in oxygen resulting in the failure to nourish the tissues at the capillary level [Although tissue perfusion problems can exist without decreased cardiac output, there may be a relationship between cardiac output and tissue perfusion.]

RELATED FACTORS: ° Hypervolemia ° Hypovolemia ° Interruption of flow ° Decreased hemoglobin concentration in blood ° Enzyme poisoning ° Altered affinity of hemoglobin for oxygen ° Impaired transport of oxygen ° Mismatch of ventilation with blood flow ° Exchange problems ° Hypoventilation

DEFINING CHARACTERISTICS
Subjective: Cardiopulmonary: ° Chest pain ° Dyspnea ° Sense of "impending doom"
Gastrointestinal: ° Nausea ° Abdominal pain or tenderness
Peripheral: ° Claudication
Objective: Renal: ° Altered blood pressure outside of acceptable parameters ° Oliguria ° Anuria ° Hematuria ° Elevation in BUN/creatine ratio
Cerebral: ° Altered mental status ° Speech abnormalities ° Behavioral changes ° [Restlessness] ° Changes in motor response ° Extremity weakness ° Paralysis ° Changes in pupillary reactions ° Difficulty in swallowing
Cardiopulmonary: ° Arrhythmias ° Capillary refill >3 sec ° Altered respiratory rate outside of acceptable parameters ° Use of accessory muscles ° Chest retraction ° Nasal flaring ° Bronchospasms ° Abnormal arterial blood gases ABGs ° [Hemoptysis]

Gastrointestinal: ° Hypoactive/absent bowel sounds ° Abdominal distention ° [Vomiting]
Peripheral: ° Altered skin characteristics (e.g., hair, nails, moisture) ° Skin temperature changes ° Skin discolorations ° Skin color pales on elevation, color does not return on lowering the leg ° Altered sensations ° Blood pressure changes in extremities ° Weak/absent pulses ° Diminished arterial pulsations ° Bruits ° Edema ° Delayed healing ° Positive Homans' sign

Transfer Ability, impaired

DEFINITION: Limitation of independent movement between two nearby surfaces Note: Specify level of independence using a standardized functional scale.

RELATED FACTORS: ° Insufficient muscle strength ° Deconditioning ° Neuromuscular impairment ° Musculoskeletal impairment (e.g., contractures) ° Impaired balance ° Pain ° Obesity ° Impaired vision ° Lack of knowledge ° Cognitive impairment ° Environment constraints (e.g., bed height, inadequate space, wheelchair type, treatment equipment, restraints)

DEFINING CHARACTERISTICS
Subjective or Objective: ° *Inability to transfer from:* ° Bed to chair/chair to bed ° Bed to standing/standing to bed ° Chair to standing/standing to chair ° Chair to floor/floor to chair ° Standing to floor/floor to standing ° Chair to car/car to chair *Inability to transfer:* ° On/off a toilet or commode ° In/out of tub or shower ° Between uneven levels

Trauma, risk for

DEFINITION: Accentuated risk of accidental tissue injury (e.g., wound, burn, fracture)

RISK FACTORS:
Internal: ° Weakness ° Balancing difficulties ° Reduced muscle coordination ° Reduced hand/eye coordination ° Poor vision ° Reduced sensation ° Lack of safety education/precautions ° Insufficient finances ° Cognitive/emotional difficulties ° History of previous trauma

External [includes but is not limited to]: ° Slippery floors (e.g., wet or highly waxed ° Unanchored rugs/electic wires ° Bathtub without antislip equipment ° Use of unsteady ladder/chairs ° Obstructed passageways ° Entering unlighted rooms ° Inadequate stair rails ° Children playing without gates at top of stairs ° High beds ° Inappropriate call-for-aid mechanisms for bed-resting client ° Unsafe window protection in homes with young children ° Pot handles facing toward front of stove ° Bathing in very hot water (e.g., unsupervised bathing of young children) ° Potential igniting gas leaks ° Delayed lighting of gas appliances ° Wearing flowing clothing around open flames ° Flammable children's clothing/toys ° Smoking in bed/near oxygen ° Grease waste collected on stoves ° Children playing with dangerous objects ° Accessability of guns ° Playing with explosives ° Experimenting with chemicals ° Inadequately stored combustibles (e.g., matches, oily rags)/ corrosives (e.g., lye) ° Contact with corrosives ° Overloaded fuse boxes ° Faulty electrical plugs ° Frayed wires ° Defective appliances ° Overloaded electrical outlets ° Exposure to dangerous machinery ° Contact with rapidly moving machinery ° Struggling with restraints ° Contact with intense cold ° Lack of protection from heat source ° Overexposure to radiotherapy ° Large icicles hanging from the roof ° Use of cracked dishware ° Knives stored uncovered ° High-crime neighborhood ° Driving a mechanically unsafe vehicle ° Driving at excessive speeds ° Driving without necessary visual aids ° Driving while intoxicated ° Children riding in the front seat of car ° Nonuse/misuse of seat restraints ° Unsafe road/walkways ° Physical proximity to vehicle pathways (e.g., driveways, lanes, railroad tracks) ° Misuse [/nonuse] of necessary headgear [e.g., for bicycles, motorcycles, skateboarding, skiing]

Urinary Elimination, impaired

DEFINITION: Disturbance in urine elimination

RELATED FACTORS: ° Multiple causality ° Sensory motor impairment ° Anatomical obstruction ° UTI ° [Mechanical trauma] ° [Fluid/volume states] ° [Psychogenic factors] ° [Surgical diversion]

DEFINING CHARACTERISTICS
Subjective: ° Frequency ° Urgency ° Hesitancy ° Dysuria ° Nocturia ° [Enuresis]
Objective: ° Incontinence ° Retention

Urinary Elimination, readiness for enhanced

DEFINITION: A pattern of urinary functions that is sufficient for meeting eliminatory needs and can be strengthened

RELATED FACTORS:° To be developed

DEFINING CHARACTERISTICS
Subjective: ° Expresses willingness to enhance urinary elimination ° Positions self for emptying of bladder
Objective: ° Urine is straw colored/odorless ° Amount of output/specific gravity is within normal limits ° Fluid intake is adequate for daily needs

Urinary Incontinence, functional

DEFINITION: Inability of usually continent person to reach toilet in time to avoid unintentional loss of urine

RELATED FACTORS: ° Altered environmental factors [e.g., poor lighting or inability to locate bathroom] ° Neuromuscular limitations ° Weakened supporting pelvic structures ° Impaired vision/cognition ° Psychological factors ° [Reluctance to request assistance/use bedpan] ° [Increased urine production]

DEFINING CHARACTERISTICS
Subjective: ° Senses need to void ° [Voiding in large amounts]
Objective: ° Loss of urine before reaching toilet ° Amount of time required to reach toilet exceeds length of time between sensing urge and

uncontrolled voiding ° Able to completely empty bladder ° May be incontinent only in early morning

Urinary Incontinence, overflow

DEFINITION: Involuntary loss of urine associated with overdistention of the bladder

RELATED FACTORS:
° Bladder outlet obstruction ° Fecal impaction ° Urethral obstruction ° Severe pelvic prolapse ° Detrusor external sphincter dyssynergia ° Detrusor hypocontractility ° Side effects of calcium channel blockers/anticholinergic/decongestant medications

DEFINING CHARACTERISTICS
Subjective: ° Reports involuntary leakage of small volumes of urine ° Nocturia
Objective: ° Bladder distention ° High post-void residual volume ° Observed involuntary leakage of small volumes of urine

Urinary Incontinence, reflex

DEFINITION: Involuntary loss of urine at somewhat predictable intervals when a specific bladder volume is reached

RELATED FACTORS: ° Tissue damage (e.g., due to radiation cystitis, inflammatory bladder conditions, or radical pelvic surgery) ° Neurological impairment above level of sacral or pontine micturition center

DEFINING CHARACTERISTICS
Subjective: ° No sensation of bladder fullness/urge to void/voiding ° Sensation of urgency without voluntary inhibition of bladder contraction ° Sensations associated with full bladder (e.g., sweating, restlessness, and abdominal discomfort)
Objective: ° Predictable pattern of voiding ° Inability to voluntarily inhibit/initiate voiding ° Complete emptying with [brain] lesion above pontine micturition center ° Incomplete emptying

with [spinal cord] lesion above sacral micturition center

Urinary Incontinence, stress

DEFINITION: Sudden leakage of urine with activities that increased intra-abdominal pressure

RELATED FACTORS: ° Degenerative changes in pelvic muscles ° Weak pelvic muscles ° High intra-abdominal pressure [e.g., obesity, gravid uterus] ° Intrinsic urethral sphincter deficiency

DEFINING CHARACTERISTICS
Subjective: ° *Reported involuntary leakage of small amounts of urine:* ° On exertion [e.g., lifting, impact aerobics] ° With sneezing, laughing, or coughing ° In the absence of detrusor contraction/an overdistended bladder
Objective: ° *Observed involuntary leakage of small amounts of urine:* On exertion [e.g., lifting, impact aerobics] ° With sneezing, laughing, or coughing ° In the absence of detrusor contraction/an overdistended bladder

Urinary Incontinence, total

DEFINITION: Continuous and unpredictable loss of urine

RELATED FACTORS: ° Neuropathy preventing transmission of reflex [signals to the reflex arc] indicating bladder fullness ° Neurological dysfunction [e.g., cerebral lesions] ° Independent contraction of detrusor reflex ° Trauma/disease affecting spinal cord nerves [destruction of sensory or motor neurons below the injury level] ° Anatomic (fistula)

DEFINING CHARACTERISTICS
Subjective: ° Constant flow of urine at unpredictable times without uninhibited bladder contractions/spasm or distention ° Nocturia ° Lack of bladder/perineal filling [awareness] ° Unawareness of incontinence
Objective: ° Unsuccessful incontinence refractory treatments

Urinary Incontinence, urge

DEFINITION: Involuntary passage of urine occurring soon after a strong sense of urgency to void

RELATED FACTORS: ° Decreased bladder capacity [e.g., history of pelvic inflammatory disease—PID, abdominal surgeries, indwelling urinary catheter] ° Bladder infection ° Atrophic urethritis/vaginitis ° Alcohol/caffeine intake ° [Increased fluids] ° Use of diuretics ° Fecal impaction ° Detrusor hyperactivity with impaired bladder contractility

DEFINING CHARACTERISTICS
Subjective: Reports: ° Urinary urgency ° Involuntary loss of urine with bladder contractions/spasms ° Inability to reach toilet in time to avoid urine loss
Objective: ° Observed inability to reach toilet in time to avoid urine loss

Urinary Incontinence, risk for urge

DEFINITION: At risk for an involuntary loss of urine associated with a sudden, strong sensation or urinary urgency

RISK FACTORS: ° Effects of medications/caffeine/alcohol ° Detrusor hyperreflexia (e.g., from cystitis, urethritis, tumors, renal calculi, CNS disorders above pontine micturition center ° Impaired bladder contractility ° Involuntary sphincter relaxation ° Ineffective toileting habits ° Small bladder capacity

Urinary Retention, [acute/chronic]

DEFINITION: Incomplete emptying of the bladder

RELATED FACTORS: ° High urethral pressure ° Inhibition of reflex arc ° Strong sphincter

° Blockage [e.g., benign prostatic hypertrophy—BPH, perineal swelling] ° [Habituation of reflex arc] ° [Infections] ° [Neurological diseases/trauma] ° [Use of medications with side effect of retention (e.g., atropine, belladonna, psychotropics, antihistamines, opiates)]

DEFINING CHARACTERISTICS
Subjective: ° Sensation of bladder fullness ° Dribbling ° Dysuria
Objective: ° Bladder distention ° Small/frequent voiding ° Absence of urine output ° Residual urine [150 mL or more] ° Overflow incontinence ° [Reduced stream]

Ventilation, impaired spontaneous

DEFINITION: Decreased energy reserves result in an individual's inability to maintain breathing adequate to support life

RELATED FACTORS: ° Metabolic factors [hypermetabolic state (e.g., infection); nutritional deficits/depletion of energy stores] ° Respiratory muscle fatigue ° [Airway size/resistance] ° [Inadequate secretion management]

DEFINING CHARACTERISTICS
Subjective: ° Apprehension ° [Difficulty breating]
Objective: ° Dyspnea ° Increased metabolic rate ° Increased heart rate ° Increased restlessness ° Decreased cooperation ° Increased use of accessory muscles ° Decreased tidal volume ° Decreased PO_2/SaO_2 ° Increased PCO_2

Ventilatory Weaning Response, dysfunctional

DEFINITION: Inability to adjust to lowered levels of mechanical ventilator support that interrupts and prolongs the weaning process

RELATED FACTORS:
Physiological: ° Ineffective airway clearance ° Sleep pattern disturbance ° Inadequate nutrition ° Uncontrolled pain ° [Muscle weakness/fatigue] ° [Inability to control respiratory muscles] ° [Immobility]
Psychological: ° Knowledge deficit of the weaning process ° Patient's perceived inefficacy about the ability to wean ° Decreased motivation ° Decreased self-esteem ° Anxiety ° Fear ° Insufficient trust in the nurse [careprovider] ° Hopelessness ° Powerlessness ° [Unprepared for weaning attempt]
Situational: ° Uncontrolled episodic energy demands ° Inappropriate pacing of diminished ventilator support ° Inadequate social support ° Adverse environment (e.g., noisy, active environment, negative events in the room, low nurse-patient ratio; unfamiliar nursing staff, [extended nurse absence from bedside]) ° History of ventilator dependence >4 days ° History of multiple unsuccessful weaning attempts

DEFINING CHARACTERISTICS
Mild DVWR
Subjective: ° Expressed feelings of increased need for O_2 ° Breathing discomfort ° Fatigue ° Warmth ° Queries about possible machine malfunction
Objective: ° Restlessness ° Slight increased respiratory rate from baseline ° Increased concentration on breathing
Moderate DVWR
Subjective: ° Apprehension
Objective: ° Slight increase from baseline blood pressure (<20 mm Hg) ° Slight increase from baseline heart rate (<20 beats/min) ° Baseline increase in respiratory rate (<5 breaths/min) ° Slight respiratory accessory muscle use ° Decreased air entry on auscultation ° Hypervigilance to activities ° Wide-eyed look ° Inability to cooperate/respond to ° Diaphoresis ° Color changes ° Pale ° Slight cyanosis
Severe DVWR
Objective: ° Agitation ° Decreased level of consciousness ° Deterioration in arterial blood gases [ABGs] from current baseline ° Increase from baseline BP (≥20 mm Hg) ° Increase from baseline heart rate (≥20 beats/min) ° Respiratory rate increases significantly

from baseline ° Full respiratory accessory muscle use ° Shallow/ gasping breaths ° Paradoxical abdominal breathing ° Adventitious breath sounds ° Audible airway secretions ° Asynchronized breathing with the ventilator ° Profuse diaphoresis ° Cyanosis

Violence, [actual/]risk for other-directed

DEFINITION: At risk for behaviors in which an individual demonstrates that he/she can be physically, emotionally, and/or sexually harmful to others

RISK FACTORS[/INDICATORS] ° *History of:* ° Violence against others (e.g., hitting, kicking, scratching, biting or spitting, throwing objects at someone; attempted rape, rape, sexual molestation; urinating/defecating on a person) ° Threats (e.g., verbal threats against property/person, social threats, cursing, threatening notes/letters, threatening gestures, sexual threats) ° Violent antisocial behavior (e.g., stealing, insistent borrowing, insistent demands for privileges, insistent interruption of meetings; refusal to eat/take medication, ignoring instructions) ° Indirect violence, (e.g., tearing off clothes, urinating/defecating on floor, stamping feet, temper tantrum; running in corridors, yelling, writing on walls, ripping objects off walls, throwing objects, breaking a window, slamming doors; sexual advances) ° Substance abuse ° Childhood abuse/witnessing family violence ° Neurological impairment (e.g., positive EEG, CT, MRI, neurological findings; head trauma; seizure disorders, [temporal lobe epilepsy]) ° Cognitive impairment (e.g., learning disabilities, attention deficit disorder, decreased intellectual functioning) ° [Organic brain syndrome] ° Pathological intoxication, [toxic reaction to medication] ° Psychotic symptomatology (e.g., auditory, visual, command hallucinations; paranoid delusions; loose, rambling, or illogical thought processes) ° [Panic states] ° [Rage reactions] ° [Catatonic/manic excitement] ° Cruelty to animals ° Firesetting ° Motor vehicle offenses (e.g., frequent traffic

violations, use of motor vehicle to release anger) ° Suicidal behavior ° Impulsivity] ° Availability of weapon(s) ° Body language (e.g., rigid posture, clenching of fists and jaw, hyperactivity, pacing, breathlessness, threatening stances) ° [Hormonal imbalance (e.g., premenstrual syndrome—PMS, postpartal depression/psychosis)] ° Prenatal/perinatal complications ° [Expressed intent/desire to harm others directly or indirectly] ° [Almost continuous thoughts of violence]

Violence, [actual]/risk for self-directed

DEFINITION: At risk for behaviors in which an individual demonstrates that he/she can be physically, emotionally, and/or sexually harmful to self

RISK FACTORS [OR INDICATORS]: ° Ages 15 to 19; over age 45 ° Marital status (single, widowed, divorced) ° Employment problems (e.g., unemployed, recent job loss/failure) ° Occupation (executive, administrator/owner of business, professional, semiskilled worker) ° Conflictual interpersonal relationships ° Family background (e.g., chaotic or conflictual, history of suicide) ° Sexual orientation (bisexual [active], homosexual [inactive]) ° Physical health problems (e.g., hypochondriac, chronic or terminal illness) ° Mental health problems (e.g., severe depression, [bipolar disorder], psychosis, severe personality disorder, alcoholism or drug abuse) ° Emotional problems (e.g., hopelessness, [lifting of depressed mood], despair, increased anxiety, panic, anger, hostility) ° History of multiple suicide attempts ° Suicidal ideation ° Suicide plan ° Lack of personal resources (e.g., poor achievement, poor insight, affect unavailable and poorly controlled) ° Lack of social resources (e.g., poor rapport, socially isolated, unresponsive family) ° Verbal clues (e.g., talking about death, "better off without me," asking questions about lethal dosages of drugs) ° Behavioral clues (e.g., writing forlorn love notes, directing angry messages at a significant other who has rejected the person, giving away personal items, taking out a large life insurance policy)

Walking, impaired

DEFINITION: Limitation of independent movement within the environment on foot (Note: Specific level of independence using a standardized functional scale)

RELATED FACTORS: ° Insufficient muscle strength ° Neuromuscular impairment ° Musculoskeletal impairment (e.g., contractures) ° Limited endurance ° Deconditioning ° Fear of falling ° Impaired balance ° Impaired vision ° Pain ° Obesity ° Depressed mood ° Cognitive impairment ° Lack of knowledge ° Environmental constraints (e.g., stairs, inclines, uneven surfaces, unsafe obstacles, distances, lack of assistive devices or person, restraints)

DEFINING CHARACTERISTICS
Subjective or Objective: ° *Impaired ability to:* ° Walk required distances ° Walk on an incline/ decline ° Walk on uneven surfaces ° Navigate curbs ° Climb stairs

Wandering, [specify sporadic or continual]

DEFINITION: Meandering, aimless or repetitive locomotion that exposes the individual to harm; frequently incongruent with boundaries, limits, or obstacles

RELATED FACTORS: ° Cognitive impairment (e.g., memory and recall deficits, disorientation, poor visuoconstructive or visuospatial ability, language defects) ° Sedation ° Cortical atrophy ° Premorbid behavior (e.g., outgoing, sociable personality; premorbid dementia) ° Separation from familiar environment ° Overstimulating environment ° Emotional state (e.g., frustration, anxiety, boredom, depression, agitation) ° Physiological state or need (e.g., hunger, thirst, pain, urination, constipation) ° Time of day

DEFINING CHARACTERISTICS
Objective: ° Frequent/continuous movement from place to place, often revisiting the same destinations ° Persistent locomotion in search of something ° Scanning/searching behaviors ° Haphazard locomotion ° Fretful locomotion/ pacing ° Long periods of locomotion without an apparent destination ° Locomotion into unauthorized or private spaces ° Trespassing ° Locomotion resulting in unintended leaving of a premise ° Inability to locate significant landmarks in a familiar setting ° Getting lost ° Locomotion that cannot be easily dissuaded ° Shadowing a caregiver's locomotion ° Hyperactivity ° Periods of locomotion interspersed with periods of nonlocomotion (e.g., sitting, standing, sleeping)

NOTE: Information appearing in [ ] has been added by the authors to clarify and facilitate the use of nursing diagnoses.

Index